Surgical Anatomy of the Lumbar Plexus

R. Shane Tubbs, PhD, PA-C
Chief Science Officer and Vice President
Seattle Science Foundation
Seattle, Washington

Marios Loukas, MD, PhD
Dean of Basic Sciences and Research
Chairman and Professor
Department of Anatomical Sciences
St. George's University School of Medicine
Grenada, West Indies

Amgad S. Hanna, MD
Associate Professor
Department of Neurological Surgery
School of Medicine and Public Health
University of Wisconsin
Madison, Wisconsin

Rod J. Oskouian, MD
Surgical Director, Spinal Tumors and Spinal Trauma
Co-Director
Spine Fellowship Program
Swedish Neuroscience Institute
Seattle, Washington

Thieme
New York • Stuttgart • Delhi • Rio de Janeiro

Executive Editor: Timothy Y. Hiscock
Assistant Managing Editor: Haley Paskalides
Director, Editorial Services: Mary Jo Casey
Production Editor: Sean Woznicki
International Production Director: Andreas Schabert
Editorial Director: Sue Hodgson
International Marketing Director: Fiona Henderson
International Sales Director: Louisa Turrell
Director of Institutional Sales: Adam Bernacki
Senior Vice President and Chief Operating Officer: Sarah Vanderbilt
President: Brian D. Scanlan

Library of Congress Cataloging-in-Publication Data

Names: Tubbs, R. Shane, editor. | Loukas, Marios, editor. | Hanna, Amgad S., editor. | Oskouian, Rod, editor.
Title: Surgical anatomy of the lumbar plexus / [edited by] R. Shane Tubbs, Marios Loukas, Amgad Hanna, Rod Oskouian.
Description: New York : Thieme, [2018] | Includes bibliographical references.
    Identifiers: LCCN 2017055657 (print) |
    LCCN 2017057244 (ebook) | ISBN
    9781626238909 (e-book) | ISBN 9781626238893 (print)
Subjects: | MESH: Lumbosacral Plexus–anatomy & histology | Lumbosacral Plexus–surgery | Lumbosacral Plexus–diagnostic imaging
Classification: LCC RD768 (ebook) | LCC RD768 (print) | NLM WL 400 | DDC
    617.5/507543–dc23
LC record available at https://lccn.loc.gov/2017055657

© 2019 by Georg Thieme Verlag KG

Thieme Publishers New York
333 Seventh Avenue, New York, NY 10001 USA
+1 800 782 3488, customerservice@thieme.com

Thieme Publishers Stuttgart
Rüdigerstrasse 14, 70469 Stuttgart, Germany
+49 [0]711 8931 421, customerservice@thieme.de

Thieme Publishers Delhi
A-12, Second Floor, Sector-2, Noida-201301
Uttar Pradesh, India
+91 120 45 566 00, customerservice@thieme.in

Thieme Publishers Rio de Janeiro, Thieme Publicações Ltda.
Edifício Rodolpho de Paoli, 25º andar
Av. Nilo Peanha, 50 - Sala 2508
Rio de Janeiro 20020-906 Brasil
+55 21 3172 2297 / +55 21 3172 1896
www.thiemerevinter.com.br

Cover design: Thieme Publishing Group
Typesetting by Thomson Digital, India

Printed in the United States by King Printing   5 4 3 2 1

ISBN 978-1-62623-889-3

Also available as an e-book:
eISBN 978-1-62623-890-9

Important note: Medicine is an ever-changing science undergoing continual development. Research and clinical experience are continually expanding our knowledge, in particular our knowledge of proper treatment and drug therapy. Insofar as this book mentions any dosage or application, readers may rest assured that the authors, editors, and publishers have made every effort to ensure that such references are in accordance with **the state of knowledge at the time of production of the book.**

Nevertheless, this does not involve, imply, or express any guarantee or responsibility on the part of the publishers in respect to any dosage instructions and forms of applications stated in the book. **Every user is requested to examine carefully** the manufacturers' leaflets accompanying each drug and to check, if necessary in consultation with a physician or specialist, whether the dosage schedules mentioned therein or the contraindications stated by the manufacturers differ from the statements made in the present book. Such examination is particularly important with drugs that are either rarely used or have been newly released on the market. Every dosage schedule or every form of application used is entirely at the user's own risk and responsibility. The authors and publishers request every user to report to the publishers any discrepancies or inaccuracies noticed. If errors in this work are found after publication, errata will be posted at www.thieme.com on the product description page.

Some of the product names, patents, and registered designs referred to in this book are in fact registered trademarks or proprietary names even though specific reference to this fact is not always made in the text. Therefore, the appearance of a name without designation as proprietary is not to be construed as a representation by the publisher that it is in the public domain.

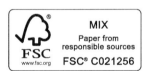

To my amazing wife, Susan, who is strong, patient, and enduring.

R. Shane Tubbs

To my late father, Dr. Saddik M. Hanna, my late mother, Dr. Aida Riad, my wife, Linda,
and my daughters, Barbara, Krista, and Cielle.

Amgad Hanna

I thank my beautiful wife, Joanna, for all of her support.

Marios Loukas

To my loving and amazing family. I would not be here today if it were not for
my incredible parents and sister, Dr. Rama, who always believed in me. The four beautiful women
in my life, you inspire me every single day, Christen, Ava, Arya, and Alina!

Rod Oskouian

Contents

Contents

Foreword

There has not yet been a book dedicated to the lumbar plexus. With the growing popularity of surgical approaches to and around this group of nerves (e.g., lateral transpsoas approaches to the lumbar spine) and increasingly sophisticated imaging methods that provide good resolution of this plexus, a book on this subject is now warranted. The current offering from these authors (two neurosurgeons and two clinical anatomists) is especially timely. With patient safety always foremost in the surgeon's mind, and accurate diagnosis always the concern of the radiologist, a book dedicated to the anatomy of the lumbar plexus is more important now than in the past. This book by Tubbs et al covers not only the detailed anatomy of each branch of the lumbar plexus but also has chapters dedicated to microscopic anatomy, comparative anatomy, anatomic variants, intraneural topography, imaging, surgical approaches, and, importantly, iatrogenic injury. Such a resource will be useful to both students (e.g., residents and fellows) first learning the clinical anatomy of the lumbar plexus and medical professionals who view images of the lumbar plexus or operate on or near the posterior abdominal wall. This book also offers original images of cadaveric dissections of the lumbar plexus and its branches, combined with excellent anatomical drawings. This combination will make learning this complicated anatomy less challenging and more rewarding.

Stephen W. Carmichael, PhD, DSc
Editor Emeritus, Clinical Anatomy
Professor Emeritus of Anatomy and Orthopaedic Surgery
Mayo Clinic

Preface

The lumbar plexus has been known since before the time of Galen. However, it has often been underrepresented in medical and surgical education. However, with recent advances in surgery to the lumbar spine such as transpsoas approaches, now more than ever, a thorough knowledge of this plexus and its branches is necessary. The primary issue with approaches to the lumbar plexus and its branches within the posterior abdominal wall is the intimate relationships that it has with surrounding anatomy. For example, many of the branches are formed within the psoas major muscle and careful dissection is necessary to liberate these nerves at surgery if damage is to be avoided. Furthermore, the iliac vessels are just medial to some of the larger branches of the plexus, e.g., femoral and obturator nerves. In the retroperitoneal space, the kidney and ureter are nearby. Lastly, due to the overlying peritoneal cavity and its contents, accessing the lumbar plexus is a challenge.

With this first textbook devoted to the lumbar plexus and its branches, we aimed to better elucidate each and every nerve, and have devoted an entire chapter to the anatomy of each of these. Additional chapters are focused on disease, imaging, anesthetic blockade, and surgery involving these nerves. In the end, the editors (two anatomists and two surgeons all with a strong background in studying/operating the peripheral nervous system) would like to thank each of the book's authors and their dedication to helping us bring the lumbar plexus to life.

R. Shane Tubbs
Marios Loukas
Amgad Hanna
Rod J. Oskouian

Acknowledgments

The editors would like to thank Thieme for their support of our project and, specifically, Haley Paskalides for her dedication to the project.

Contributors

Nihal Apaydin, MD, PhD
Professor
Department of Anatomy
Ankara University Brain Research Center
Ankara University
Ankara, Turkey

Fabio Barroso, MD
Head
Neuromuscular Disorders
Foundation for Neurological Research
  "Dr. Raúl Carrea" (FLENI)
Buenos Aires, Argentina

Garvin Bowen, MD
Teaching Fellow
Department of Anatomical Sciences
St. George's Unviersity
Grenada, West Indies

Inés Tatiana Escobar Buitrago, MD
Medical Doctor, Radiologist
Radiology Department
San Rafael University Hospital Clinic
Bogota, Colombia

Claudia Cejas, MD
Professor of Radiology
Head of Radiology Department
Foundation of Neurological Research, FLENI
Buenos Aires, Argentina

Parthasarathi Chamiraju, MD
Neurosurgery Chief House Staff Officer
Department of Neurosurgery
Wayne State University
Detroit, Michigan

Peter G. Collin, BS
Clinical Anatomy Research Fellow
New York University School of Medicine
New York, New York

Marcus Cox, MD
Internal Medicine Residency Program
Saint Michael's Medical Center
Newark, New Jersey

Michele Davis, MD
Resident Physician
The Brooklyn Hospital Center
Brooklyn, New York

Javier Moratinos-Delgado, MD
Institute of Applied Molecular Medicine
CEU-San Pablo University School of Medicine
Madrid, Spain

Bryan Edwards, MD
Post-Graduate Fellow
St. George's University
British Columbia, Canada

Manuel Fernández-Domínguez, MD
Head of Maxiofacial and Oral Department
Hospital Monteprincipe
Madrid, Spain

Virginia García-García, MD
Institute of Applied Molecular Medicine
CEU-San Pablo University School of Medicine
Madrid, Spain

Rachel A. Graham, BS
Clinical Anatomy Research Fellow
New York Medical College
School of Medicine
Valhalla, New York

Peter Grunert, MD
Department of Neurosurgery
Swedish Neuroscience Institute
Seattle, Washington

Arunprasad Gunasekaran, BS
Medical Student
Department of Neurosurgery
University of Arkansas for Medical Sciences
Little Rock, Arkansas

Amgad S. Hanna, MD
Associate Professor
Department of Neurosurgery
School of Medicine and Public Health
University of Wisconsin
Madison, Wisconsin

Jaspreet Johal, MD
Clinical Anatomy Research Fellow
Department of Anatomical Sciences
School of Medicine
St. George's University
Grenada, West Indies

Mohammad W. Kassem, MD
Clinical Anatomy Research Fellow
Seattle Science Foundation
St. George's University School of Medicine
Seattle Science Foundation
Seattle, Washington
Department of Anatomical Science
St. George's University School of Medicine
Grenada, West Indies
Mercy Health- Neuroscience Institute
Mercy St. Vincent Street Medical Center
Toledo, Ohio

Noojan Kazemi, MD, FACS
Assistant Professor
Department of Neurosurgery
University of Arkansas for Medical Sciences
Little Rock, Arkansas

Shehzad Khalid, MD
Assistant Professor
Department of Anatomical Sciences
St. George's University
Grenada, West Indies

Fabiola Machés, MD
Assistant Professor
Anesthesiology CEU-San Pablo
  University School of Medicine
Madrid, Spain

Prasanthi Maddali, MD, DNP
  (Diplomate of National Board, India)
Seattle Science Foundation
Grosse Pointe, Michigan

Malcon Andrei Martinez-Pereira
Adjunct Professor
Animal Anatomy Laboratory
Campus Curitibanos
Federal University of Santa Catarina
Rio Grande do Sul, Brazi

Lexian McBain, MD
Teaching Fellow
Department of Anatomical Sciences
St. George's University School of Medicine
True Blue, St. George's
Grenada, West Indies

S. Ali Mirjalili, MD, PhD, PGDipSurgAnat,
  PGCertCPU, PGDipSci
Senior Lecturer
Faculty of Medical and Health Sciences
Anatomy and Medical Imaging Department
University of Auckland
Auckland, New Zealand

Marc D. Moisi, MD
Department of Neurological Surgery
Wayne State University
Detroit, Michigan

Michael Montalbano, MD
Clinical Anatomy Research Fellow
St. George's University
Grenada, West Indies

Garrett Ng, BS
Clinical Anatomy Research Fellow
Department of Molecular, Cellular, and Biomedical Sciences
The CUNY School of Medicine
New York, New York

Chidinma Nwaogbe, BS
Clinical Anatomy Research Fellow
Department of Molecular, Cellular & Biomedical Sciences
CUNY School of Medicine, Seattle Science Foundation
New York, New York

Peter Oakes, BS
Clinical Anatomy Research Fellow
Seattle Science Foundation
Birmingham, Alabama

Naomi Ojumah, MD
Instructor
Department of Anatomical Sciences
St. George's University
Missouri City, Texas

Diego Leonardo Pineda Ordóñez, MD, MSC
Radiologist, Neuroradiology
Neuroradiology Unit
Resonancia Magnética del Country
Clìnica del Country
Bogotá, Colombia

Vikas Parmar, MD
Resident Physician
Department of Neurosurgery
University of Wisconsin Health Clinics
Madison, Wisconsin

Matthew Protas, MD
Clinical Anatomy Research Fellow
Department of Anatomical Sciences
Saint George's University School of Medicine
Grenada, West Indies

Rebecca C. Ramdhan, MD
Demonstrator
Teaching Fellow of Anatomical Sciences
St. George's University School of Medicine
Grenada, West Indies

Miguel Angel Reina, MD PhD
Professor
Department of Anesthesiology
School of Medicine
Madrid Monteprincipe University Hospital
CEU San Pablo University
Madrid, Spain

Cameron Schmidt, BS
Clinical Anatomy Research Fellow
Seattle Science Foundation
Seattle, Washington

Maria Mercedes Serra, MD
Radiology Department
Foundation of Neurological Research, FLENI
Buenos Aires, Argentina

Susan I. Toth, MD
General Surgeon
Department of Surgery
UnityPoint Health
Meriter-UnityPoint Health Hospital
Madison, Wisconsin

R. Shane Tubbs, PhD, PA-C
Chief Science Officer and Vice President
Seattle Science Foundation
Seattle, Washington

Joy M. H. Wang, MD
Clinical Anatomy Research Fellow
Department of Anatomical Sciences
St. George's University
Grenada, West Indies

Denise Maria Zancan, PhD
Biologist
Associate Professor
Physiology Department and Neuroscience Graduate
  Program
Laboratory of Comparative Neurobiology
Institute of Basic Health Sciences
Universidade Federal do Rio Grande do Sul
Porto Alegre, RS, Brazil

1 An Overview of the Lumbar Plexus

Jaspreet Johal, S. Ali Mirjalili

Abstract

Knowledge of the lumbar plexus and its branches is important to those imaging or operating on this collection of peripheral nerves. In this chapter, the general anatomy of this plexus and its branches is reviewed. A better understanding of the lumbar plexus can aid in improved diagnoses and surgical outcomes.

Keywords: anatomy, surgery, complications, lateral approaches, spine, peripheral nerves, approaches, surgery, operations

1.1 Introduction

The lumbar plexus forms within the psoas major muscle, and is derived from contributions arising from the first three lumbar ventral rami, along with additional contributions from parts of the 4th lumbar ventral ramus and 12th thoracic ventral ramus (▸ Fig. 1.1, ▸ Fig. 1.2, ▸ Fig. 1.3).

1.2 Iliohypogastric Nerve (T12, L1)

The iliohypogastric nerve forms within the lumbar plexus, and arises from contributions from the 12th thoracic ventral ramus and 1st lumbar ventral ramus. It courses past the psoas major and exits from the upper lateral border of psoas major, at a point between the anterior surface of quadratus lumborum and the posterior aspect of the kidney. The iliohypogastric nerve then traverses past the posterior part of the transversus abdominis, traveling superior to the iliac crest. Near the iliac crest, it divides into anterior and lateral branches between the transversus abdominis and internal oblique. The anterior branch of the iliohypogastric nerve supplies surrounding muscles, such as the internal oblique and transversus abdominis, while also supplying sensory innervation of the suprapubic skin. The lateral cutaneous branch supplies the posterolateral gluteal skin.[1,2] In the presence of a pyramidalis muscle, it is likely to be innervated by the iliohypogastric nerve.

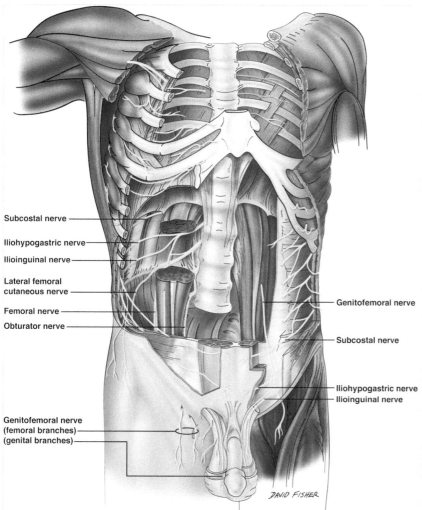

Fig. 1.1 Schematic drawing of the lumbar plexus. Note that the right side has had a section of the psoas major and minor muscles removed to show the course of the underlying lumbar plexus branches.

Subcostal nerve

Iliohypogastric nerve

Ilioinguinal nerve

Lateral femoral cutaneous nerve

Femoral nerve

Obturator nerve

Genitofemoral nerve (femoral branches) (genital branches)

Genitofemoral nerve

Subcostal nerve

Iliohypogastric nerve
Ilioinguinal nerve

DAVID FISHER

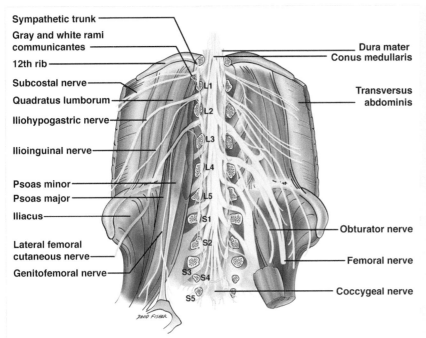

Sympathetic trunk
Gray and white rami communicantes
12th rib
Subcostal nerve
Quadratus lumborum
Iliohypogastric nerve
Ilioinguinal nerve
Psoas minor
Psoas major
Iliacus
Lateral femoral cutaneous nerve
Genitofemoral nerve

Dura mater
Conus medullaris
Transversus abdominis
Obturator nerve
Femoral nerve
Coccygeal nerve

L1
L2
L3
L4
L5
S1
S2
S3 S4
S5

DAVID FISHER

Fig. 1.2 Schematic drawing of the lumbar plexus following removal of the vertebral bodies and after opening of the anterior dura mater. The psoas muscles on the left side have been removed.

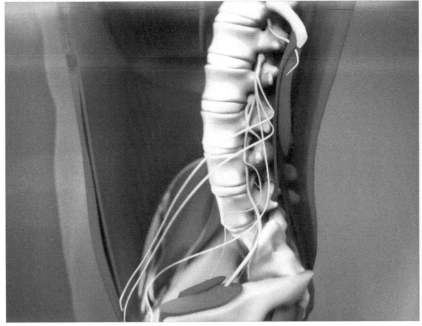

Fig. 1.3 Lateral view of the branches of the left lumbar plexus following removal of the psoas muscles and partial removal of the iliac crest.

1.3 Ilioinguinal Nerve (L1)

The ilioinguinal nerve exists as a collateral branch of the first lumbar ventral ramus, and it emerges from along the lateral border of the psoas major alongside or just below the iliohypogastric nerve. It then proceeds down the anterior surface of the quadratus lumborum toward the upper portion of iliacus. It travels through transversus abdominis near the iliac crest, and then pierces the internal oblique to supply it. During its descent, it passes 3 cm medial and 3.5 cm inferior to the anterior superior iliac spine. At this point, the ilioinguinal nerve is located in the plane between the internal and external abdominal obliques and travels through the inguinal canal. It then exits the superficial inguinal ring on the anterior aspect of the round ligament/spermatic cord. The ilioinguinal nerve goes on to supply sensory innervation of the medial thigh, along with the root of the penis and anterior scrotum in males or the mons pubis and labium majus in females.[1]

1.4 Genitofemoral Nerve (L1, L2)

The genitofemoral nerve forms within the psoas major from contributions arising from the first and second lumbar ventral rami. It is first seen at the anterior surface of psoas major. It then proceeds downward along the psoas major, traveling within the fascia iliaca and posteriorly to the ureter and peritoneum. The genitofemoral nerve then travels along the lateral border of the common and external iliac arteries, and divides into genital and femoral branches at a point above the inguinal ligament. The genital branch enters the deep inguinal ring by traveling through the transverse and spermatic fasciae. It then descends down the inguinal canal deep to the round ligament/spermatic cord and provides innervation of the cremaster muscle. Finally, it exits through the superficial inguinal ring and gives off sensory branches to the lateral aspect of the scrotum in males or the mons pubis and labium majus in females along with surrounding parts of the thigh. The femoral branch of the genitofemoral nerve travels alongside the femoral artery underneath the inguinal ligament and travels through the femoral sheath at a point superficial and lateral to the femoral artery and distal to the inguinal ligament. It then emerges from the sheath and fascia lata to provide sensory innervation of the skin of the upper anterior part of the femoral triangle.[3]

1.4.1 Variation

The iliohypogastric nerve may be absent from the lumbar plexus in up to 20% of cases. The ilioinguinal nerve is not seen in less than 3% of the population, and in 25% of cases, it may emerge with the iliohypogastric nerve. Within the inguinal canal, the ilioinguinal nerve is usually seen anterior to the spermatic cord but it may also lie within or posterior to the cord, or outside the inguinal canal entirely. The genitofemoral nerve arises from two separate branches in 20% of cases, and in some instances either of its branches or the entire nerve may be absent.

1.4.2 General Mechanisms of Injury

The iliohypogastric, ilioinguinal, and genitofemoral nerves may be injured along their course through the anterior and posterior abdominal wall either directly by trauma (e.g., surgical injury or during suture ligation) or indirectly by ischemic damage secondary to reduced perfusion or stretch. These nerves may be most prone to injury during certain portions of their course through the abdomen and surrounding regions. The anterior branch of the iliohypogastric nerve may be most vulnerable to injury during its course through the internal and external obliques. The ilioinguinal nerve appears to be prone to injury during its descent along the anterior abdominal wall, and the genitofemoral nerve is vulnerable to injury throughout its entire course but this risk is most pronounced in the retroperitoneum and within the inguinal canal.

1.4.3 Context of Injury

These nerves may undergo iatrogenic injury during abdominal and pelvic surgery (e.g., appendectomy, repair of inguinal hernia, gynecologic procedures through transverse incision, femoral artery catheterization, fascial closure, and procedures for urinary incontinence such as needle suspension and tension-free vaginal tape). Surgery to repair an inguinal hernia commonly results in injury to the ilioinguinal nerve. Laparoscopic inguinal hernia repair also may cause injury to the femoral branch of the genitofemoral nerve, whereas open inguinal hernia repair may damage the genital branch. The femoral branch may also be injured during femoral artery catheterization procedures.

1.4.4 Effects of Injury

Clinical manifestations of injury to the iliohypogastric nerve appear to differ based on whether injury occurs above or below the anterior superior iliac spine. In injuries occurring below the anterior superior iliac spine, some loss of sensory innervation of suprapubic skin may be observed; however, this is rarely seen due to collateral sensory innervation of this region. Injuries occurring above the anterior superior iliac spine may, however, weaken muscles such as the internal oblique, and transversus abdominis. A direct hernia may form secondary to this loss of muscle innervation. Injury to the ilioinguinal nerve may lead to numbness and paresthesia over skin of the genitalia, and entrapment injuries during surgery may lead to the development of recurrent pain along its area of distribution. Injury to the genitofemoral nerve will also produce paresthesia and anesthesia along its area of distribution.

1.5 Lateral Cutaneous Nerve of the Thigh (L2, L3)

The lateral cutaneous nerve of the thigh is derived from contributions arising at the second and third ventral rami of the lumbar nerve, and is seen emerging from the lateral margin of psoas major. It then proceeds downward and deep to the fascia that covers the iliacus, and passes underneath or less commonly through the inguinal ligament at a point medial to the anterior superior iliac spine. In its course through the thigh, the lateral cutaneous nerve of the thigh initially runs deep to the fascia lata and over the surface of the sartorius muscle. It then pierces the fascia lata to supply sensory innervation to the lateral aspect of the thigh. At this point, it divides into anterior and posterior branches. The anterior branch serves to provide sensory innervation of skin along the anterolateral thigh and goes on to contribute to the patellar plexus. The patellar plexus is formed by the anterior branch of the lateral cutaneous nerve of the thigh, anterior cutaneous branches of the femoral nerve, and infrapatellar branches of the saphenous nerve. The posterior branch of the lateral cutaneous nerve of the thigh provides sensory innervation of skin from the greater trochanter to the middle of the thigh.[4,5]

1.5.1 Variation

Anatomical variations of the lateral cutaneous nerve of the thigh are observed in around 25% of the population, and the nerve may be completely absent in around 10% of individuals.

1.5.2 General Mechanisms of Injury

The lateral cutaneous nerve of the thigh is most prone to injury either around the inguinal ligament or along the anterior or anterolateral proximal thigh by direct trauma. Commonly indicated mechanisms of injury include iatrogenic injury secondary to incision, transection, or suture ligation along with prolonged use of belts and braces, and accidental trauma. Iatrogenic injury to the lateral cutaneous nerve of the thigh has been reported as the eighth most common cause of iatrogenic injury during surgical and medical procedures in New Zealand.[6]

1.5.3 Context of Injury

Iatrogenic injury of the lateral cutaneous nerve of the thigh may occur during surgical procedures involving the abdomen and pelvis. Implicated procedures include any involving an anterior or anterolateral approach to the hip, ilioinguinal approach to the acetabulum, inguinal hernia repair, inguinal lymph node biopsy, discectomy, ovarian cystectomy, and femoral artery catheterization performed by radiologists.

1.5.4 Effects of Injury

Injury to the lateral cutaneous nerve of the thigh can result in a spectrum of clinical disability that can range from a sensory defect of the lateral thigh to painful neuromas in its area of distribution. Injury to the nerve is implicated in the development of meralgia paresthetica, which is a clinical syndrome characterized by itching, burning, pain, and numbness over the anterolateral aspects of the thigh.

1.6 Obturator Nerve (L2, L3, L4)

The obturator nerve is derived from the anterior divisions of the ventral rami of the second to fourth lumbar nerves. It initially proceeds to posterior to psoas major to appear at the medial side of psoas major at a point near the pelvic brim. This point of emergence is localized medial to the lumbosacral trunk, and posterior to the common iliac vessels. The obturator nerve then descends down the lateral pelvic wall to exit the pelvis via the obturator foramen. During its course down the lateral pelvic wall, it runs alongside the obturator artery and travels on the obturator internus muscle. At this point, there are several anatomical significant structures that lie in close proximity to the obturator nerve. From posterior to anterior, these structures are the iliac vessels, the ureter, rarely a pelvic appendix on the right and a sigmoid colon on the left, the ovary and infundibulum of the fallopian tube in females, and the ductus deferens in males.

As the obturator nerve passes through the obturator foramen, it will divide into anterior and posterior branches (▶ Fig. 1.3). The anterior branch of the obturator nerve travels in a plane formed by adductor longus anteriorly and adductor brevis posteriorly. A branch of the anterior division supplies the hip joint and the majority of the adductor muscles, and an arterial branch travels to the femoral artery. It also communicates with cutaneous branches of the femoral nerve within the adductor canal, forming the subsartorial plexus and also provides innervation of the medial aspect of the thigh. The posterior branch of the obturator nerve pierces through the obturator externus and innervates this muscle. It then proceeds downward behind adductor brevis and travels on adductor magnus. The posterior division will innervate the adductor magnus, and may occasionally supply the adductor brevis muscle. It then travels through the adductor hiatus to reach the popliteal fossa, where it

transmits an articular branch to the knee joint that runs alongside the middle genicular artery.

1.6.1 Variation

The accessory obturator nerve is a variation seen in 15 to 30% of individuals. It is commonly formed from contributions arising from the ventral rami of the third and fourth lumbar nerves. This nerve often traverses past the medial border of psoas major, crossing past the superior pubic ramus and running behind the pectineus muscle. Depending on its exact trajectory, it may supply the pectineus muscle and/or the hip joint. Its point of origin may be the trunk of obturator nerve, or it may connect with the anterior division of the obturator nerve.[7]

1.6.2 General Mechanisms of Injury

During its course, the obturator nerve is prone to either direct injury as a result of trauma (e.g., compression, iatrogenic damage during incision or transection, or accidental) or indirect injury secondary to ischemic damage. Some mechanisms such as a pelvic mass (e.g., ovarian tumor or obturator hernia) may produce both direct traumatic and indirect ischemic injury. The most vulnerable aspect of this nerve is the intrapelvic segment.

1.6.3 Context of Injury

Iatrogenic injury of the obturator nerve may occur during abdominopelvic procedures, hip joint repair, regional anesthesia delivery, and urological surgery. Implicated procedures include radical prostatectomy, total hip arthroplasty, labor and delivery of a neonate, abdominal aortic aneurysm repair, and obturator hernia repair.

1.6.4 Effects of Injury

Obturator nerve injury may produce pain and sensory abnormalities of the medial thigh and these symptoms may occasionally extend below the knee. Loss of sensory innervation may be limited as its area of distribution overlaps with neighboring cutaneous branches. Loss of motor innervation may result in atrophy of muscles within the medial thigh, but impaired functionality will be limited to the adductor magnus muscle. This will result in muscle disability characterized by limited adduction, which will not impact walking but may make crossing of the legs more difficult.

1.7 Femoral Nerve (L2, L3, L4)

The femoral nerve forms from the posterior division of the ventral rami from the second to fourth lumbar nerves. It first exits from along the lateral border of psoas major within the iliac fossa at a point around 4 cm above the inguinal ligament. The femoral nerve then enters the femoral triangle. Within the thigh, the femoral nerve gives off a number of sensory and muscular branches, and its sole branch, the saphenous nerve, goes on to course below the knee.

Within the iliac fossa, it courses alongside the external iliac artery as it exits the abdomen. It runs posterior to the ileocecal portion of the bowel on the right and posterior to the sigmoid colon on the left. The femoral nerve gives off small branches to the femoral artery and iliacus muscle within the iliac fossa. It also innervates the pectineus muscle. As it enters the femoral triangle, the femoral nerve runs lateral to the femoral sheath and the vessels within it segregated from them by psoas fibers. It lies upon the iliacus with the fascia lata serving as the roof of the femoral triangle. After giving off a number of small branches, the femoral nerve divides into anterior and posterior divisions at a point about 1 to 4 cm below the inguinal ligament. These divisions may often be separated by the lateral circumflex femoral artery, or this artery will lie deep to both divisions.[8]

The anterior division of femoral nerve is relatively short and immediately gives off a branch to sartorius and two sensory branches after forming below the inguinal ligament. The two sensory nerves are the intermediate and medial cutaneous nerves of the thigh.

The intermediate cutaneous nerve of the thigh travels through the fascia lata at a point about 8 cm below the inguinal ligament and further divides into two branches. These branches then descend down the thigh and innervate the skin down to the knee where they contribute to the peripatellar plexus. The more laterally located of these two branches communicates with the femoral branch of the genitofemoral nerve and may also supply the sartorius muscle.

The medial cutaneous nerve of the thigh descends laterally past the femoral artery and gives off small branches that pierce through the fascia lata and provide innervation to the superior part of the medial thigh. At the apex of the femoral triangle, the medial cutaneous nerve of the thigh will pass anterior to the femoral artery and divides into anterior and posterior branches. The anterior branch descends down sartorius and pierces through the fascia lata at around the middle length of the thigh, where it further divides into two branches. One of these branches supplies the skin of the medial knee and another connects with the infrapatellar branch of the saphenous nerve. The posterior branch travels down the posterior border of sartorius to the knee, where it goes through the fascia lata and connects with the saphenous nerve. It goes on to contribute to the subsartorial plexus and also provides innervation to the medial aspect of the leg just below the knee.

The posterior division of the femoral nerve gives off the saphenous nerve and also provides innervation to the quadriceps femoris and articularis genus. In the groin, it runs lateral to the femoral artery before crossing over to the medial side via the adductor canal. As it leaves the adductor canal alongside the saphenous branch of the descending genicular artery, the saphenous nerve gives off an infrapatellar branch that pierces the sartorius and supplies skin surrounding the knee. It then descends further downward to pierce the fascia lata between the tendons of sartorius anteriorly and gracilis posteriorly, and communicates with the great saphenous vein at a point behind the medial aspect of the knee. It travels alongside the vein in the leg and divides into two branches at a variable point.[9] The larger of these branches, the anterior branch, courses alongside the great saphenous vein at the medial surface of the tibia and goes on to supply skin on the medial aspect of the foot down to the first metatarsophalangeal joint. The posterior branch descends down the medial border of the tibia to terminate at the ankle and supply cutaneous sensation to the medial aspect of the leg.

Muscular branches of the posterior division of the femoral nerve supply the rectus femoris, vastus lateralis, vastus medialis, vastus intermedius, and articularis genus. The branch to rectus femoris enters through the posterior surface of the muscle and also supplies the hip joint. Vastus lateralis is supplied by a larger branch that descends alongside the lateral circumflex femoral artery and enters through the muscle through its anterior border while also supplying the knee joint. An even larger branch supplies the vastus medialis and is seen to travel alongside the femoral vessels and saphenous nerve within the adductor canal. It gives off branches to upper and lower segments of the muscle, and also sends a long filamentous branch to the knee. A few branches to vastus intermedius enter through that muscle's anterior surface at around the midthigh level and a small branch descends to supply the articularis genus and the knee joint.

The femoral nerve is supplied by the iliolumbar artery within the pelvis, by the deep circumflex iliac artery in the inguinal area, and by the lateral circumflex femoral artery within the thigh. On the right side, the deep circumflex iliac artery gives more arterial branches to the femoral nerve relative to the left side, and also forms a richer anastomosis with the iliolumbar and fourth lumbar arteries. The left femoral nerve is therefore more prone to ischemic injury than the right side. The intrapelvic segment of the nerve also appears to be more vulnerable to ischemia than other segments of the nerve.[10]

1.7.1 Variations

Around one-third of individuals appear to show some degree of variability in femoral nerve anatomy. Of these variations, the only one of any clinical significance is within the femoral triangle where the nerve is reported to enter the thigh at some point between the femoral artery and femoral vein.[11]

1.7.2 General Mechanisms of Injury

The femoral nerve can be involved in both open and closed injury resulting from penetrating trauma and gunshot wounds, blunt trauma, and injury secondary to disease and iatrogenic causes. Penetrating trauma can cause injury at any point along the course of the femoral nerve, but is most likely to occur during wounding of the anterior aspect of the femoral triangle. Blunt injury may occur following an automobile accident, sports injury, or a severe fall. Injury can also occur directly through trauma (e.g., transection following pubic fracture) or secondary to ischemic damage following stretch or impaired perfusion (e.g., hemorrhage into the iliacus compartment following rupture of iliacus or iliopsoas). Some disease processes may damage the nerve directly via inflammation and toxic injury or indirectly due to ischemic damage (e.g., tumors, renal or appendiceal abscess, and hemorrhagic diseases).

1.7.3 Context of Iatrogenic Injury

Iatrogenic injury of the femoral nerve can be reported after procedures involving the abdomen and pelvis, hip surgery, femoral artery puncture, and delivery of regional anesthesia.[12] Several causes of nerve injury exist during procedures of the abdomen and pelvis, including compression, ischemia, and direct injury from utilization of surgical instruments (e.g., trocars). Risk factors for iatrogenic injury include thin or obese body habitus, and the use of Pfannenstiel incisions. Compression injuries usually occur during the use of retractors, as they may compress the nerve against the pelvic wall or the tip of the blade may directly exert pressure on the nerve. Stretching and compression of the femoral nerve may also occur during procedures in which a patient is placed in a lithotomy position with extreme flexion, abduction, and external rotation of the thighs for a prolonged period of time. During this positioning, the femoral nerve can become sharply angulated underneath the inguinal ligament. Nerve compression can also occur due to formation of a hematoma in anticoagulated patients undergoing vascular procedures.[12]

The femoral nerve can also experience iatrogenic damage during orthopaedic procedures, especially those involving lateral and anterolateral approaches to the hip joint. Causes of femoral nerve injury during hip surgery include (1) prolonged or extreme retraction of the nerve during surgery by instruments, bone, or prosthesis; (2) compression and stretching from hyperextension and limb lengthening; (3) formation of a hematoma around the femoral vein or iliacus; (4) cement extrusion; and (5) laceration or transection.[12] Iatrogenic injury can also occur during delivery of regional anesthesia, particularly during femoral nerve block. The etiology appears to be direct needle penetration of the nerve due to ischemia intraneural injection and neural toxicity caused by large doses of local anesthetic agent.[12]

Transient neuropathy of the femoral nerve has also been reported during the use of regional anesthesia during inguinal hernia repair and iliac crest bone harvest. This occurs because anesthetic agents delivered into the plane between transversus abdominis and the transversalis fascia can easily diffuse posteriorly into the space iliacus and its overlying fascia, where the femoral nerve is located.[13] The femoral nerve can also be injured when blood is obtained from the femoral artery for arterial blood gas analysis or angiography through the femoral artery. This occurs either due to direct injury or indirectly due to compression from hematoma or pseudo aneurysm.

Injury to the saphenous nerve may be the subject of surgical management, as the nerve may be sectioned or damaged during surgical procedures. Iatrogenic injury to the saphenous nerve has commonly been reported during total stripping of the great saphenous vein. This is due to the course of the nerve and the close proximity in which it follows the vein below the knee. It has also been reported that the saphenous nerve can be compressed on the operating table due to improper application of supporting braces. Iatrogenic injury has been reported during utilization of peripheral nerve blocks as well; however, there appears to be no indication of saphenous nerve injury secondary to adductor canal blockade.[14]

1.7.4 Effects of Injury

The femoral nerve is most vulnerable to injury at the lower abdomen and upper thigh due to its relatively superficial course in that region and its close proximity to the acetabular rim. It may also be compressed by tumors or hematomas within the pelvis. Severe injury to the femoral nerve within the pelvis may result in weakness of ipsilateral hip flexion, knee extension, sensory impairment over the anterior thigh and medial aspect of leg and foot, loss of knee jerk reflex, and atrophy of the quadriceps with loss of patellar reflex. Destabilization of the lower limb can lead to difficulty performing activities such as walking uphill or on uneven ground, and climbing stairs. Sensory impairments seen are limited to hyperesthesia, paresthesia, and numbness over the anteromedial aspect of the thigh and leg, and pain in the thigh or groin.

Injury to the femoral nerve occurring within the thigh can produce a range of clinical presentations, including complete or isolated motor or sensory deficit. Physical symptoms include reduced or completely absent patellar reflex, and partial or complete atrophy of the quadriceps femoris. An incomplete lesion of the femoral nerve may be indicated by sweating within its autonomous cutaneous distribution. Lesions of the femoral nerve may be more common on the left side than on the right due to relatively less blood supply on the left.[10] Patients who experience a postoperative fall with subsequent alteration and impairment of cutaneous sensation in the distribution of femoral nerve should be examined for femoral nerve injury.[15] Injury to the saphenous nerve will result in sensory disturbances over the medial aspect of the leg extending along the inner border of the foot to the big toe.

References

[1] Klaassen Z, Marshall E, Tubbs RS, Louis RG, Jr, Wartmann CT, Loukas M. Anatomy of the ilioinguinal and iliohypogastric nerves with observations of their spinal nerve contributions. Clin Anat. 2011; 24(4):454–461

[2] Wijsmuller AR, Lange JF, Kleinrensink GJ, et al. Nerve-identifying inguinal hernia repair: a surgical anatomical study. World J Surg. 2007; 31(2):414–420, discussion 421–422

[3] Rab M, Ebmer And J, Dellon AL. Anatomic variability of the ilioinguinal and genitofemoral nerve: implications for the treatment of groin pain. Plast Reconstr Surg. 2001; 108(6):1618–1623

[4] Aszmann OC, Dellon ES, Dellon AL. Anatomical course of the lateral femoral cutaneous nerve and its susceptibility to compression and injury. Plast Reconstr Surg. 1997; 100(3):600–604

[5] Carai A, Fenu G, Sechi E, Crotti FM, Montella A. Anatomical variability of the lateral femoral cutaneous nerve: findings from a surgical series. Clin Anat. 2009; 22(3):365–370

[6] Moore AE, Zhang J, Stringer MD. Iatrogenic nerve injury in a national no-fault compensation scheme: an observational cohort study. Int J Clin Pract. 2012; 66(4):409–416

[7] Katritsis E, Anagnostopoulou S, Papadopoulos N. Anatomical observations on the accessory obturator nerve (based on 1000 specimens). Anat Anz. 1980; 148(5):440–445

[8] Orebaugh SL. The femoral nerve and its relationship to the lateral circumflex femoral artery. Anesth Analg. 2006; 102(6):1859–1862

[9] Wilmot VV, Evans DJ. Categorizing the distribution of the saphenous nerve in relation to the great saphenous vein. Clin Anat. 2013; 26(4):531–536

[10] Boontje AH, Haaxma R. Femoral neuropathy as a complication of aortic surgery. J Cardiovasc Surg (Torino). 1987; 28(3):286–289

[11] Bergman RA, Thompson SA, Afifi AK. Catalog of Human Variation. Baltimore, MD: Urban & Schwarzenberg; 1984:159

[12] Moore AE, Stringer MD. Iatrogenic femoral nerve injury: a systematic review. Surg Radiol Anat. 2011; 33(8):649–658

[13] Rosario DJ, Jacob S, Luntley J, Skinner PP, Raftery AT. Mechanism of femoral nerve palsy complicating percutaneous ilioinguinal field block. Br J Anaesth. 1997; 78(3):314–316

[14] Henningsen MH, Jaeger P, Hilsted KL, Dahl JB. Prevalence of saphenous nerve injury after adductor-canal-blockade in patients receiving total knee arthroplasty. Acta Anaesthesiol Scand. 2013; 57(1):112–117

[15] Feibel RJ, Dervin GF, Kim PR, Beaulé PE. Major complications associated with femoral nerve catheters for knee arthroplasty: a word of caution. J Arthroplasty. 2009; 24(6) Suppl:132–137

2 Subcostal Nerve

Rachel A. Graham and Rebecca C. Ramdhan

Abstract

The branches of the lumbar plexus are frequently encountered in various invasive procedures. Therefore, a thorough knowledge of each of its branches is important to the clinician who performs such procedures. This chapter reviews the clinical anatomy and associated pathologies of the subcostal nerve. It is hoped that a better understanding of this nerve and its distribution will decrease patient morbidity.

Keywords: anatomy, posterior abdominal wall, nerves, complications, surgery, subcostal

2.1 Anatomy of the Subcostal Nerve

The subcostal nerve has been acknowledged as an anatomical feature since the 1800s (▶ Fig. 2.1 and ▶ Fig. 2.2).[1] There are 12 pairs of thoracic spinal nerves originating from the spinal cord. The first 11 thoracic nerves (T1–T11) lie between the ribs and are called intercostal nerves, whereas the 12th thoracic nerve (T12) lies below the last rib and is called the subcostal nerve.[2] Generally, there are four main branches of intercostal nerves: collateral, lateral cutaneous, anterior cutaneous, and muscular.[2] Each thoracic spinal nerve is formed from the dorsal and ventral roots from each segment of the spinal cord, and each spinal nerve then gives rise to a dorsal and ventral ramus. The ventral ramus receives postganglionic sympathetic fibers from the sympathetic trunk via the gray rami. The ventral rami of T6 to L1 emit branches at each segment of the vertebral column.[2,3] The ventral ramus of T12 (subcostal nerve) is larger than the other ventral rami, and gives off a communicating branch to the first lumbar ventral ramus. This communicating branch is also called the dorsolumbar nerve. Shortly after, it gives off a collateral branch, which helps to supply the intercostal muscles and the parietal pleura,[2,4] and then continues to accompany the subcostal vessels along the inferior border of the 12th rib. From superior to inferior, the subcostal vein, artery, and nerve run alongside one another at the lower border of the 12th rib. The subcostal vein and artery are hidden within the costal groove, leaving the subcostal nerve vulnerable to risk for iatrogenic injury during surgical procedures. The subcostal nerve then courses posterior to the lateral arcuate ligament and kidney, and anterior to the upper region of the quadratus lumborum.[2] It then perforates the aponeurosis of the origin of the transversus abdominis and continues to course between the transversus abdominis and internal oblique[2] and is then distributed in the same manner as the lower intercostal nerves.[4] It imparts muscular branches to the muscles of the anterior abdominal wall.[1,5] Its innervation to the most inferior part of the external oblique, the rectus abdominis, and the transversus abdominis[6,7,8] attests to its role in respiration. The subcostal nerve then joins with the first spinal nerve of the lumbar plexus, the iliohypogastric

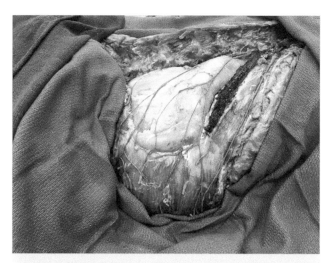

Fig. 2.1 Right lateral dissection of the subcostal nerve. The right 12th rib is colored in blue and the lumbar spine is seen at the top of the image. Also note the 11th intercostal nerve just superior (right) to the 12th rib. The subcostal in this specimen shows three large branches that, here, are traveling superficial to the transversus abdominis muscle. Inferior to the subcostal nerve (left), the L1 ventral ramus is shown dividing into a superior iliohypogastric nerve and inferior ilioinguinal nerve.

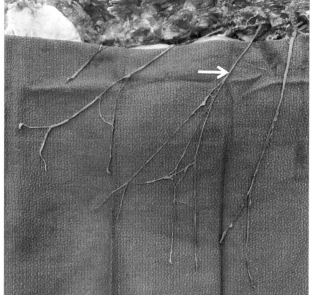

Fig. 2.2 Another right-sided lateral dissection of the subcostal nerve (*arrow*). The midline spine is shown at the top of the image. Also note the 11th intercostal nerve just superior (right) to the subcostal nerve. Inferior to the subcostal nerve (left), the L1 ventral ramus is shown dividing into a superior iliohypogastric nerve and inferior ilioinguinal nerve. Below (left) the L1 nerve, the L2 ventral ramus is seen.

nerve, and sends a branch to the pyramidalis (a muscle of the anterior wall that attaches to the pubic symphysis and crest). Innervation by the subcostal nerve allows this muscle to tense the linea alba.[2,9] As with each intercostal nerve, the subcostal nerve has a branch called the lateral cutaneous branch, which pierces the internal and external oblique muscles. It then usually descends over the iliac crest approximately 5 cm posterior to the anterior superior iliac spine (ASIS) and innervates the anterior gluteal skin, but some filaments can descend as low as the greater trochanter of the femur.[2,4,8]

2.2 Variations of the Subcostal Nerve

It has been shown in the literature that the subcostal nerve does not always contribute to the lumbar plexus.[5,10] In addition, the literature highlights variations in the innervation of the pyramidalis muscle.[8,11] Tokita reported that the anterior rami of T12, L1, and L2 can all give branches to the pyramidalis muscle.[8] D'Souza et al. also found variations in the thickness of the lateral cutaneous branch of the subcostal nerve.[7]

2.3 Pathology of the Subcostal Nerve

The subcostal nerve has been implicated in several pathological conditions. One is called intercostal neuralgia, which is described in the literature as a strong, shooting pain over the corresponding dermatome. It can be caused by a nerve entrapment, a tumor, thoracotomy, breast surgery, or other conditions such as herpes zoster virus.[12,13,14] Furthermore, Nasseh et al performed a cross-sectional study on 68 patients who experienced ipsilateral abdominal pain or upper thigh numbness after a percutaneous nephrolithotomy.[13] They reported that the most commonly affected area is that supplied by the subcostal nerve, or T12, dermatome.[14] In some situations, patients can develop a postoperative neuroma of the subcostal nerve. A retrospective study by Williams et al reported that a neuroma of the 12th thoracic spinal nerve could occur after an open nephrectomy.[11] Also, during a nephrectomy, postoperative abdominal wall bulging (also known as a pseudohernia or a flank bulge) can occur if the subcostal nerve has been injured.[9] Flank bulge is a common complication after lumbotomy for renal surgery. This is often a direct result of iatrogenic damage to the intercostal and subcostal nerves supplying the abdominal wall muscles due to initial incision or closing sutures after the procedure. The damage of these nerves and subsequent denervation results in paralysis and atrophy of parts of the abdominal wall.[15] Tumors of the subcostal nerve can also compress the conus medullaris of the spinal cord, affecting the normal function of the bladder and anus, producing symptoms similar to a saddle anesthesia.[16] The close proximity of the posteriorly positioned subcostal nerve to the kidney, and the fact that it is exposed, unlike the subcostal vein and artery, increases the likelihood of injury when operating on the kidney.

In a clinical condition known as slipping rib syndrome, malposition of the costovertebral joint can cause compression of the intercostal nerve. The name of the condition arises from patients' descriptions of their symptoms, particularly the feeling that their rib had "slipped" away from its conventional position. This syndrome, also known as 12th rib syndrome,[17,18] is associated with extensive movement of the rib, such that the rib can impinge on the subcostal nerve and cause severe pain.[16] Furthermore, the subcostal nerve can become entrapped as it pierces the aponeurosis of the rectus sheath, producing a condition known as rectus abdominis syndrome.[2,19] This most often occurs as a result of a desmoid tumor, which is a tumor of the aponeurosis of skeletal muscle.[18] Clinically, this can present with significant pain and numbness in the abdominal region.[2]

It was reported that some "pseudocoxalgias" may be a result of neuralgia of the lateral rami exiting the subcostal and iliohypogastric nerves above the lateral edge of the iliac crest.[20] Maigne et al performed an anatomic study of the nerves pathways and pattern of distribution. The rami arising from the subcostal and iliohypogastric nerves cross close together, which creates a bony groove that is palpable in thin patients and is transformed into an osseomembranous tunnel by the aponeurosis of these muscles. This region is directly subcutaneous and therefore exposed to possible friction and microtrauma (tight clothes). As a result, this arrangement can give rise to an entrapment syndrome.[20]

2.4 Surgical Procedures

The subcostal nerve is involved in different procedures, including ultrasound-guided transversus abdominis nerve block, in which the lumbar triangle is used for injections to anesthetize spinal nerves T11–L1.[21] Furthermore, the literature shows that the subcostal nerve is at risk for iatrogenic injury during certain surgical approaches. D'Souza et al discovered a variation in the distance between the ASIS and the lateral cutaneous branch of the subcostal nerve while performing an osteotomy.[7] Using the modified Smith-Peterson approach, they found that the lateral cutaneous branch of the subcostal nerve crossed 2 to 5 cm behind the ASIS.[7] This difference would be relevant for avoiding sensory loss or disturbances while operating in the gluteal region.[7] Another study by Chou et al reported that the subcostal nerve was highly likely to be injured during the harvesting of bone from the iliac crest, as injury to the subcostal nerve branches may occur with incision over the iliac crest posterior to the ASIS.[21] It was recommended that the surgeon should dissect carefully after reaching 6 cm posterior to the ASIS to avoid injury. It is a general rule that the nerve may be encountered as early as four fingerbreadths behind the ASIS and, therefore, surgeons should be extremely cautious when dissecting in this region. However, if the nerve is accidently cut, it is best to allow the nerve to fall back into healthy tissues and avoid including the nerve with closing the fascia.[22] Furthermore, it is at risk for iatrogenic injury during minimally invasive approaches to the lateral spine, specifically during exposure of the upper lumbar vertebrae or even while suturing the abdominal wall.[9,22] Because of this increased likelihood, the authors suggest making an incision parallel to the subcostal nerve to reduce the risk of injury.[22]

Naturally, one could assume that because the subcostal nerve gives branches to the muscles of the anterior wall, injury to it could also impair the function of those muscles. However, Standring stated that the anterolateral wall of the abdomen is innervated by several branches of segmented spinal nerves.[2] Therefore, injury to one spinal nerve is very unlikely to produce any notable loss in muscle tone.[2] To reduce the function of the anterolateral wall muscles effectively, it would be necessary to injure more than one spinal nerve.[2]

References

[1] Harman NB. The caudal limit of the lumbar visceral efferent nerves in man. J Anat Physiol. 1898; 32(Pt 3):403–421

[2] Standring S. Gray's Anatomy: The Anatomical Basis of Clinical Practice. 41st ed. New York, NY: Elsevier Health Sciences; 2015

[3] Lykissas MG, Kostas-Agnantis IP, Korompilias AV, Vekris MD, Beris AE. Use of intercostal nerves for different target neurotization in brachial plexus reconstruction. World J Orthop. 2013; 4(3):107–111

[4] Moore KL, Daly AF, Agur AMR. Clinically Oriented Anatomy. 6th ed. Philadelphia, PA: Lippincott Williams & Wilkins; 2010

[5] Dakwar E, Vale FL, Uribe JS. Trajectory of the main sensory and motor branches of the lumbar plexus outside the psoas muscle related to the lateral retroperitoneal transpsoas approach. J Neurosurg Spine. 2011; 14(2):290–295

[6] Fahim DK, Kim SD, Cho D, Lee S, Kim DH. Avoiding abdominal flank bulge after anterolateral approaches to the thoracolumbar spine: cadaveric study and electrophysiological investigation. J Neurosurg Spine. 2011; 15(5):532–540

[7] D'Souza L, Jagannathan S, McManus F. The subcostal nerve (ouch!): anatomical awareness in Salter's innominate osteotomy. J Pediatr Orthop. 1994; 14(5):660–661

[8] Tokita K. Anatomical significance of the nerve to the pyramidalis muscle: a morphological study. Anat Sci Int. 2006; 81(4):210–224

[9] Tubbs RS, Rizk E, Shoja MM, Loukas M, Barbaro N, Spinner RJ. Nerves and Nerve Injuries. Vol 2: Pain, Treatment, Injury, Disease, and Future Directions. 1st ed. New York, NY: Elsevier; 2015

[10] Lovering RM, Anderson LD. Architecture and fiber type of the pyramidalis muscle. Anat Sci Int. 2008; 83(4):294–297

[11] Williams EH, Williams CG, Rosson GD, Heitmiller RF, Dellon AL. Neurectomy for treatment of intercostal neuralgia. Ann Thorac Surg. 2008; 85(5):1766–1770

[12] Kim KS, Ji SR, Kim HM, Kwon YJ, Hwang JH, Lee SY. Intercostal nerve schwannoma encountered during a rib-latissimus dorsi osteomyocutaneous flap operation. Arch Plast Surg. 2015; 42(6):800–802

[13] Nasseh H, Pourreza F, Saberi A, Kazemnejad E, Kalantari BB, Falahatkar S. Focal neuropathies following percutaneous nephrolithotomy (PCNL)–preliminary study. Ger Med Sci. 2013; 11(7):Doc07

[14] Ombregt L. Disorders of the thoracic spine: pathology and treatment. In: A System of Orthopaedic Medicine. 3rd ed. Edinburgh: Churchill Livingstone; 2013:169–184

[15] van der Graaf T, Verhagen PC, Kerver AL, Kleinrensink GJ. Surgical anatomy of the 10th and 11th intercostal, and subcostal nerves: prevention of damage during lumbotomy. J Urol. 2011; 186(2):579–583

[16] Cranfield KA, Buist RJ, Nandi PR, Baranowski AP. The twelfth rib syndrome. J Pain Symptom Manage. 1997; 13(3):172–175

[17] Machin DG, Shennan JM. Twelfth rib syndrome: a differential diagnosis of loin pain. Br Med J (Clin Res Ed) 1983; 287(6392):586

[18] CCNY Libraries. http://web.b.ebscohost.com.ccny-proxy1.libr.ccny.cuny.edu/ehost/pdfviewer/pdfviewer?sid=4013f1ba-a541-4843-92a2-8eac0f199bb4%40sessionmgr102&vid=1&hid=1070

[19] Tran TM, Ivanusic JJ, Hebbard P, Barrington MJ. Determination of spread of injectate after ultrasound-guided transversus abdominis plane block: a cadaveric study. Br J Anaesth. 2009; 102(1):123–127

[20] Maigne JY, Maigne R, Guérin-Surville H. Anatomic study of the lateral cutaneous rami of the subcostal and iliohypogastric nerves. Surg Radiol Anat. 1986; 8(4):251–256

[21] Chou D, Storm PB, Campbell JN. Vulnerability of the subcostal nerve to injury during bone graft harvesting from the iliac crest. J Neurosurg Spine. 2004; 1(1):87–89

[22] Cahill KS, Martinez JL, Wang MY, Vanni S, Levi AD. Motor nerve injuries following the minimally invasive lateral transpsoas approach. J Neurosurg Spine. 2012; 17(3):227–231

3 Iliohypogastric Nerve

Garvin Bowen, Bryan Edwards

Abstract

The branches of the lumbar plexus are frequently encountered in various invasive procedures. Therefore, a thorough knowledge of each of its branches is important to the clinician who performs such procedures. This chapter reviews the clinical anatomy and associated pathologies of the iliohypogastric nerve. It is hoped that a better understanding of this nerve and its distribution will decrease patient morbidity.

Keywords: anatomy, posterior abdominal wall, nerves, complications, surgery

3.1 Introduction

The iliohypogastric nerve (▶ Fig. 3.1, ▶ Fig. 3.2, ▶ Fig. 3.3) measures approximately 210 mm in length[1] and is a mixed nerve that provides both motor and sensory innervation to numerous structures in the lower abdominopelvic regions. The motor component contributes to the innervation of both the transversus abdominis

and internal oblique muscles that function to maintain abdominal tone, increase intra-abdominal pressure, and, particularly for the internal oblique, cause lateral flexion.[2] The sensory component supplies the skin over the hypogastric region, as well as the upper lateral aspect of the thigh and gluteal region.[3,4,5,6] The clinical relevance of this nerve lies in its vulnerability to injury, most commonly intraoperatively during attempts to gain access to the peritoneal cavity, pelvis, or perineum. This can result in motor dysfunction of the lower abdominal wall and sensory disturbances in the aforementioned regions.

3.2 Anatomy

The origin of the iliohypogastric nerve is the ventral ramus of the L1 spinal nerve,[5] measuring approximately 4 mm in diameter.[1] After leaving the L1–L2 intervertebral foramen, the L1 spinal nerve root bifurcates into the iliohypogastric and ilioinguinal nerve posterior to the psoas major.[2,4] Then, emerging from the superior lateral margin of the psoas major and posterior to the medial arcuate ligament at the level of L1–L2,[6] the iliohypogastric nerve, measuring 2.2 mm in diameter, enters the abdominal cavity and descends laterally between the anterior surface of the quadratus lumborum and the posterior surface of the inferior pole of the kidney to continue onto the transversus abdominis.[2,4,7,8,9,10,11,12,13] The iliohypogastric nerve subsequently pierces the surface of the posterior aspect of the transversus abdominis and travels parallel to the iliac crest between the transversus abdominis and the internal oblique. The nerve then divides into two branches—the lateral cutaneous (iliac) nerve and the hypogastric (anterior) nerve.[3,4] The iliac branch pierces the internal oblique muscles and travels across the tubercle superior to the iliac crest, where, just above this, it pierces the external oblique aponeurosis and splits into two cutaneous branches—one traveling and providing sensory innervation of the skin over the tensor fasciae latae on the lateral aspect of the upper thigh, while the second cutaneous branch provides sensory information of the integument over the gluteus medius and lateral third of gluteus maximus muscles at the level of the greater trochanter. The hypogastric branch continues to travel between the transversus abdominis and internal oblique muscles, providing motor innervation to both muscles, until reaching the level of the anterior superior iliac spine, where it pierces the internal oblique muscle to run parallel to the inguinal ligament ventromedially between the internal and external oblique muscles. Along a vertical line drawn from the midpoint of the outer margin of the superficial inguinal ring, the hypogastric nerve pierces the external oblique aponeurosis, providing sensory innervation to the suprapubic integument.[3]

The location in which the iliohypogastric nerve pierces the internal oblique is 1.5 to 8 cm medial to the anterior superior iliac spine on the left and 2.3 to 3.6 cm medial to the anterior superior iliac spine on the right.[14] The iliohypogastric nerve pierced the abdominal wall 2.8 ± 1.3 cm (range, 1.1–5.5 cm) medial and 1.4 ± 1.2 cm (range, 0.6–5.1 cm) inferior to the anterior superior iliac spine, and then coursed on a straight

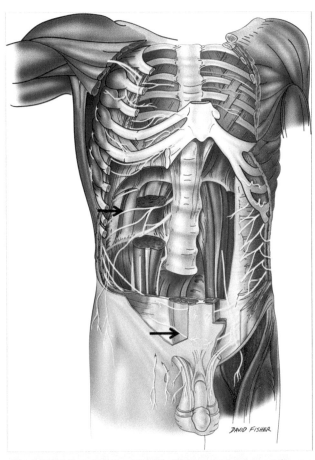

Fig. 3.1 Drawing of the course of the iliohypogastric nerve on the posterior abdominal wall (*upper arrow*) and on the anterior abdominal wall (*lower arrow*). This nerve's iliac branch is also seen crossing over the iliac crest.

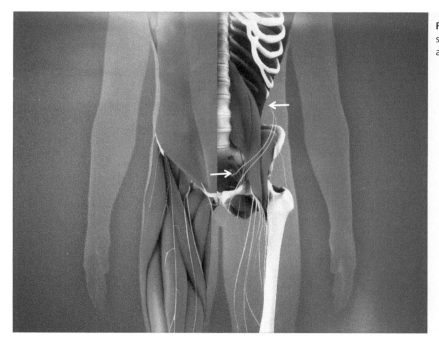

Fig. 3.2 The course of the iliohypogastric nerve shown on the left side with the anterolateral abdominal muscles removed.

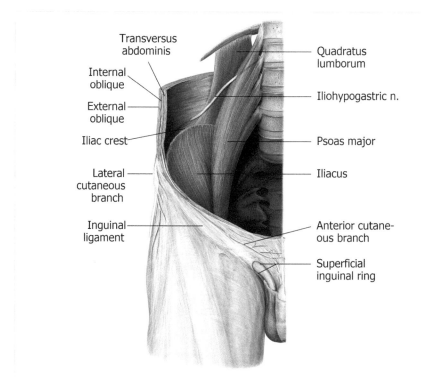

Transversus abdominis

Internal oblique

External oblique

Iliac crest

Lateral cutaneous branch

Inguinal ligament

Quadratus lumborum

Iliohypogastric n.

Psoas major

Iliacus

Anterior cutaneous branch

Superficial inguinal ring

Fig. 3.3 The intramuscular course of the iliohypogastric nerve on the right side. Also note its lateral cutaneous branch coursing over the iliac crest. (Reproduced with permission from Gilroy AM, MacPherson BR, Ross LM, Schuenke M, Schulte E, Schumacher U. Atlas of Anatomy. 2nd ed. New York, NY: Thieme Medical Publishers; 2012. Illustration by Karl Wesker.)

path to terminate 4.0 ± 1.3 cm (range, 2.0–12.6 cm) lateral to the linea alba.[5]

The pubic symphysis is innervated by branches from the iliohypogastric, ilioinguinal, and pudendal nerves.

3.3 Variations

The iliohypogastric nerve can exhibit variability in several ways. First, the iliohypogastric nerve may be absent in up to 20% of lumbar plexuses. Interestingly, this absence of the iliohypogastric leads to minimal sensory deficits as the sensory regions of the genitofemoral and ilioinguinal nerves largely overlap with that of the iliohypogastric.[4] Secondly, the iliohypogastric nerve can vary in its point of origin and can be classified into morphological types I–IV. In 7%, the iliohypogastric nerve arose at T12 and was classed as type I. Type II, noted in 14%, arose conjointly from T12 and L1. Type III, which occurred in 10%, had its origin from L1, while type IV (6%) started from both T11 and T12.[5] Thirdly, the iliohypogastric nerve can communicate with other nerves in the lumbar plexus including the lateral femoral cutaneous and ilioinguinal via small accessory nerve branches over the surface of the transverus abdominis muscle in 5 and 55%, respectively.[5,15,16,17,18,19,20,21,22] Additionally, the subcostal nerve can directly contribute to the iliohypogastric nerve.[4,5,17,23,24] Fourthly, morphological variability of the nerve has also been observed. For example, the ilioinguinal nerve can be found in place of the hypogastric branch of the iliohypogastric nerve prior to exiting the superficial inguinal ring.[4] A common trunk between the iliohypogastric and subcostal nerves can be found in as many as 30% of cases. In such cases, the division of the nerve can have three locations: posterior to the kidneys, between the internal oblique muscles and the transversus abdominis, and in a few cases between the internal and external oblique muscles. These common trunks of the iliohypogastric and subcostal nerves can be located behind the lateral arcuate ligament, the nerves separating either within the vicinity of the quadratus lumborum and transversus abdominis muscles or laterally between the internal oblique and transversus abdominis.

3.4 Landmarks

It is important that surgeons know the relevant landmarks of the iliohypogastric nerve while operating so as to avoid intraoperative injury, which is most common during appendectomy, inguinal hernia repair, hysterectomy, or cesarean section. The nerve first appears ventrally on the surface of the quadratus lumborum muscle near the lateral border of the psoas muscle at the L1–L2 vertebral level approximately 1 cm paravertebrally. On the right, the iliohypogastric nerve travels posterior to the central portion of the right kidney, appearing 2 cm superior to the inferior pole on the lateral aspect of the kidney. The left iliohypogastric nerve travels 2 cm higher than the right, at the level of the kidney in 66% of cases. It then traverses the fibers of the transversus abdominis aponeurosis superior to the iliac crest, equidistant from the crest and the tip of the 12th rib. The nerve can be located up to 3 cm medial at the level of the anterior superior iliac spine between the layers of the transversus abdominis and internal oblique muscles. At this level, it pierces the internal oblique muscle and courses 4 cm superior and parallel to the inguinal ligament, deep to the aponeurosis of the external oblique muscle, with its terminal branches penetrating its aponeurosis 4 cm lateral to the midline. At the lateral peak of the iliac crest between the transversus abdominis and the internal oblique muscles, the lateral cutaneous branch of the iliohypogastric nerve is given off and innervates the integument superficial to the tensor fasciae latae.[25]

3.5 Pathology

Iliohypogastricus syndrome results from injury to the iliohypogastric nerve and can cause abdominal dysfunction, including weakened flexion and rotation, and sensory dysfunction associated with episodic pain aggravated by walking or sitting, as well as stabbing, burning, shooting, or pricking sensation in the lower abdominal region, upper thigh, or pelvic area.[26,27,28,29] The injury may be traumatic in nature such as iatrogenically during surgical procedures or from traction. The most common surgical causes of iliohypogastric nerve injury are incisions within the lower abdominal wall, suture entrapment, ilium

harvesting for grafting, lymph node dissection within the inguinal region, femoral catheterization, orchiectomy,[25,30] and trocar placement during laparoscopic surgery within the lower abdominal wall.[31] Tractional or entrapment injuries can also occur due to the pathway the nerve takes between muscular layers and the potential for it to be pulled and stretched.[6,26] In contrast, injury of the iliohypogastric nerve may be induced by compressive forces such as from tumors arising in the lower kidney or lower lumbar region that can directly impinge the nerve given the close proximity the nerve has with these structures or from hematomas from blunt abdominal trauma.[26]

3.5.1 Surgery

As previously noted, the major cause of iliohypogastric nerve injury is following surgical intervention within the lower abdominal wall. One study using univariate and multivariate analysis showed that failure to identify the iliohypogastric nerve was significantly correlated with presence of chronic pain and the risk of developing inguinal pain.[32] This further emphasizes the need for proper anatomical knowledge of the course of the iliohypogastric nerve to preclude such injuries. The particular surgical incision used can determine the pathology encountered. Several surgical incisions of the abdominal wall can affect the iliohypogastric nerve. For example, particular care should be taken to avoid injuring the anterior branch of this nerve during an appendectomy using a lateral incisional approach.[33] Surgeons can do this by avoiding incising the area 3 cm superior and medial to the anterior superior iliac spine to ensure the safety of the nerve. The iliohypogastric nerve can also be compromised during inguinal hernia repair. When an oblique incision is performed, the anterior branches of the nerve can be injured as the incision is expanded medially.[34] Incisions of the abdominal wall endanger the iliohypogastric nerve 4 cm superior to the inguinal ligament. Finally, in an oblique lumbar incision (Pfannenstiel's incision), the iliohypogastric nerve can be harmed if the dissection is too close to the lateral border of the rectus abdominis muscle. This can potentially lead to the development of a neuroma.[35]

3.6 Imaging

Although no studies have been conducted to ascertain which imaging modality is best for visualizing the iliohypogastric nerve and associated nerve pathology, several image modalities can be used to guide therapy and identify pathology. In preparation for various surgical procedures of the lower abdominal or suprapubic region, iliohypogastric nerve block can be performed with ultrasound guidance. Variations of the nerve were better appreciated using an ultrasound-guided nerve block technique, which resulted in an increased effectiveness of the anesthetics characterized by a decrease in the required dose of anesthetic preoperatively and a reported decrease in postoperative pain levels.[4,6,25,36,37] Magnetic resonance neurography can reveal an entrapped or enlarged iliohypogastric nerve, although its main function is to visualize tumors along the anatomical course of the iliohypogastric nerve. Electrophysiological data are insufficiently accurate for diagnostic purposes, and to confirm a diagnosis, it can be necessary to achieve nerve block with local anesthesia.[28]

3.7 Treatment

The primary presentation associated with iliohypogastric nerve injury is chronic postoperative pain. There are several approaches to treating postsurgical pain, ranging from conservative management to surgical excision of the nerve, depending on the severity of the pain and the patient's preference. In one study of 5,506 patients undergoing herniography for repair of inguinal hernia, 125 patients reported severe to extremely severe pain, remaining long term in as many as 25%.[38] Antidepressants and antiepileptics seem to be more efficacious in relieving the neuropathic groin pain associated with nerve injury than conventional analgesics such as nonsteroidal anti-inflammatory drugs, opioids, and muscle relaxants. However, in most cases, patients experience recurrence because they develop tolerance to analgesics.[39] Ultrasound-guided nerve blockade has been used to treat the pain associated with iliohypogastric neuropathy with high accuracy and selectivity.[37]

It is recommended that surgical intervention be considered at least 6 months postoperatively to allow neuropraxia to disappear on its own or be medically treated. Surgery is indicated when pain is refractory to the aforementioned treatment options. Neurectomy should be only used when substantial to complete alleviation of pain can be achieved by nerve blockade.[39] There is still debate as to whether only the iliohypogastric nerve should be excised in cases of iliohypogastric neuropathy associated with the groin or if all three nerves supplying the groin (iliohypogastric, ilioinguinal, and genitofemoral nerves) should be involved. This is because the remaining nerves can still transmit pain signals.

References

[1] Izci Y, Gurkanlar D, Ozan H, Gonul E. The morphological aspects of lumbar plexus and roots: an anatomical study. Turk Neurosurg. 2005; 15:87–92
[2] Standring S. Gray's Anatomy: The Anatomical Basis of Clinical Practice. 41st ed. London: Elsevier; 2016
[3] Griffin M. Some varieties of the last dorsal and first lumbar nerves. J Anat Physiol. 1891; 26(Pt 1):48–55
[4] Anloague PA, Huijbregts P. Anatomical variations of the lumbar plexus: a descriptive anatomy study with proposed clinical implications. J Manual Manip Ther. 2009; 17(4):e107–e114
[5] Klaassen Z, Marshall E, Tubbs RS, Louis RG, Jr, Wartmann CT, Loukas M. Anatomy of the ilioinguinal and iliohypogastric nerves with observations of their spinal nerve contributions. Clin Anat. 2011; 24(4):454–461
[6] Papadopoulos NJ, Katritsis ED. Some observations on the course and relations of the iliohypogastric and ilioinguinal nerves (based on 348 specimens). Anat Anz. 1981; 149(4):357–364
[7] Mahadevan V. Pelvic girdle and lower limb. In: Standring S, ed. Gray's Anatomy: The Anatomical Basis of Clinical Practice. 40th ed. New York, NY: Elsevier; 2008:1327–1429
[8] Williams A. Pelvic girdle and lower limb. In: Standring S, ed. Gray's Anatomy: The Anatomical Basis of Clinical Practice. 39th ed. New York, NY: Elsevier; 2005:1456–1499
[9] Moore KL, Dalley AF. Clinically Oriented Anatomy. 4th ed. Baltimore, MD: Lippincott, Williams & Wilkins; 1999
[10] Palastanga N, Field D, Soames R. Anatomy & Human Movement: Structure & Function. 3rd ed. Boston, MA: Butterworth Heinemann; 1998
[11] Sauerland EK. Grant's Dissector. 11th ed. Baltimore, MD: Williams & Wilkins; 1994
[12] Linder HH. Clinical Anatomy. East Norwalk, CT: Appleton & Lange; 1989
[13] Pratt NE. Clinical Musculoskeletal Anatomy. New York, NY: Lippincott; 1991
[14] Avsar FM, Sahin M, Arikan BU, Avsar AF, Demirci S, Elhan A. The possibility of nervus ilioinguinalis and nervus iliohypogastricus injury in lower abdominal incisions and effects on hernia formation. J Surg Res. 2002; 107(2):179–185
[15] Bardeen CR. A statistical study of the abdominal and border nerves in man. Am J Anat. 1902; 1:203–228
[16] Bardeen CR. Development and variation of the nerves and the musculature of the inferior extremity and of the neighboring regions of the trunk in man. Am J Anat. 1906; 6:259–390
[17] Hollinshead WH. Anatomy for Surgeons: Vol. 2. The Thorax, Abdomen and Pelvis. New York, NY: Hoeber-Harper; 1956:850–870
[18] Webber RH. Some variations in the lumbar plexus of nerves in man. Acta Anat (Basel). 1961; 44:336–345
[19] Moosman DA, Oelrich TM. Prevention of accidental trauma to the ilioinguinal nerve during inguinal herniorrhaphy. Am J Surg. 1977; 133(2):146–148
[20] Moore KL, Agur AMR. Abdomen: Essential Clinical Anatomy. 2nd ed. Baltimore, MD: Lippincott Williams & Williams; 2002:128
[21] Netter FH. Abdomen: Atlas of Human Anatomy. 3rd ed. Teterboro, NJ: Icon Learning Systems; 2003:259
[22] Sasaoka N, Kawaguchi M, Yoshitani K, Kato H, Suzuki A, Furuya H. Evaluation of genitofemoral nerve block, in addition to ilioinguinal and iliohypogastric nerve block, during inguinal hernia repair in children. Br J Anaesth. 2005; 94(2):243–246
[23] Bergman RA, Thompson SA, Afifi AK. Catalogue of Human Variations. Baltimore, MD: Urban & Schwarzenberg; 1984:158–161
[24] Mandelkow H, Loeweneck H. The iliohypogastric and ilioinguinal nerves. Distribution in the abdominal wall, danger areas in surgical incisions in the inguinal and pubic regions and reflected visceral pain in their dermatomes. Surg Radiol Anat. 1988; 10(2):145–149
[25] Pecina MM, Krmptoc-Nemanic J, Markiewitz AD. Tunnel Syndromes: Peripheral Nerve Compression Syndromes. 2nd ed. Boca Raton, FL: CRC Press; 1997
[26] Vuilleumier H, Hübner M, Demartines N. Neuropathy after herniorrhaphy: indication for surgical treatment and outcome. World J Surg. 2009; 33(4):841–845
[27] Soldatos T, Andreisek G, Thawait GK, et al. High-resolution 3-T MR neurography of the lumbosacral plexus. Radiographics. 2013; 33(4):967–987
[28] Whiteside JL, Barber MD, Walters MD, Falcone T. Anatomy of ilioinguinal and iliohypogastric nerves in relation to trocar placement and low transverse incisions. Am J Obstet Gynecol. 2003; 189(6):1574–1578, discussion 1578
[29] Choi PD, Nath R, Mackinnon SE. Iatrogenic injury to the ilioinguinal and iliohypogastric nerves in the groin: a case report, diagnosis, and management. Ann Plast Surg. 1996; 37(1):60–65
[30] van Ramshorst GH, Kleinrensink GJ, Hermans JJ, Terkivatan T, Lange JF. Abdominal wall paresis as a complication of laparoscopic surgery. Hernia. 2009; 13(5):539–543
[31] Alfieri S, Rotondi F, Di Giorgio A, et al. Groin Pain Trial Group. Influence of preservation versus division of ilioinguinal, iliohypogastric, and genital nerves during open mesh herniorrhaphy: prospective multicentric study of chronic pain. Ann Surg. 2006; 243(4):553–558
[32] Stulz P, Pfeiffer KM. Postoperative nerve irritation syndromes of peripheral nerves after routine interventions in the lower abdomen and the inguinal region [in German]. Chirurg. 1980; 51(10):664–667
[33] Condon RE, Nyhus LM. Complications of groin hernia and of hernial repair. Surg Clin North Am. 1971; 51(6):1325–1336
[34] Loos MJA, Scheltinga MRM, Roumen RMH. Surgical management of inguinal neuralgia after a low transverse Pfannenstiel incision. Ann Surg. 2008; 248(5):880–885
[35] Khedkar SM, Bhalerao PM, Yemul-Golhar SR, Kelkar KV. Ultrasound-guided ilioinguinal and iliohypogastric nerve block, a comparison with the conventional technique: an observational study. Saudi J Anaesth. 2015; 9(3):293–297
[36] Eichenberger U, Greher M, Kirchmair L, Curatolo M, Moriggl B. Ultrasound-guided blocks of the ilioinguinal and iliohypogastric nerve: accuracy of a selective new technique confirmed by anatomical dissection. Br J Anaesth. 2006; 97(2):238–243
[37] Courtney CA, Duffy K, Serpell MG, O'Dwyer PJ. Outcome of patients with severe chronic pain following repair of groin hernia. Br J Surg. 2002; 89(10):1310–1314
[38] Hakeem A, Shanmugam V. Current trends in the diagnosis and management of post-herniorraphy chronic groin pain. World J Gastrointest Surg. 2011; 3(6):73–81
[39] Amid PK, Hiatt JR. New understanding of the causes and surgical treatment of postherniorrhaphy inguinodynia and orchalgia. J Am Coll Surg. 2007; 205(2):381–385

4 Ilioinguinal Nerve

Peter G. Collin, Bryan Edwards

Abstract

The branches of the lumbar plexus are encountered in various invasive procedures. Therefore, a thorough knowledge of each of its branches is important to the clinician who performs such procedures. This chapter reviews the clinical anatomy of the ilioinguinal nerve. It is hoped that a better understanding of this nerve and its distribution will decrease patient morbidity.

Keywords: anatomy, posterior abdominal wall, nerves, complications, surgery

4.1 Anatomy and Variations

The ilioinguinal nerve (▶ Fig. 4.1, ▶ Fig. 4.2, ▶ Fig. 4.3) originates from the anterior rami of the L1 spinal nerve but can often receive contributions from T12, L2, and L3.[1,2,3,4,5,6] Its diameter is 2.2 mm with a range from 1.3 to 3.3 mm, inversely proportional to that of the iliohypogastric nerve to which it runs lateral and inferior.[3,7] In a minority of cases, 20% according to Klaassen et al, the ilioinguinal nerve forms a common trunk with the iliohypogastric nerve but separates shortly after exiting the intervertebral foramen.[3,8] Communicating branches with the subcostal, and lateral femoral cutaneous nerves have been reported.[1]

The ilioinguinal nerve continues laterally as it courses past the proximal and lateral border of the psoas major muscle approximately 4.4 to 8.6 cm cranial to the posterior superior iliac spine, and more generally passing posterior to the inferior

pole of the kidney.[6,8,9] Continuing to descend inferolaterally,[1,2] it travels anterior to the quadratus lumborum and transversus abdominis, passing inferiorly to the lower pole of the kidney and posterior to the ascending colon if describing the right orientation of ilioinguinal nerve or descending colon if describing the left orientation. It then pierces the transversus abdominis cranially to the midpoint between the anterior superior iliac spine and the iliac crests, up to 3.0 cm, and in 13% of cases, according to Reinpold et al, it passes slightly inferior to the midpoint of the superior iliac spines.[5,9] In this area between the transversus abdominis and internal oblique known as the transversus abdominis plane, the ilioinguinal nerve may communicate with the hypogastric branch of the iliohypogastric nerve through small accessory fibers.[1,2] After traveling for a short distance between the transversus abdominis and internal oblique muscles and supplying the inferior fibers of the transversus abdominis with motor innervation, it penetrates the internal oblique and supplies it.[6,8,10,11] According to Avsar et al, this penetration occurs 4.85 cm inferomedially (range, 3–6.4 cm) from the anterior superior iliac spine on the right and 3.37 cm inferomedially (range, 2–5 cm) on the left, 2.99 cm (range, 0.2–6.1 cm) from McBurney's point on the right and 3.74 cm (range, 1.8–7.5 cm) on the left.[12] Whiteside et al found a similar proximity to the anterior superior iliac spine[13]; in pediatric patients, this proximity is much closer.[14] On a line connecting the anterior superior iliac spine to the umbilicus, the ilioinguinal nerve is 1.9 mm from the former (range, 0.61–4.01 mm) on the left and 2.0 mm (range, 0.49–3.44 mm) on the right.[14]

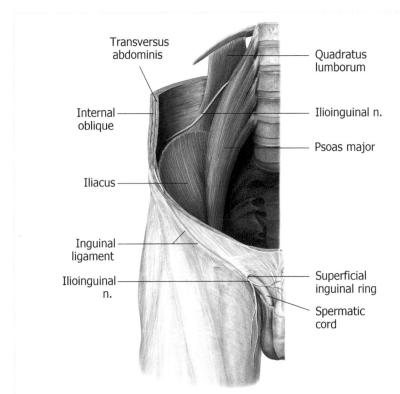

Fig. 4.1 Intramuscular course of the ilioinguinal nerve. (Reproduced with permission from Gilroy AM, MacPherson BR, Ross LM, Schuenke M, Schulte E, Schumacher U. Atlas of Anatomy. 2nd ed. New York, NY: Thieme Medical Publishers; 2012. Illustration by Karl Wesker.)

Transversus abdominis

Internal oblique

Iliacus

Inguinal ligament

Ilioinguinal n.

Quadratus lumborum

Ilioinguinal n.

Psoas major

Superficial inguinal ring

Spermatic cord

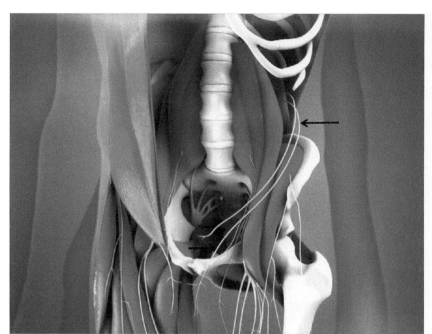

Fig. 4.2 Course of the left ilioinguinal nerve with anterolateral muscles removed.

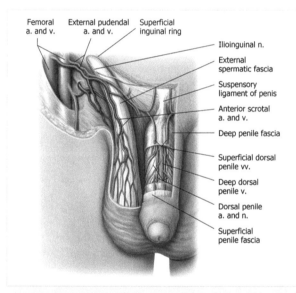

Femoral a. and v. — External pudendal a. and v. — Superficial inguinal ring

Ilioinguinal n.

External spermatic fascia

Suspensory ligament of penis

Anterior scrotal a. and v.

Deep penile fascia

Superficial dorsal penile vv.

Deep dorsal penile v.

Dorsal penile a. and n.

Superficial penile fascia

Fig. 4.3 Termination of the ilioinguinal nerve as the anterior scrotal nerve. (Reproduced with permission from Gilroy AM, MacPherson BR, Ross LM, Schuenke M, Schulte E, Schumacher U. Atlas of Anatomy. 2nd ed. New York, NY: Thieme Medical Publishers; 2012. Illustration by Karl Wesker.)

Between the external and internal oblique muscles, the ilioinguinal nerve is concealed by the fascia of the external oblique until it reaches the round ligament or spermatic cord.[3,7] According to Ndiaye et al, it perforates the external oblique muscle fascia before reaching the spermatic cord or round ligament in 28.72% of cases, so it is extra-aponeurotic. As it passes over the superficial aspect of the internal oblique muscle, it is on average about 1.015 cm (range, 0–4 cm) from the inguinal ligament, but the distance is less than 1 cm in 66% of cases.[7]

As it passes between the external and internal oblique muscles, it does not enter the inguinal canal through the deep inguinal ring but rather by piercing the canal wall.[15] The ilioinguinal nerve and its sensory aspect course in the inguinal canal with two distinct patterns according to Rab et al.[5] In type A (43.7%), the cutaneous aspect of the nerve joins the genitofemoral nerve either between the internal and external oblique muscles lateral to the deep inguinal ring, within the deep inguinal ring, or near the lateral aspect of the inguinal canal; the genital branch of the genitofemoral nerve runs ventrally on the spermatic cord or round ligament.[5] In types B (28.1%), C (20.3%), and D (7.8%), the genital branch of the genitofemoral nerve and the cutaneous portion of the ilioinguinal nerve enter the deep inguinal canal, and the ilioinguinal nerve courses on the ventral aspect of the round ligament or spermatic cord.[5] Types B, C, and D differ mainly in how the genital branch of the genitofemoral nerve and genitofemoral branch to the cremaster muscle course compared to the round ligament or spermatic cord, but the placement of the ilioinguinal nerve ventral to the spermatic cord is consistent.[5,10,16] The classification by Rab et al is supported by earlier work by Moosman and Oelrich. In the "aberrant" course described by Moosman and Oelrich, the sensory component of the ilioinguinal nerve was incorporated into the genital branch of the genitofemoral nerve in 35% of cases, posteriorly located within the spermatic cord (or posterior to the round ligament) and coursing downward deep to the cremasteric layer.[15,16] This "aberrant" path matches the type A classification by Rab et al, types B–D mirroring the "classical" course.[5,15,16] However, other literature has reported fewer instances of the "aberrant" course.[17]

As it exits the inguinal canal through the superficial inguinal ring, it lies superior to the spermatic cord or round ligament.[17] After emerging from the superficial inguinal ring with the spermatic cord, the cutaneous aspect of the ilioinguinal nerve supplies the proximal medial thigh, external genitalia, skin over the inguinal canal, anterior hemiscrotum, and the root of the penis in males or the mons pubis and lateral aspect of the labia majora in females.[1,2,4,6,8,10,11,16] The distribution of the genital branch of the genitofemoral nerve overlaps with this area and also provides cutaneous innervation to the anteromedial thigh, anterior hemiscrotum, or mons pubis and labia majora.[5,10] The overlapping cutaneous distributions of these two nerves were also classified by Rab et al: type A (43.7%) having contributions only from the genital branch of the genitofemoral nerve, type B (28.1%) only from the cutaneous aspect of the ilioinguinal nerve, and the remainder from both nerves. Type C (20.3%) also has cutaneous branches of the ilioinguinal nerve to the mons pubis, inguinal crease, and root of the penis or labia majora, while the genital branch of the genitofemoral nerve innervates the inferior aspects of the inguinal and anteromedial thigh regions. In type D (7.8%), both nerves contribute to these regional distributions.[5]

It should be noted that Ndiaye et al, Salama et al, Wijsmuller et al, and Al-dabbagh all found the ilioinguinal nerve to be absent, often unilaterally, in about 7% of inguinal dissections.[7,15,17,18] Distal anastomotic terminal branches with the iliohypogastric nerve have also been reported.[5]

The pubic symphysis is innervated by branches from the iliohypogastric, ilioinguinal, and pudendal nerves.

4.2 Pathology

Injury to the ilioinguinal nerve is commonly iatrogenic in origin, incurred during lower abdominal surgery or by nerve entrapment owing to scarring following surgery and pathological impingement.[6,19,20,21] The surgeries that frequently injure the ilioinguinal nerve are herniorrhaphy (most common), laparoscopic procedures in abdomen, treatment of stress incontinence in women, and surgeries using a Pfannenstiel incision such as cesarean section births, appendectomy, prostatectomy, inguinal hernioplasty, and abdominal hysterectomy.[6,13,22,23,24,25]

The nerve can be directly injured during surgery if the path of the incision crosses the nerve or stretches it while the surgical field is being manipulated, as in the Pfannenstiel incision and open hernia repairs.[15,20,22,26,27] A Pfannenstiel incision is made 2 to 3 cm superior to the pubic symphysis, followed by stretching 8 to 15 cm and cutting through the skin, subcutaneous fat, rectus sheath, and laterally through the fasciae of the transversus abdominis and internal and external oblique muscles. The anterior fascia and linear alba are separated from the rectus and pyramidalis muscles to allow for their separation at the midline and to gain access to the peritoneum.[20,21,22] This incision and surgical field passes through the area occupied by the ilioinguinal nerve, which can therefore be injured directly or through scarring. Open hernia repair can cause ilioinguinal neuralgia specifically due to stretching of the abdominal wall, accidental incising of the nerve, or the use of a mesh causing a neuroma to form.[7,26,28,29] Direct iatrogenic injury to the nerve is most likely when splitting the internal oblique aponeurosis, manipulating the spermatic cord, or manipulating the surgical field, as the ilioinguinal nerve runs parallel to the inguinal canal.[7,30] Caution should also be observed when approaching or operating in the triangle of doom, between the ductus deferens and the spermatic vessels, and the triangle of pain, the space created by the overlapping courses of the femoral, genitofemoral,

and lateral femoral cutaneous nerves, owing to the high chance of ilioinguinal nerve injury.[9,31,32]

Ilioinguinal nerve entrapment can arise from fibrosis and scarring of the region subjected to surgery, or the nerve simply being caught on the sutures, surgical staples, prosthetic materials, or mesh from the surgery.[6,21,28,32,33,34] This can lead to the formation of a neuroma or, when a mesh is involved, a "meshoma."[6,19,21,26,31] The nerve can also become injured or entrapped because of nonsurgical trauma to the lower quadrants of abdominal wall or inguinal region, or stretching of the abdominal walls following pregnancy, endometriosis, or tumors.[23,25,29] In regard to muscular entrapment, the ilioinguinal nerve is most often entrapped at the iliac crest, the paravertebral area, and the rectus border, specifically classified as an abdominal cutaneous nerve entrapment.[6,21,35] "Spontaneous entrapment" resulting from trauma to the abdominal wall usually involves the transverse abdominis and internal oblique muscles as the nerve courses in a "zig-zag fashion" through them.[6,19,35]

The symptoms of ilioinguinal nerve injury, e.g., from entrapment or incision, can be characterized generally as sensory changes throughout the nerve distribution.[4,5,6,23,34] The clinical triad of symptoms to confirm ilioinguinal nerve injury has some variations, but is most often reported as (1) hyperesthesia and/or dysesthesia of the medial aspect of the superior thigh and scrotum or labia majora, (2) pain exacerbated by hip extension and pressure applied to or medially to the anterior superior iliac spine, lateral rectus muscle, or the likely area of entrapment, and (3) pain relieved by injections of the ilioinguinal nerve.[5,6,19,29,36,37] Other symptoms include motor weakness, alterations in the cremasteric reflex, chronic "difficult to pin down" pelvic, abdominal, or suprapubic pain, burning pain from the incision to the nerve distribution, a bulge of the abdomen, or a "stabbing pain" during walking due to the extension of the hip joint.[6,25,36,38] The ilioinguinal pain or discomfort is diminished by hip flexion and lateral recumbent positioning.[4,6]

The different locations of entrapment can be detected through palpation, which elicits tenderness. Rectus border entrapment is detected with palpation of the rectus border inferior to the umbilicus.[6] For entrapment around the iliac crest, palpate the free edge of the external oblique muscle near the iliac crest, and for paravertebral entrapment, palpate the paravertebral space of L1.[6]

The symptoms of ilioinguinal nerve neuralgia are frequently confused with those of appendicitis, tendonitis of the abdominal muscles, lumbar radiculopathy, endometriosis, myofascial pain, upper lumbar facet pathology, interstitial cystitis, rectus sheath neuromas, and irritable bowels.[6] These alternative diagnoses must therefore be excluded, while the clinical triad of the diagnosis and a history of abdominal or pelvic surgeries are kept in mind.[6] Further complicating a proper diagnosis is the overlap of the distributions of the genitofemoral, ilioinguinal, and iliohypogastric nerves, and the possibility that more than one of them is injured.[5,6,25]

4.3 Surgery

The main operations involving the ilioinguinal nerve are performed either to prevent ilioinguinal neuralgia from presenting postoperatively or to resolve it. During repairs of inguinal hernias through a Lichtenstein herniorrhaphy or laparoscopic approach, the ilioinguinal nerve can be excised in order to avoid postoperative neuralgia, but the long-term effectiveness of this method is doubtful.[15,27,39,40,41,42,43,44,45] For laparoscopic surgeries, Kingman et al suggest excision of the ilioinguinal nerve as it transverses over the quadratus lumborum muscle, with clips secured proximally and distally to the site of excision. This potentially prevents neuroma formation and also provides a radiographic identifier if nerve block procedures are required postoperatively.[40] For open hernia repair, Malekpour et al and Khoshmohabat et al recommend neurectomy 1 to 2 cm lateral to the deep inguinal ring, with 3 to 4 cm of nerve excised.[41,45] Mui et al recommend excising the ilioinguinal nerve from its entrance to the rectus abdominis muscle to "as lateral of the deep ring as possible."[44] However, it should be noted that there are no standard guidelines for ilioinguinal neurectomy due to the lack of evidence.[15,39,42,43]

Alternatively, nerve blocks and resections are the most common methods for relieving ilioinguinal neuralgia resulting from pelvic or abdominal surgery. Ilioinguinal nerve blocks can be performed either blind using landmarks or more commonly with ultrasound guidance. When landmarks alone are used, an imaginary line is made between the anterior superior iliac spine and umbilicus and the needle inserted along the lateral one-fourth to one third of this line.[11,46] However, van Schoor et al suggested 2.5 mm from the anterior superior iliac spine as a more accurate injection site in a pediatric patient.[11,14] The needle, inserted either at a 45-degree angle or perpendicularly, produces a "click" after piercing the internal oblique muscle.[11] A first "click" may be heard when the external oblique muscle is initially pierced, but in this location it could be an aponeurosis. Levobupivacaine or bupivacaine is injected after the fascial "click" of the internal oblique muscle is detected, the injection being positioned as the nerve courses between the transversus abdominis and internal oblique muscles.[11,46] For the injection, either the angle of the needle toward the groin or umbilicus can be altered, or the needle angle can be maintained while applying the anesthetic first after feeling the "click" of the internal oblique fascia, secondly injecting superficial to this layer, and then continuing to withdraw the needle after the "click" of the external oblique fascia.[11] This procedure is complicated by the risk of falsely identifying the fascia planes or improper needle placement leading to colonic puncture, femoral nerve block, or injection into the peritoneum.[46]

To increase the accuracy of ilioinguinal nerve blocks, ultrasound is frequently used. For an ultrasound-guided nerve block, a high-frequency linear probe, 6 to 15 MHz, is used with the patient lying supine.[11,47] For obese patients, a medium-frequency and a curved probe can also be used, and recent literature detailed by Mathers et al demonstrates that a lateral decubitus position is beneficial.[11,48] The anterior superior iliac spine is identified and the probe is used to trace the imaginary line from there to the umbilicus.[6,11,47,49] The abdominal wall layers are identified, and the iliohypogastric and ilioinguinal nerves should be identified between internal oblique muscle and either the external oblique or the transversus abdominis muscle.[11,49] This visualization is easier in pediatric patients; fluid may be required for contrast in adults.[11] However, if visualization is unsuccessful, anesthetic can be placed in the planes superficial and deep to the internal oblique muscle.[11] The needle can be inserted either "in-plane," medial to lateral at a shallow angle toward the anterior superior iliac spine, or "out-of-plane" at a 45-degree angle with the probe positioned obliquely.[11] In both approaches, the location of the needle is confirmed by the ultrasound. The anesthetic that surrounds the nerves will appear hypoechoic.[11,50] Fluoroscopy can also be used to provide a nerve block, and this mirrors the procedures of a nerve root block or transforaminal epidural rather than that of the ultrasound-guided technique.[6] A peripheral nerve stimulator is used to identify the pathology. When approaching for paravertebral injections, fluoroscopy is used on a prone patient to distinguish the foramen, and a peripheral nerve stimulator is used to identify the ilioinguinal nerve from a selective nerve root technique.[6]

The other main solution to ilioinguinal neuralgia is neurectomy. There are various procedures for approaching the ilioinguinal nerve, but they all start with a nerve block using the procedures previously highlighted.[29,51] Kline et al describe a method using vital blue dye along with the anesthetic during the nerve block in order to stain the relevant areas. The incision is made above the injection site and then through the external oblique aponeurosis, where the dye should be found.[52] The stained tissue, including the external oblique fascia, subcutaneous fat, and potentially the internal oblique muscle, is resected with the accompanying nerve portion.[52] Hanna utilizes preoperative ultrasound-guided wire placement for more precise localization of the ilioinguinal nerve.[54] Alternatively, Campanelli et al suggest approaching anteriorly with a transverse incision over the inguinal canal, if opening the scar tissue superior to the external oblique aponeurosis is not an option. This approach advocates identifying the surgical equipment most likely to be responsible, such as sutures or mesh from previous abdominal or pelvic surgery, removing the ilioinguinal nerve from its entrapment, and then excising the nerve. Using a similar incision, the ilioinguinal nerve can be accessed for resection as it crosses either the anterior superior iliac spine or the quadratus lumborum muscle, cranial to the psoas major.[53] Hahn suggests an incision in a similar area with a 6- to 8-cm oblique incision from the anterior iliac spine, which allows the external oblique fascia to be accessed and incised. The ilioinguinal nerve, identified medial and deep to the iliac spine, can be electrocauterized and then transected.[29] Alternative methods of nerve ablation utilize radiofrequency or microwave energy.

References

[1] Schaeffer JP. Morris' Human Anatomy: A Complete Systematic Treatise. 11th ed. New York, NY: McGraw-Hill Book Company, Inc.; 1953

[2] Thane GD. Quain's Elements of Anatomy, Vol. 3, Part 2: The Nerves. 10th ed. London: Longmans, Green, and Co.; 1895

[3] Klaassen Z, Marshall E, Tubbs RS, Louis RG, Jr, Wartmann CT, Loukas M. Anatomy of the ilioinguinal and iliohypogastric nerves with observations of their spinal nerve contributions. Clin Anat. 2011; 24(4):454–461

[4] Vanetti TK, Luba ATR, Assis FD, de Oliveira CA. Genitofemoral nerve entrapment: pelvic. In: Trescot AM, ed. Peripheral Nerve Entrapments. Cham: Springer; 2016:479–489

[5] Rab M, Ebmer And J, Dellon AL. Anatomic variability of the ilioinguinal and genitofemoral nerve: implications for the treatment of groin pain. Plast Reconstr Surg. 2001; 108(6):1618–1623

[6] Amin N, Krashin D, Trescot AM. Ilioinguinal and iliohypogastric nerve entrapment: abdominal. In: Trescot AM, ed. Peripheral Nerve Entrapments. Cham: Springer; 2016:413–424

[7] Ndiaye A, Diop M, Ndoye JM, et al. Anatomical basis of neuropathies and damage to the ilioinguinal nerve during repairs of groin hernias. (about 100 dissections). Surg Radiol Anat. 2007; 29(8):675–681

[8] Walji AH, Tsui BC. Clinical anatomy of the lumbar plexus. In: Tsui BCH, Suresh S, eds. Pediatric Atlas of Ultrasound- and Nerve Stimulation-Guided Regional Anesthesia. New York, NY: Springer; 2016:165–175

[9] Reinpold W, Schroeder AD, Schroeder M, Berger C, Rohr M, Wehrenberg U. Retroperitoneal anatomy of the iliohypogastric, ilioinguinal, genitofemoral, and lateral femoral cutaneous nerve: consequences for prevention and treatment of chronic inguinodynia. Hernia. 2015; 19(4):539–548

[10] Standring S. Gray's Anatomy: The Anatomical Basis of Clinical Practice. 41st ed. New York, NY: Elsevier Health Sciences; 2015

[11] Tsui BC. Ilioinguinal and iliohypogastric nerve blocks. In: Tsui BCH, Suresh S, eds. Pediatric Atlas of Ultrasound- and Nerve Stimulation-Guided Regional Anesthesia. New York, NY: Springer; 2016:477–483

[12] Avsar FM, Sahin M, Arikan BU, Avsar AF, Demirci S, Elhan A. The possibility of nervus ilioinguinalis and nervus iliohypogastricus injury in lower abdominal incisions and effects on hernia formation. J Surg Res. 2002; 107(2):179–185

[13] Whiteside JL, Barber MD, Walters MD, Falcone T. Anatomy of ilioinguinal and iliohypogastric nerves in relation to trocar placement and low transverse incisions. Am J Obstet Gynecol. 2003; 189(6):1574–1578, discussion 1578

[14] van Schoor AN, Boon JM, Bosenberg AT, Abrahams PH, Meiring JH. Anatomical considerations of the pediatric ilioinguinal/iliohypogastric nerve block. Paediatr Anaesth. 2005; 15(5):371–377

[15] Wijsmuller AR, Lange JF, Kleinrensink GJ, et al. Nerve-identifying inguinal hernia repair: a surgical anatomical study. World J Surg. 2007; 31(2):414–420, discussion 421–422

[16] Moosman DA, Oelrich TM. Prevention of accidental trauma to the ilioinguinal nerve during inguinal herniorrhaphy. Am J Surg. 1977; 133(2):146–148

[17] Al-dabbagh AK. Anatomical variations of the inguinal nerves and risks of injury in 110 hernia repairs. Surg Radiol Anat. 2002; 24(2):102–107

[18] Salama J, Sarfati E, Chevrel J. The anatomical bases of nerve lesions arising during the reduction of inguinal hernia. Anat Clin. 1983; 5(2):75–81

[19] Knockaert DC, D'Heygere FG, Bobbaers HJ. Ilioinguinal nerve entrapment: a little-known cause of iliac fossa pain. Postgrad Med J. 1989; 65(767):632–635

[20] Luijendijk RW, Jeekel J, Storm RK, et al. The low transverse Pfannenstiel incision and the prevalence of incisional hernia and nerve entrapment. Ann Surg. 1997; 225(4):365–369

[21] Murinova N, Krashin D, Trescot AM. Ilioinguinal nerve entrapment: pelvic. In: Trescot AM, ed. Peripheral Nerve Entrapments. Cham: Springer; 2016:467–477

[22] Loos MJ, Scheltinga MR, Mulders LG, Roumen RM. The Pfannenstiel incision as a source of chronic pain. Obstet Gynecol. 2008; 111(4):839–846

[23] Poobalan AS, Bruce J, Smith WCS, King PM, Krukowski ZH, Chambers WA. A review of chronic pain after inguinal herniorrhaphy. Clin J Pain. 2003; 19(1):48–54

[24] Purves JK, Miller JD. Inguinal neuralgia: a review of 50 patients. Can J Surg. 1986; 29(1):43–45

[25] McCrory P, Bell S. Nerve entrapment syndromes as a cause of pain in the hip, groin and buttock. Sports Med. 1999; 27(4):261–274

[26] Gaines RD. Complications of groin hernia repair: their prevention and management. J Natl Med Assoc. 1978; 70(3):195–198

[27] Dittrick GW, Ridl K, Kuhn JA, McCarty TM. Routine ilioinguinal nerve excision in inguinal hernia repairs. Am J Surg. 2004; 188(6):736–740

[28] Vernadakis AJ, Koch H, Mackinnon SE. Management of neuromas. Clin Plast Surg. 2003; 30(2):247–268, vii

[29] Hahn L. Treatment of ilioinguinal nerve entrapment - a randomized controlled trial. Acta Obstet Gynecol Scand. 2011; 90(9):955–960

[30] Stark E, Oestreich K, Wendl K, Rumstadt B, Hagmüller E. Nerve irritation after laparoscopic hernia repair. Surg Endosc. 1999; 13(9):878–881

[31] Rosenberger RJ, Loeweneck H, Meyer G. The cutaneous nerves encountered during laparoscopic repair of inguinal hernia: new anatomical findings for the surgeon. Surg Endosc. 2000; 14(8):731–735

[32] Demirer S, Kepenekci I, Evirgen O, et al. The effect of polypropylene mesh on ilioinguinal nerve in open mesh repair of groin hernia. J Surg Res. 2006; 131(2):175–181

[33] Amid PK. Causes, prevention, and surgical treatment of postherniorrhaphy neuropathic inguinodynia: triple neurectomy with proximal end implantation. Hernia. 2004; 8(4):343–349

[34] Miller JP, Acar F, Kaimaktchiev VB, Gultekin SH, Burchiel KJ. Pathology of ilioinguinal neuropathy produced by mesh entrapment: case report and literature review. Hernia. 2008; 12(2):213–216

[35] Kopell HP, Thompson WA, Postel AH. Entrapment neuropathy of the ilioinguinal nerve. N Engl J Med. 1962; 266:16–19

[36] Stulz P, Pfeiffer KM. Peripheral nerve injuries resulting from common surgical procedures in the lower portion of the abdomen. Arch Surg. 1982; 117(3):324–327

[37] Starling JR, Harms BA. Diagnosis and treatment of genitofemoral and ilioinguinal neuralgia. World J Surg. 1989; 13(5):586–591

[38] Acar F, Ozdemir M, Bayrakli F, Cirak B, Coskun E, Burchiel K. Management of medically intractable genitofemoral and ilioingunal neuralgia. Turk Neurosurg. 2013; 23(6):753–757

[39] Barazanchi AWH, Fagan PVB, Smith BB, Hill AG. Routine neurectomy of inguinal nerves during open onlay mesh hernia repair: a meta-analysis of randomized trials. Ann Surg. 2016; 264(1):64–72

[40] Kingman SA, Amid PK, Chen DC. Laparoscopic triple neurectomy. In: Jacob B, Chen D, Ramshaw B, Towfigh S, eds. The SAGES Manual of Groin Pain. Cham: Springer; 2016:333–342

[41] Malekpour F, Mirhashemi SH, Hajinasrolah E, Salehi N, Khoshkar A, Kolahi AA. Ilioinguinal nerve excision in open mesh repair of inguinal hernia–results of a randomized clinical trial: simple solution for a difficult problem? Am J Surg. 2008; 195(6):735–740

[42] Alfieri S, Amid PK, Campanelli G, et al. International guidelines for prevention and management of post-operative chronic pain following inguinal hernia surgery. Hernia. 2011; 15(3):239–249

[43] Picchio M, Palimento D, Attanasio U, Matarazzo PF, Bambini C, Caliendo A. Randomized controlled trial of preservation or elective division of ilioinguinal nerve on open inguinal hernia repair with polypropylene mesh. Arch Surg. 2004; 139(7):755–758, discussion 759

[44] Mui WL, Ng CS, Fung TM, et al. Prophylactic ilioinguinal neurectomy in open inguinal hernia repair: a double-blind randomized controlled trial. Ann Surg. 2006; 244(1):27–33

[45] Khoshmohabat H, Panahi F, Alvandi AA, Mehrvarz S, Mohebi HA, Shams Koushki E. Effect of ilioinguinal neurectomy on chronic pain following herniorrhaphy. Trauma Mon. 2012; 17(3):323–328

[46] Bugada D, Peng PWH. Ilioinguinal, iliohypogastric, and genitofemoral nerve blocks. In: Jankovic D, Peng PWH, eds. Regional Nerve Blocks in Anesthesia and Pain Therapy: Cham: Springer; 2015:707–715

[47] Hong JY, Kim WO, Koo BN, Kim YA, Jo YY, Kil HK. The relative position of ilioinguinal and iliohypogastric nerves in different age groups of pediatric patients. Acta Anaesthesiol Scand. 2010; 54(5):566–570

[48] Mathers J, Haley C, Gofeld M. Ilioinguinal nerve block in obese patients: description of new technique. J Med Ultrasound. 2015; 23(4):185–188

[49] Thomassen I, van Suijlekom JA, van de Gaag A, Ponten JE, Nienhuijs SW. Ultrasound-guided ilioinguinal/iliohypogastric nerve blocks for chronic pain after inguinal hernia repair. Hernia. 2013; 17(3):329–332

[50] Gofeld M, Christakis M. Sonographically guided ilioinguinal nerve block. J Ultrasound Med. 2006; 25(12):1571–1575

[51] Aasvang E, Kehlet H. Surgical management of chronic pain after inguinal hernia repair. Br J Surg. 2005; 92(7):795–801

[52] Kline CM, Lucas CE, Ledgerwood AM. Directed neurectomy for treatment of chronic postsurgical neuropathic pain. Am J Surg. 2013; 205(3):246–248, discussion 248–249

[53] Campanelli G, Bertocchi V, Cavalli M, et al. Surgical treatment of chronic pain after inguinal hernia repair. Hernia. 2013; 17(3):347–353

[54] Hanna A, Ehlers M, Lee K. Preoperative ultrasound-guided wire location of the lateral femoral cutaneous nerve. Oper Neurosurg. 2017; 13(3):402–408

5 Lateral Femoral Cutaneous Nerve

Jaspreet Johal

Abstract

The branches of the lumbar plexus are encountered in various invasive procedures. Therefore, a thorough knowledge of each of its branches is important to the clinician who performs such procedures. This chapter reviews the clinical anatomy of the lateral femoral cutaneous nerve. It is hoped that a better understanding of this nerve and its distribution will decrease patient morbidity.

Keywords: anatomy, posterior abdominal wall, nerves, complications, surgery, lumbar plexus, lateral approaches, spine, peripheral nerves, lateral femoral cutaneous nerve

5.1 Anatomy and Function

The lateral femoral cutaneous nerve (LFCN) is formed by contributions from the ventral rami of the L2 and L3 spinal nerves (▶ Fig. 5.1 and ▶ Fig. 5.2). It is a cutaneous nerve serving the lateral aspect of the thigh. Along its highly variable course, it initially emerges from beneath the lateral border of the psoas muscle and traverses the pelvis by running obliquely past the iliacus muscle. It then approaches the anterior superior iliac spine (ASIS) parallel to the iliac crest as it exits the pelvis. At this point, the LFCN supplies sensory innervation to the parietal peritoneum of the iliac fossa. On the left side, it passes behind the lower segment of the descending colon, and on the right side it courses posterolaterally past the cecum. It exits the pelvis and enters the thigh region by piercing through the fascia lata beneath the inguinal ligament.[1,2]

As it travels through the thigh beneath the inguinal ligament, the LFCN courses subcutaneously in a lateral and distal direction. During its descent through the thigh, it divides into anterior and posterior branches. At a point 10 cm distal to the ASIS, its anterior branch becomes superficial and provides sensory innervation to the skin of the anterolateral thigh down to the knee. The anterior branch also connects with cutaneous branches of the anterior femoral nerve and the infrapatellar branch of the saphenous nerve to form the peripatellar plexus. The posterior branch pierces through the fascia lata at a point higher than the anterior branch and further divides to provide innervation to the lateral skin from the greater trochanter to mid-distance along the thigh, and can also supply the gluteal skin.[1,2] Hanna described a complete fascial canal surrounding the LFCN in the thigh.[28]

An analysis of the LFCN by Ray et al revealed that it is usually flattened at the inguinal ligament, where it is encompassed by a concentrically arranged thick perineurium.[3] Its mean cross-sectional area at this point was recorded as 1.921 ± 0.414 mm^2. The LFCN was also found to contain three to six fascicles at this point, with a mean of 4.5 fascicles per nerve and a mean fascicular area of 0.647 ± 0.176 mm^2. The cadaveric study by Ray et al also reported that the mean distance from the ASIS to the point at which the LFCN passes the inguinal ligament is 1.87 ± 0.48 cm, and the mean distance from the ASIS to the point at which it crosses the lateral border of the sartorius muscle is 6.15 ± 1.79 cm.[3]

5.2 Variations

As mentioned earlier, the exact path taken by the LFCN during its descent through the pelvis and anterolateral thigh can vary greatly. de Ridder et al found some degree of anatomical variation in the LFCN in at least 25% of the patient population.[4] This variability could contribute to the occurrence of iatrogenic injury to the nerve during surgical procedures secondary to difficulty in predicting its exact course.[5,6,7] The first source of variability lies in the nerves that contribute to the formation of the LFCN. Normally, it arises from the posterior divisions of L2 and L3, but it can also arise from L1 and L2 ("high form") and from L3 and L4 ("low form"). It can also emerge from the femoral nerve or as a distinct branch of the lumbar plexus.[2] Sim and Webb found that the LFCN arose from the first two lumbar nerves in 22 of 60 patients, solely from the L2 ventral ramus in 1, and from the femoral nerve in 6, with almost half showing some variation in the nerves from which the LFCN was derived.[8] Webber observed at least eight distinct patterns of neural origin and contributions to the LFCN.[9] Carai et al found that the LFCN was absent in almost 9% of patients who required operative intervention for meralgia paresthetica.[5] Other variations include an absence of the nerve on either side and its replacement by a contribution from the anterior femoral cutaneous nerve.[10]

Another significant area of variability is the point at which the LFCN exits the pelvis and enters the thigh region. Normally, it exits medial to the ASIS and runs underneath the inguinal ligament.[11] Aszmann et al distinguished five categories of anatomical variation in the LFCN's exit from the pelvis and entry to the thigh during their cadaveric studies, and these findings have been corroborated by other studies.[12,13,14,15] Aszmann et al defined type A as the LFCN running posterior to the ASIS and across the iliac crest, type B as anterior to the ASIS and superficial to the sartorius muscle but within the inguinal ligament, type C as medial to the ASIS and enclosed fully within the tendinous origin of the sartorius muscle, type D as medial to the sartorius muscle and deep to the inguinal ligament while running between the tendon of the sartorius and the thick fascia of the iliopsoas muscle, and type E as the most medial, deep to the inguinal ligament, and embedded within a sheet of loose connective tissue. Type E was also observed to contribute to the femoral branch of the genitofemoral nerve.[12,16]

Finally, there is a variety of branching patterns with bifurcations being reported within the pelvis, in the thigh, and near the exit of the nerves from the pelvis. Grothaus et al found that the LFCN bifurcates into additional branches before traveling underneath the inguinal ligament in 27.6% of 29 cadavers studied.[17] Rudin et al recently proposed a classification system for the various branching patterns seen when the LFCN travels past the ASIS. In the sartorius-type pattern, a dominant anterior branch travels along the lateral border of the sartorius muscle with only a very thin posterior branch. The posterior-type is defined as having a posterior branch at least as thick as the anterior branch. This posterior branch leaves laterally and travels across the medial border of the tensor fasciae latae muscle, which lies distal to the ASIS. Finally, the fan-type pattern

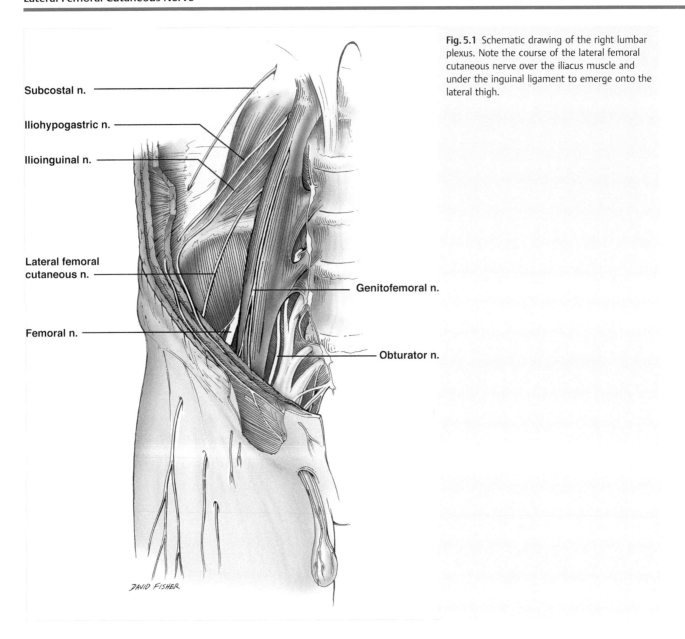

Subcostal n.

Iliohypogastric n.

Ilioinguinal n.

Lateral femoral
cutaneous n.

Femoral n.

Genitofemoral n.

Obturator n.

DAVID FISHER

Fig. 5.1 Schematic drawing of the right lumbar plexus. Note the course of the lateral femoral cutaneous nerve over the iliacus muscle and under the inguinal ligament to emerge onto the lateral thigh.

displays many branches of similar thickness that fan out across the anterolateral thigh, traveling across the lateral border of the sartorius and the tensor fasciae latae muscles.[18] Trifurcation and quadrification have also been reported.[11,13]

5.3 Pathology and Surgery

Given the unpredictable path of the LFCN and the many anatomical variations reported in the literature, the nerve is highly vulnerable to iatrogenic or accidental injury. This risk is greatest along the anterior or anterolateral proximal thigh or during its course alongside the inguinal ligament. Mechanisms of iatrogenic injury include accidental damage to the nerve during incision, suture ligation, and transection. This occurs most often during procedures involving the abdomen, pelvis, or hip. Surgeries that can injure the LFCN include inguinal hernia repair, inguinal lymph node biopsy, femoral artery catheterization, and any procedure involving an anterior or anterolateral approach

to the hip or an ilioinguinal approach to the acetabulum. The nerve can also be injured during iliac crest bone graft harvesting. Noniatrogenic injury can occur secondary to use of belts and braces, or due to trauma.[1]

Irritation of the LFCN produces a syndrome referred to as meralgia paresthetica (Bernhardt–Roth syndrome). This syndrome occurs secondary to entrapment of the LFCN as it exits the pelvis and passes deep to or through the inguinal ligament.[3] Meralgia paresthetica produces a symptomology of pain, paresthesias, and loss of sensory functionality within the distribution of the LFCN along the anterolateral thigh.[16] The syndrome was first described by Hager and further defined and named by Roth.[19,20] Its incidence may be higher in diabetic patients and those with a long-term history of strenuous activities such as soccer or gymnastics.[16,21,22] Other associated factors include obesity, constricting garments, postural alterations, and activities or physical states such as pregnancy that place greater demands on the abdominopelvic region. The LFCN is believed

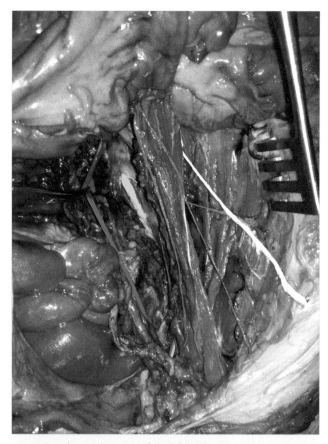

Fig. 5.2 Cadaveric dissection of the left lumbar plexus. The two branches of the genitofemoral nerve (purple) are seen exiting the anterior surface of the psoas major muscle and the large femoral nerve (purple) is seen leaving the pelvis on the lateral border of psoas major. The white colored nerve leaving the lateral side of psoas major and traveling over iliacus toward the anterior superior iliac spine is the lateral femoral cutaneous nerve. The obturator nerve (red) is pulled medially to show the L5 ventral ramus (green).

to be most susceptible to compression and iatrogenic injury at its emergence from the pelvis, and the high variability in that region contributes to the occurrence of meralgia paresthetica following surgical procedures within this area.[23]

Meralgia paresthetica seems especially common in hip replacement procedures and spine surgeries.[16] Analyses of patients undergoing hip surgery have revealed a high incidence of postoperative LFCN neuropraxia. Goulding et al found that 91% of patients who underwent anterior approach hip resurfacing and 67% of those who underwent anterior approach total hip arthroplasty had such complications.[24] Rudin et al concluded that iatrogenic injury to the LFCN during anterior hip procedures could be avoided depending on the type of branching pattern it displays as it passes the ASIS. For a sartorius-type branching pattern, a more lateral incision further from the lateral border of the sartorius muscle is indicated. The posterior-type and fan-type branching patterns are more susceptible to incisions, and incisions made even more lateral might not prevent injury. Rudin et al recommended restricting skin incisions to superficial levels of the subcutaneous tissue. They also posit that injury to the posterior branch could be prevented by blunt

dissection techniques and proximal mobilization of the branch and its accompanying vessels.[18] Gupta et al found that 12% of their patients who underwent posterior lumbar spine surgery had postoperative neuropraxia within the region innervated by the LFCN.[25] They went on to hypothesize that because patients are placed in a prone position for prolonged periods during this procedure, the resultant compression of the anterior hip leads to development of meralgia paresthetica.[16,25] Others have reported a similar incidence of LFCN neuropraxia following spinal procedures involving the patient being placed in a prone position.[26,27] In order to release the LFCN, Hanna proposes using preoperative ultrasound-guided wire placement; due to the variability in the course of the nerve [29]. He also proposes mobilizing the nerve away from the ASIS through medial transposition [30].

References

[1] Mirjalili SA. Anatomy of the lumbar plexus. In: Tubbs RS, Rizk E, Shoja MM, Loukas M, Barbaro N, Spinner RJ, eds. Nerves and Nerve Injuries. Vol. 1. San Diego, CA: Elsevier; 2015:614–617

[2] Apaydin N. Variations of the lumbar and sacral plexuses and their branches. In: Tubbs RS, Rizk E, Shoja MM, Loukas M, Barbaro N, Spinner RJ, eds. Nerves and Nerve Injuries. Vol. 1. San Diego: Elsevier; 2015:614–617

[3] Ray B, D'Souza AS, Kumar B, et al. Variations in the course and microanatomical study of the lateral femoral cutaneous nerve and its clinical importance. Clin Anat. 2010; 23(8):978–984

[4] de Ridder VA, de Lange S, Popta JV. Anatomical variations of the lateral femoral cutaneous nerve and the consequences for surgery. J Orthop Trauma. 1999; 13(3):207–211

[5] Carai A, Fenu G, Sechi E, Crotti FM, Montella A. Anatomical variability of the lateral femoral cutaneous nerve: findings from a surgical series. Clin Anat. 2009; 22(3):365–370

[6] Williams PH, Trzil KP. Management of meralgia paresthetica. J Neurosurg. 1991; 74(1):76–80

[7] Dibenedetto LM, Lei Q, Gilroy AM, Hermey DC, Marks SC, Jr, Page DW. Variations in the inferior pelvic pathway of the lateral femoral cutaneous nerve: implications for laparoscopic hernia repair. Clin Anat. 1996; 9(4):232–236

[8] Sim IW, Webb T. Anatomy and anaesthesia of the lumbar somatic plexus. Anaesth Intensive Care. 2004; 32(2):178–187

[9] Webber RH. Some variations in the lumbar plexus of nerves in man. Acta Anat (Basel). 1961; 44:336–345

[10] Bergman RA, Thompson SA, Afifi AK, Saddeh FA. Compendium of human anatomical variations. Baltimore, MD: Urban and Schwarzenburg; 1988:143–148

[11] Tomaszewski KA, Popieluszko P, Henry BM, et al. The surgical anatomy of the lateral femoral cutaneous nerve in the inguinal region: a meta-analysis. Hernia. 2016; 20(5):649–657

[12] Aszmann OC, Dellon ES, Dellon AL. Anatomical course of the lateral femoral cutaneous nerve and its susceptibility to compression and injury. Plast Reconstr Surg. 1997; 100(3):600–604

[13] Sürücü HS, Tanyeli E, Sargon MF, Karahan ST. An anatomic study of the lateral femoral cutaneous nerve. Surg Radiol Anat. 1997; 19(5):307–310

[14] Majkrzak A, Johnston J, Kacey D, Zeller J. Variability of the lateral femoral cutaneous nerve: an anatomic basis for planning safe surgical approaches. Clin Anat. 2010; 23(3):304–311

[15] Ropars M, Morandi X, Huten D, Thomazeau H, Berton E, Darnault P. Anatomical study of the lateral femoral cutaneous nerve with special reference to minimally invasive anterior approach for total hip replacement. Surg Radiol Anat. 2009; 31(3):199–204

[16] Cheatham SW, Kolber MJ, Salamh PA. Meralgia paresthetica: a review of the literature. Int J Sports Phys Ther. 2013; 8(6):883–893

[17] Grothaus MC, Holt M, Mekhail AO, Ebraheim NA, Yeasting RA. Lateral femoral cutaneous nerve: an anatomic study. Clin Orthop Relat Res. 2005(437):164–168

[18] Rudin D, Manestar M, Ullrich O, Erhardt J, Grob K. The anatomical course of the lateral femoral cutaneous nerve with special attention to the anterior approach to the hip joint. J Bone Joint Surg Am. 2016; 98(7):561–567

[19] Hager W. Neuralgia Femoris. Resection des Nerv. Cutan. Femoris anterior externus Heilung. Dtsch Med Wochenschr. 1885; 11:218

[20] Roth VK. Meralgia paresthetica. Med Obozr Mosk. 1895; 43:678

[21] Parisi TJ, Mandrekar J, Dyck PJ, Klein CJ. Meralgia paresthetica: relation to obesity, advanced age, and diabetes mellitus. Neurology. 2011; 77(16):1538–1542

[22] Ulkar B, Yildiz Y, Kunduracioğlu B. Meralgia paresthetica: a long-standing performance-limiting cause of anterior thigh pain in a soccer player. Am J Sports Med. 2003; 31(5):787–789

[23] Sunderland S. Anatomical features of nerve trunks in relation to nerve injury and nerve repair. Clin Neurosurg. 1970; 17:38–62

[24] Goulding K, Beaulé PE, Kim PR, Fazekas A. Incidence of lateral femoral cutaneous nerve neuropraxia after anterior approach hip arthroplasty. Clin Orthop Relat Res. 2010; 468(9):2397–2404

[25] Gupta A, Muzumdar D, Ramani PS. Meralgia paraesthetica following lumbar spine surgery: a study in 110 consecutive surgically treated cases. Neurol India. 2004; 52(1):64–66

[26] Cho KT, Lee HJ. Prone position-related meralgia paresthetica after lumbar spinal surgery : a case report and review of the literature. J Korean Neurosurg Soc. 2008; 44(6):392–395

[27] Yang SH, Wu CC, Chen PQ. Postoperative meralgia paresthetica after posterior spine surgery: incidence, risk factors, and clinical outcomes. Spine. 2005; 30 (18):E547–E550

[28] Hanna A. The lateral femoral cutaneous nerve canal. J Neurosurg. 2017; 126 (3):972–978

[29] Hanna A, Ehlers M, Lee K. Preoperative ultrasound-guided wire location of the lateral femoral cutaneous nerve. Oper Neurosurg. 2017; 13(3): 402–408

[30] Hanna A. Lateral femoral cutaneous nerve transposition: renaissance of an old concept in the light of new anatomy. Clin Anat. 2017; 30(3): 409–412

6 Genitofemoral Nerve

Marcus Cox, Jaspreet Johal

Abstract

The branches of the lumbar plexus are frequently encountered in various invasive procedures. Therefore, a thorough knowledge of each of its branches is important to the clinician who performs such procedures. This chapter reviews the clinical anatomy and associated pathologies of the genitofemoral nerve. It is hoped that a better understanding of this nerve and its distribution will decrease patient morbidity.

Keywords: anatomy, posterior abdominal wall, nerves, complications, surgery, inguinal, anatomy, lumbar plexus, lateral approaches, spine, peripheral nerves, genitofemoral nerve

6.1 Introduction

The genitofemoral nerve (historically known as the genitocrural nerve) arises from the lumbar plexus (▶ Fig. 6.1 and ▶ Fig. 6.2). It is formed by the union of spinal nerve branches from L1 and L2 ventral rami within the psoas major muscle. The second lumbar nerve provides the majority of the contributions to this nerve, although it is also partly derived from the first lumbar nerve and the connective fibers between the first and second lumbar nerves.[1,2,3] Although the anatomy of this nerve is well described, a wide range of diversity exists in its anatomical form and many different variations can be observed.[4] The nerve is often described as functionally innervating components of both the external genital organs and parts of the thigh.[1,5,6] Awareness of its variations is important, especially for surgeons who operate in the lower abdominal, pelvic, and upper leg areas. This understanding helps to avoid iatrogenic injury to fibers of the genitofemoral nerve.[5,7]

6.2 Anatomy and Variations

The genitofemoral nerve is formed within the psoas major muscle, and is derived from both the first and second lumbar nerves. When comparing these contributions, the vast majority arise from the second lumbar nerve, although the genitofemoral nerve does receive some input from the first lumbar nerve as well as connecting fibers between L1 and L2.[1,3] Once having formed within the psoas muscle, the genitofemoral nerve emerges from the psoas muscle at the L3–L4 vertebral level and travels obliquely and inferiorly. At this point, the genitofemoral nerve lies on fascia that covers the anterior surface of the psoas muscle.[1,8] It then divides into an internal or genital branch, and an external or femoral (crural) branch. This point of division can occur at variable heights, but most often is at a point proximal to the inguinal ligament and shortly after crossing the ureter posteriorly.[1,2,3] In some cases, it divides closer to its origin from the plexus, in which case the two separate branches will travel through the psoas muscle along varying trajectories.[1,3,4]

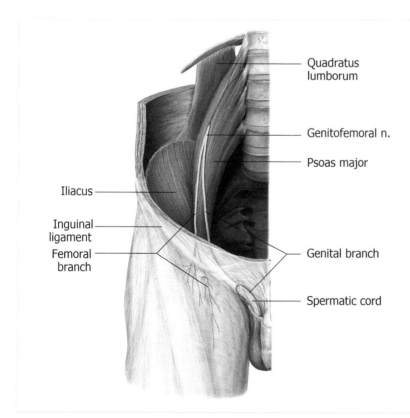

Fig. 6.1 Schematic drawing of the right genitofemoral nerve and its course. (Reproduced with permission from Gilroy AM, Ross LM, MacPherson BR, Schuenke M, Schulte E, Schumacher U. Atlas of Anatomy. New York, NY: Thieme Medical Publishers; 2008. Illustration by Karl Wesker.)

Quadratus lumborum

Genitofemoral n.

Psoas major

Iliacus

Inguinal ligament

Femoral branch

Genital branch

Spermatic cord

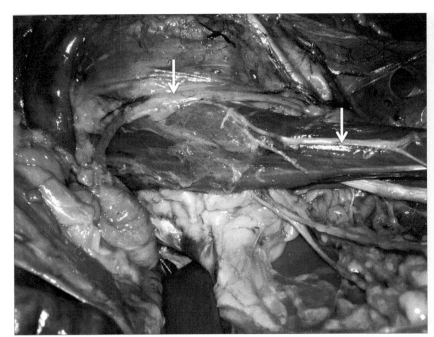

Fig. 6.2 Right-sided cadaveric dissection noting the genitofemoral nerve (*right arrow*). The arrow is at the nerve just prior to its branching into genital and femoral branches. Note the psoas fascia over psoas major and the right ureter (*left arrow*). For reference, the inferior vena cava is just medial to the ureter, and lateral to the psoas major muscle are the larger femoral nerve and smaller lateral femoral cutaneous nerve.

The genital branch of the genitofemoral nerve (also termed the external spermatic nerve in males) is found upon or near the external iliac artery where it crosses the lower part of that vessel. It then enters the deep inguinal ring after perforating the transversalis fascia and follows the spermatic cord in males or the round ligament in females. At this point, the genital branch goes on to supply the cremaster muscle in males and supplies cutaneous innervation of the external genitalia in both males and females.[1,2,3] The femoral branch (crural branch) descends down the psoas muscle and lateral to the external iliac artery. It then crosses over the deep circumflex iliac artery and passes behind the inguinal ligament on its descent to enter the femoral sheath, which lies lateral to the femoral artery.[1,2,3,4,5] The femoral branch has been shown to have communications with the middle cutaneous branch of the anterior femoral nerve, and some supporting filaments may connect it to the femoral artery.[1]

It is important to be aware of the anatomical variations that can exist in the origin, course, and point of division of the genitofemoral nerve as it can be affected by iatrogenic injury during certain procedures, especially abdominal incisions.[8] Variations may exist in the division of this nerve, as the genital and femoral branches may arise independently from the lumbar plexus in certain individuals. Occasionally, the genital branch may be derived from the last thoracic and first lumbar nerves.[1] Another variation that may be seen is the absence of one division completely, or the whole nerve altogether. In these cases, the fibers that normally contribute to the genitofemoral branch will have instead joined another nerve. The fibers that usually form the genital branch may be associated with the ilioinguinal nerve, and the fibers that normally contribute to the femoral nerve may be connected with the cutaneous branches of the femoral nerve.[1,3]

The genitofemoral nerve may also penetrate the psoas major muscle at varying distances and locations. An analysis by Rab and colleagues showed that in roughly two-thirds of sampled specimens, the nerve is seen as a single nerve trunk penetrating the psoas muscle at a distance between 4 to 12 cm from the sacral prominence. After traveling an average of 7 cm (±3.5 cm), it divides into its two branches. In the remaining one-third of specimens, the branches were observed to penetrate the psoas muscle separately and descend as separate nerve fibers. In these cases, the distance between the site of penetration and the sacral prominence ranged from 1.5 to 13 cm for the femoral branch, and from 4 to 13 cm for the genital branch.[4]

Of particular significance for surgeons are variations in the course of the genitofemoral nerve as it courses through the lower abdominal and pelvic regions. Three varying trajectories of the genitofemoral nerve have been distinguished on the basis of the nerve's course along the psoas major muscle.[9] In the first category, the genitofemoral nerve emerges from the psoas muscle as a single trunk and divides into the genital and femoral branches. In the second category, it again emerges from the psoas muscle as a single trunk but this time continues inferiorly as a single trunk to the inguinal ligament. Lastly, in the third category, the genital and femoral branches emerge separately from the psoas muscle. It was found that the first category was most common, seen in around 50% of cases. The second category comprised 30% and the third category was 20% of specimens observed.[9] The vertebral level at which the genitofemoral nerve emerges from the psoas muscle is also of clinical and surgical significance. Using the transverse process of L2 and the iliac crest as landmarks, it has been shown that the nerve can emerge superior to the L2 transverse process, from between the L2 transverse process and the iliac spine, or inferior to the iliac crest. A recent analysis found that the nerve emerges from between the L2 transverse process and the iliac spine in 70% of specimens, inferior to the iliac crest in 20% of cases, and superior to the L2 transverse process in 10%.[9] Knowledge of these anatomical variations is important to avoid unintended iatrogenic injury.

6.3 Innervation and Functional Variations

The genitofemoral branch carries both sensory and motor fibers. Via the genital branch, it supplies motor innervations to the cremaster muscle and sensory innervation to the anterior third of the scrotum in males and the mons pubis and labium majora in females. The femoral branch is responsible for cutaneous innervation to the anteromedial thigh.[2,3,4,5] Although the innervation and function of the genitofemoral branch have been well established, variations do exist in the innervation patterns observed across individuals. Four different cutaneous branching patterns have been observed in the inguinal region, with a high degree of variability in the source of innervations. Adding further complexity, a recent analysis by Rab et al showed that only 40.6% of cases studied displayed bilateral symmetry.[4]

The first pattern of innervation was seen in 43.7% of cases, and was described as having a dominant genitofemoral nerve, with no sensory contributions from the ilioinguinal nerve. The skin of the pubis, ventral scrotum/labia, and ventromedial thigh were innervated by the genital branch of the genitofemoral nerve, which entered the inguinal canal through the deep inguinal ring and coursed along the ventral surface of the spermatic cord, supplying motor innervations to the cremaster muscle in the male specimens. The cutaneous division of the genital branch coursed along the dorsal aspect of the spermatic cord/round ligament as it exited through the superficial inguinal ring.[4]

The second pattern of innervation was observed in 28.1% of specimens, and was described as having a dominant ilioinguinal nerve, with the genitofemoral nerve sharing a branch with the ilioinguinal nerve and supplying motor innervation to the cremaster muscle but giving no sensory contributions to the groin area. The skin of the pubis, ventral scrotum/labia, and ventromedial thigh was innervated by the cutaneous component of the ilioinguinal nerve. The genital branch of the genitofemoral nerve entered the inguinal canal through the deep inguinal ring and coursed along the ventral side of the spermatic cord, supplying motor innervation to the cremaster muscle. In male cadavers, it shared several branches with the cutaneous division of the ilioinguinal nerve within the inguinal canal. In contrast, the genital branch became integrated into the ilioinguinal nerve in the female cadavers. In the end, no cutaneous branches could be observed from the genital branch of the genitofemoral nerve.[4]

The third pattern of innervation was observed in 20.3% of specimens, and was described as having a dominant genitofemoral branch. In these cases, the ilioinguinal nerve supplied sensory fibers to the mons pubis and inguinal crease together with the root of the penis or labium majus. The cutaneous division of the genital branch of the genitofemoral nerve supplied the remaining lower parts of the inguinal and ventromedial thigh areas. The genital branch and the ilioinguinal nerve both entered the inguinal canal as described previously for the second pattern of innervation. The genital branch contained both motor fibers for the cremaster muscle and cutaneous fibers. The cutaneous division of the ilioinguinal nerve and motor supply to the cremaster muscle from the genitofemoral nerve both coursed ventrally to the spermatic cord. The cutaneous division of the genital branch of the genitofemoral nerve coursed dorsally. In females, it ran on the dorsal side of the round ligament.[4]

The fourth pattern of innervation was observed in 7.7% of specimens, and was described as having cutaneous branches emerging from both the genitofemoral and ilioinguinal nerves. In these individuals, the ilioinguinal nerve supplied the mons pubis and inguinal crease together with the anteroproximal part of the root of the penis and labia majora. The pattern of entrance into the inguinal canal and the relationship of the motor and cutaneous divisions of both the genitofemoral and ilioinguinal nerves to the spermatic cord/round ligament were similar to the third pattern of innervation described previously. However, in the fourth category, the ilioinguinal nerve contributed cutaneous innervations to the pubis and inguinal and ventromedial thigh regions.[4]

6.3.1 Clinical Significance and Injury

The genitofemoral nerve is at risk during abdominal procedures, particularly those involving the left and/or right lower quadrants, or the psoas major muscle.[1,2,3,4,5] The resulting condition is termed genitofemoral neuralgia and is characterized by a pattern of chronic neuropathic pain that can become debilitating.[5] The condition results in constant or intermittent pain in the regions supplied by the genitofemoral nerve and its terminal branches. This pain and discomfort is usually intensified by walking, standing, stooping, or hip extension, and relieved by recumbency. Among the noted clinical symptoms are groin pain, paresthesias, and a burning sensation extending from lower abdomen to the medial aspect of the thigh.[5,10] Most commonly, this neuropathy results from iatrogenic injury to the genitofemoral nerve during surgical procedures such as femoral or inguinal herniorrhaphy. Because of the overlap of the cutaneous distribution of the genitofemoral nerve with the other inguinal nerves and the variability in cutaneous innervations described previously, selective nerve blocking is often necessary to establish a definitive diagnosis. Genitofemoral neuralgia can be treated by both invasive and noninvasive procedures ranging from a combination of analgesic and anesthetic injections to radiofrequency ablation, microwave ablation, cryoablation, nerve blocking techniques, and neurectomy.[5,11,12] In some cases, it may be difficult to identify a single nerve as the cause of neuropathy, and a paravertebral block of the L1 and L2 nerve plexus or triple neurectomy will be necessary.[5,8]

The genitofemoral nerve is also thought to play a role in the inguinoscrotal phase of testicular descent.[3,13] Studies on animal models have highlighted the important role this nerve may play in successful descent of the testes.[14,15] Hutson and colleagues detailed the different stages of testicular descent and extrapolated data from murine to human males. They observed that calcitonin gene–related peptide (CGRP) is critical for testicular descent. CGRP, which is released by the genitofemoral nerve, induces rhythmic contractility in the developing cremaster muscle of the gubernaculum and provides a chemotactic gradient that stimulates gubernacular migration toward the scrotum. It was also proposed that exposure of the genitofemoral nerve to androgens is essential for its masculinization and for preprogramming the gubernacular proliferative response to CGRP.[13,14,15]

References

[1] Schafer EA, Thane GD. Quain's Elements of Anatomy, Vol III-Part II: The Nerves. 10th ed. London: Longmans, Green, and Co; 1895

[2] Schaeffer JP. Morris' Human Anatomy: A Complete Systematic Treatise. 11th ed. New York, NY: McGraw-Hill; 1953

[3] Standring S, Anand N, Birch R, et al. Gray's Anatomy: The Anatomical Basis of Clinical Practice. 41st ed. Philadelphia, PA: Elsevier; 2016

[4] Rab M, Ebmer And J, Dellon AL. Anatomic variability of the ilioinguinal and genitofemoral nerve: implications for the treatment of groin pain. Plast Reconstr Surg. 2001; 108(6):1618–1623

[5] Cesmebasi A, Yadav A, Gielecki J, Tubbs RS, Loukas M. Genitofemoral neuralgia: a review. Clin Anat. 2015; 28(1):128–135

[6] Maldonado PA, Slocum PD, Chin K, Corton MM. Anatomic relationships of psoas muscle: clinical applications to psoas hitch ureteral reimplantation. Am J Obstet Gynecol. 2014; 211(5):563.e1–563.e6

[7] Tagliafico A, Bignotti B, Cadoni A, Perez MM, Martinoli C. Anatomical study of the iliohypogastric, ilioinguinal, and genitofemoral nerves using high-resolution ultrasound. Muscle Nerve. 2015; 51(1):42–48

[8] Brown JS, Butrick CW, Carter JE, et al. Pelvic Pain Diagnosis and Management. Philadelphia, PA: Lippincott Williams and Wilkins; 2000

[9] Geh N, Schultz M, Yang L, Zeller J. Retroperitoneal course of iliohypogastric, ilioinguinal, and genitofemoral nerves: A study to improve identification and excision during triple neurectomy. Clin Anat. 2015; 28(7):903–909

[10] Verstraelen H, De Zutter E, De Muynck M. Genitofemoral neuralgia: adding to the burden of chronic vulvar pain. J Pain Res. 2015; 8:845–849

[11] Acar F, Ozdemir M, Bayrakli F, Cirak B, Coskun E, Burchiel K. Management of medically intractable genitofemoral and ilioingunal neuralgia. Turk Neurosurg. 2013; 23(6):753–757

[12] Shanthanna H. Successful treatment of genitofemoral neuralgia using ultrasound guided injection: a case report and short review of literature. Case Rep Anesthesiol. 2014; 2014:371703

[13] Hutson JM, Southwell BR, Li R, et al. The regulation of testicular descent and the effects of cryptorchidism. Endocr Rev. 2013; 34(5):725–752

[14] Cousinery MC, Li R, Vannitamby A, Vikraman J, Southwell BR, Hutson JM. Neurotrophin signaling in a genitofemoral nerve target organ during testicular descent in mice. J Pediatr Surg. 2016; 51(8):1321–1326

[15] Su S, Farmer PJ, Li R, et al. Regression of the mammary branch of the genitofemoral nerve may be necessary for testicular descent in rats. J Urol. 2012; 188(4) Suppl:1443–1448

7 Femoral Nerve

Peter Oakes, Michele Davis

Abstract

The branches of the lumbar plexus are encountered in various invasive procedures. Therefore, a thorough knowledge of each of its branches is important to the clinician who performs such procedures. This chapter reviews the clinical anatomy of the femoral nerve. It is hoped that a better understanding of this nerve and its distribution will decrease patient morbidity.

Keywords: anatomy, posterior abdominal wall, nerves, complications, surgery

7.1 Anatomy

The femoral nerve (▶ Fig. 7.1, ▶ Fig. 7.2, ▶ Fig. 7.3, ▶ Fig. 7.4), the largest branch of the lumbar plexus, runs laterally and caudally through the psoas major muscle and anterior to the iliacus muscle (the latter of which it supplies) at a mean sagittal angle of approximately 27.78 degrees.[1,2,3,4,5] It originates from the posterior divisions of the ventral rami of the second, third, and fourth lumbar spinal nerves within the psoas major muscle (~ 9 cm from the skin surface) and runs between the lateral femoral cutaneous nerve and the obturator nerve from the lumbar plexus.[6,7,8] The femoral nerve emerges from the lateral border of the psoas major muscle 4 cm superior to the inguinal ligament but still beneath the fascia of the iliacus muscle.[6] It enters the thigh with the iliacus muscle while passing under the inguinal ligament and through the lateral space of the lacuna musculorum, approximately half the medial–lateral distance between the anterior superior iliac spine and the pubic symphysis.[4,5,6] It enters the thigh lateral to the femoral artery and therefore outside the femoral sheath.[1,6] The femoral nerve emerges from under cover of the inguinal ligament about half-way between the anterior superior iliac spine and the pubic tubercle. The femoral neurovascular bundle is contained within the femoral triangle at the level of the inguinal crease, where it is covered by layers of skin, fat, and fascia lata.[9] The femoral triangle is formed laterally by the sartorius muscle, medially by the adductor longus muscles, and superiorly by the inguinal ligament.[9] Approximately 1.50 ± 0.47 cm distal to the inguinal ligament (others have reported a distance of 3–5 cm), before the femoral crease, the femoral nerve splits into numerous posterior and anterior branches, which are observed in 80% of cases to be divided by the lateral circumflex femoral artery.[4,6,7,10,11] One anatomical study showed that most cadavers (83.3%) possessed a femoral nerve located anterior to the profunda femoris artery, while the femoral nerves in the remainder were posterior to this structure (16.7%).[1]

The nerve receives its blood supply from the iliolumbar artery when travelling through the pelvis, the deep circumflex iliac artery when traversing the inguinal region, and the lateral circumflex femoral artery upon entering the thigh.[7] Interestingly, some have discovered that the deep circumflex iliac artery on the left side gives fewer branches than its equivalent on the right, potentially rendering the femoral nerve on that side more susceptible to ischemic injury.[7] Three different lymphatic routes are known to drain the femoral nerve. In the iliac fossa, one or two routes drain, which then move to lymph nodes near the external iliac artery.[12] The third lymphatic route drains into the lymph nodes near the femoral canal after leaving the nerve where the femoral nerve passes under the inguinal ligament.[12]

The femoral nerve displays multiple subtle changes in its structure and relationship with other structures as it descends into the leg. It is nearly 50% wider and significantly closer to the

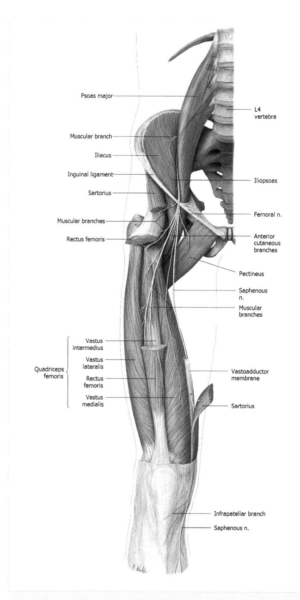

Fig. 7.1 Schematic drawing of the course of the femoral nerve and the muscles it innervates. (Reproduced with permission from Gilroy AM, MacPherson BR, Ross LM, Schuenke M, Schulte E, Schumacher U. Atlas of Anatomy. 2nd ed. New York, NY: Thieme Medical Publishers; 2012; ░Fig. 29.16▒. Illustration by Karl Wesker.)

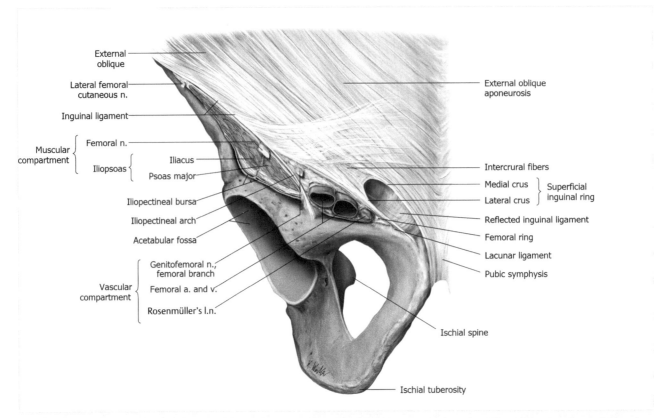

Fig. 7.2 Course of the femoral nerve under inguinal ligament and into the thigh. Note its position lateral to the femoral sheath and superficial to the iliacus muscle. (Reproduced with permission from Gilroy AM, MacPherson BR, Ross LM, Schuenke M, Schulte E, Schumacher U. Atlas of Anatomy. 2nd ed. New York, NY: Thieme Medical Publishers; 2012; ▓Fig. 29.31▓. Illustration by Karl Wesker.)

fascia lata (6.8 vs. 26.4 mm) at its location in the inguinal crease than at the inguinal ligament.[9] It is partially covered by the femoral artery at the level of the inguinal crease in approximately 70% of cases, but in only 11.7% of cases in the inguinal ligament region.[9] Interestingly, the spatial arrangement within the femoral neurovascular bundle seems more consistent at the level of the inguinal crease (where the nerve is also more superficial) than at the level of the inguinal ligament.[9] Ultrasound imaging has shown that as the nerve travels distally, it becomes generally flatter, wider, and less compact.[11] Below the inguinal ligament, the branch free length of the nerve is approximately 1.0 to 1.5 cm.[6] Cross-sections of the compound femoral nerve (i.e., the portion of the nerve between the inguinal ligament and the first branch formed in the thigh) are oval, with average major and minor diameters of approximately 10.5 and 2.3 mm, respectively.[6] Closer to the lumbar plexus, before the flattening of the nerve, the thickness is between approximately 4.52 and 4.85 mm.[2] The medial cutaneous branches and nerves of the vastus medialis, vastus intermedius, vastus lateralis, and rectus femoris were dissected and found to be arranged in that order from a medial to lateral direction.[6] Within the femoral nerve, a muscular branch to the sartorius muscle and two sensory branches (the intermediate and medial cutaneous branches of the thigh) make up the anterior division, while the posterior division comprises the motor nerves to the quadriceps femoris and articularis genus, and the saphenous nerve.[7] In the thigh, the most medial branch is that to the pectineus muscle, some

authors contending that this is the most anterior portion of the nerve and others suggesting that the branch to the sartorius muscle holds this distinction.[6] One other point of contention is that while some claim that the medial cutaneous nerve and adductor longus branch of the femoral nerve are the first to branch away in the thigh, others claim that the medial cutaneous nerve branches more distal to the pectineus and sartorius innervating branches.[6] Some variations in these structures may be due to the capacity of the obturator nerve to give rise to several of these muscle-bound branches.[6]

Another study showed the femoral nerve was found to be made up of three-layered intrinsic divisions sorted from superficial to deep.[13] The first division was an intrinsic structure in the femoral nerve. The middle layer or second division was predominately connected to the sartorius muscle. The deepest layer or third division included the saphenous nerve and muscular branches to the quadriceps femoris. The most superficial layer contained the cutaneous branches crossing over the proximal part of the sartorius muscle. These often communicated with the lateral femoral cutaneous nerve with some moving out toward the lateral aspect of the thigh instead of the main trunk of the lateral femoral cutaneous nerve. These branches were always the most superficial layer of the femoral nerve before it divided into several branches as it passed under the inguinal ligament. These cutaneous branches usually divided containing both cutaneous branches and muscular branches. The cutaneous branches penetrated the sartorius muscle. The muscular

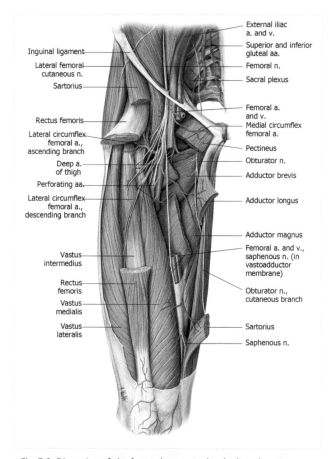

Fig. 7.3 Dissection of the femoral nerve in the thigh and noting its long saphenous branch. (Reproduced with permission from Gilroy AM, MacPherson BR, Ross LM, Schuenke M, Schulte E, Schumacher U. Atlas of Anatomy. 2nd ed. New York, NY: Thieme Medical Publishers; 2012; Fig. 29.34b. Illustration by Karl Wesker.)

branches that supplied the sartorius muscle were in the middle layer of the femoral nerve. The most superficial layer also contained muscular branches going to the pectineus muscle and cutaneous branches headed toward the medial aspect of the thigh. These cutaneous branches showed a close correlation with the lateral femoral cutaneous nerve.[13]

One key facet of the fascicular anatomy of the femoral nerve is branches with individual fascicles or groups of fascicles within the compound femoral nerve can be traced to their branching points and into the subsequently formed nerves (▶ Fig. 7.4).[6] Such branches with their own traceable fascicles include those to the sartorius, pectineus, vastus medialis, vastus intermedius, vastus lateralis, and rectus femoris muscles, as well as the medial cutaneous and saphenous nerves.[6] Fascicles that formed the branches to the vastus medialis, vastus intermedius, and vastus lateralis distally were consistently observed to be in the center and dorsally within the proximal femoral nerve.[6] Fascicles for the sensory nerves, such as the saphenous and medial cutaneous, as well as the nerve innervating the rectus femoris, were consistently located on the periphery.[6] Whereas the fascicles making up the sartorius nerve generally branch away in a ventral fashion, they are often located in the lateral, medial, or central portions of the nerve.[6] Fascicles that become the pectineus nerve are often located in a ventral position.[6] Few fascicular anastomoses are seen between the distal nerve branches and the proximal compound femoral nerve, and no interfascicular plexus are formed either.[6]

Tracing the femoral nerve to the various structures it innervates should indicate the purpose of these branches. The muscles that the femoral nerve innervates are primarily responsible for leg extension at the knee joint and flexion of the thigh, ultimately making this nerve of key importance in standing up (for which the three vasti muscles are primarily designed) and stepping.[6] Other muscles innervated by this nerve include the biarticulate rectus femoris and sartorius,

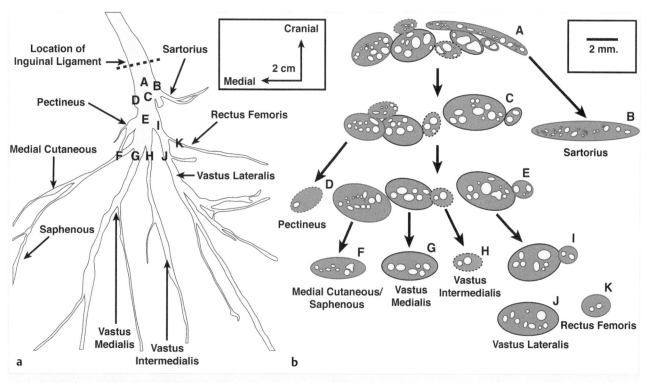

Fig. 7.4 Branching pattern of the (a) femoral nerve and its (b) fascicular patterns.

which are involved in the motion needed to progress from sitting to standing.[6] The nerve also has several sensory branches: one carries sensation from the anteromedial thigh (medial cutaneous nerve) and another dictates sensation in the medial side of the leg and foot (saphenous nerve).[3,6,7]

With all the advances in knowledge of the fascicular anatomy of the femoral nerve, some have ventured to try applying new therapies involving functional electrical stimulation to spinal cord injuries.[6] Owing to their large size and importance in essential bodily movements, the vastus lateralis and vastus intermedius are most commonly targeted by neural prostheses with the ultimate goal of allowing ambulation following spinal cord injury.[6] Currently, neural prostheses target muscles rather than nerves.[6] Two surgically implanted functional electrical stimulation systems that have shown promise in improving hand grip in patients with midcervical tetraplegia entail using either epimysial electrodes attached to the muscle at the point of nerve entry or intramuscular electrodes near the innervating neural structure.[6] Mapping of specific branch fascicles within the compound femoral nerve potentially allows a nerve cuff electrode to be placed.[6]

One of the most clinically relevant applications of the anatomy of the femoral nerve is femoral nerve block. Despite the many scenarios that call for a femoral nerve block, it remains a relatively underused procedure.[9] Some have speculated that this could be due to inconsistency in the literature concerning which site of needle insertion is preferable.[9] One study established that there was no evidence of a femoral nerve sheath substantial enough to communicate methylene blue to the lumbar plexus or the obturator nerve, suggesting that the three-in-one block is limited generally to the lateral femoral cutaneous nerve and femoral nerve, but not the lumbar plexus or obturator nerve.[14] Ignorance of the anatomy of the femoral nerve during this procedure can lead to various sequelae, such as needle penetration of the nerve or creation of a hematoma or pseudoaneurysm, which could compress the nerve over time.[15] Traditionally, the femoral artery has been considered an important marker for needle insertion, and it is usually suggested that the needle be inserted immediately lateral to this structure.[10] With such topography, it should come as no surprise that vascular puncture (often that of the lateral circumflex femoral artery) is sometimes associated with the procedure (approximately 6% of the time according to some reports).[10] Any injury to the nerve itself can lead to permanent motor and/or sensory deficits in these patients.[7] It can also disrupt sensation to the anteromedial thigh and medial leg, prejudice the ability to extend the knee, and cause atrophy of the quadriceps muscle.[7] Unexpectedly, variant anatomy is not a leading cause of such injury.[7] While this iatrogenic injury is considered rare because it is often self-limiting, many have speculated that its incidence is underreported.[7] Several studies have been performed with a view to decreasing the incidence of sequelae from this particular procedure. In one such study involving cadavers, it was found that the generally accepted insertion point of the needle (at the level of the inguinal crease, and next to the lateral border of the femoral artery) caused the greatest frequency of contact with the femoral nerve (71%) of all methods attempted.[9] This may be due to various previously discussed anatomical characteristics of the nerve at this location, such as its greater width.[9] Other methods include insertion of the needle at the level of

the inguinal ligament, but detractors claim that this location has more anatomical variation.[9] Many trials have shown that instead of inserting the needle on the lateral border of the femoral artery, inserting it at the level of the inguinal crease but 20 mm lateral to the femoral artery (which proved to be lateral to the femoral nerve) caused no needle–femoral nerve contact.[9] Such a distance is consistent with a second study, which found that the lateral circumflex femoral artery and its equivalent vein were within 1 cm of the inguinal crease in 50% of cases.[10] Others have documented the use of ultrasound scanning at the femoral crease before inserting the needle, and have found that some patients have branching vessels lateral to the main femoral artery. This suggests that it is important to deploy the imaging technique before inserting the needle.[16] Not surprisingly, similar injuries can be induced by drawing blood from the femoral artery or during angiography.[15]

Optimal visualization of the femoral nerve calls for a specific method of imaging. Ultrasound cannot consistently follow the branching of the femoral nerve at the femoral crease and generates more inconsistent measurements than gross anatomy.[11] On full-volume maximum intensity projection MRI (magnetic resonance imaging), the lumbosacral plexus and its branches are more effectively visualized at 3.0 Tesla (T) than at 1.5 T.[17] Specifically, the branches of the lumbosacral plexus could be traced significantly further at 3.0 T, and the sharpness of the nerves was increased by 97 to 169%.[17]

7.2 Pathologic Involvement

Several pathological states can injure the femoral nerve. One such state is metabolic syndrome.[18] Rats with elevated plasma glucose, mild hypertension, and polyneuropathy consistent with metabolic syndrome have a decreased axonal cross-sectional area, myelin thickness, and myelin fiber count specifically in the femoral nerve.[18] These rats also have granules of lipofuscin in their unmyelinated fiber axons, and a higher rate of injury in large myelinated fibers than controls.[18] Overall, it was determined that rats with metabolic syndrome express changes in their peripheral nerves consistent with early-onset aging of the structure.[18]

Another pathology involving the femoral nerve is compression due to impingement by surrounding muscle. Slippage of the iliacus muscle has even been implicated in splitting of the femoral nerve.[19] The slippage of this muscle in particular, because it is close to the nerve, was as high as 7.9% in one cadaveric study, and has been correlated with nerve entrapment.[19] This muscle-related splitting caused the nerve to enter the thigh as several branches instead of a single unit.[19] A second study found that in 68 cadavers, 4 (5.9%) had slippages of the iliacus and psoas major muscles.[20] In three cadavers, the femoral nerve was actually pierced by the slippage.[20] One anomaly found to cause tension on the nerve was an accessory slip of the iliacus muscle due to an iliolumbar ligament passing inferiorly and anterior to it and traversing the nerve, with its tendon splitting and attaching proximally to the lesser trochanter.[20]

Iliacus tunnel syndrome can also present with femoral nerve compression.[4] The cause could range from arteriovenous malformation and vascular aneurysm to iatrogenic causes such as femoral vessel catheterization.[4] The location of the lesion (high vs. low) can be estimated on the basis of the patient's presenting symptoms.[4] For example, patients with high lesions will present with difficulty standing up when seated.[4] Those with a lower injury of the nerve will be unable to extend their knee without difficulty and will experience atrophy of the anterior thigh.[4] Losses in sensation can also accompany iliacus tunnel syndrome.[4] Difficulty in walking also occurs in any pathology that causes compression of the nerve.[15] If sweating is retained, a complete lesion of the nerve can be ruled out.[15]

Injury to the nerve can cause a series of events leading to fibrosis within the nerve itself.[21] Any injury that causes compression of the nerve is accompanied by some element of ischemia.[21] A progressive or repetitive force causes the nerve to become "ribbonlike" and the increase in intraneural pressure can cause retardation of venous flow, resulting in edema and increased pressure.[21] This in turn can cause fibroblasts to respond and increase epineural and perineural fibrosis.[21] Endoneurial fluid pressure also increases and endoneurial fibrosis can soon occur.[21] Blood flow can then be affected and ischemic injury can result, reducing the nerve's ability to repair and regenerate axons.[21] Treatment is indicated under the following conditions: (1) the symptoms are bothersome to the patient and do not resolve within a "reasonable period" with postural treatment and anti-inflammatory medications; or (2) the symptoms include severe motor/sensation deficits or pain.[21] Surgery is often the course of action for impingement or pressure on the nerve, and fortunately it tends to have a good prognosis in cases with iatrogenic causes, and typically a 12-month recovery in "pure" entrapment cases.[21] However, many are opposed to surgical intervention as the risks are considered too high, and conservative therapy such as physical therapy and reversal of coagulopathies causing compression of the nerve should be pursued instead if possible.[4]

7.3 Surgery Involving the Femoral Nerve

Surgeries close to the femoral nerve have sometimes caused iatrogenic injury to it. A recent study suggested that the transpsoas lateral surgical approach, which had been proposed as an alternative to the anterior approach to the L4–L5 disc space, can cause postoperative thigh pain, paresthesia, and/or weakness secondary to femoral nerve injury.[22] It has been speculated that the exact cause during surgery is retractor dilation due to self-retaining ring retractors.[15,22] Surgery in the pelvis, in general, has also been implicated in femoral nerve injury, and is in fact the most common cause of femoral nerve compression.[4] Other surgeries that can injure the nerve include those involving the abdomen and hip, including appendectomies, inguinal hernia repairs, biopsies or removal of lymph nodes for malignancies in the inguinal region, and hip arthroplasties.[12,15] Compression of the nerve or the vessels supplying it and direct injury from instruments such as trocars have been implicated especially in very thin or obese patients.[15] Pfannenstiel' incisions have also been correlated with femoral nerve injuries.[15] Certain positionings of the body can also exert stress on the nerve, such as the lithotomy position, extreme flexion, extreme abduction, and extreme external rotation at the hip joint.[15] Specifically in the lithotomy position, the femoral nerve can be damaged by the

inguinal ligament.[15] To protect against nerve injury, it is recommended to palpate the femoral arteries before and after positioning the patient, and if there is a significant change in the pulse, it indicates there is pressure on the femoral arteries and therefore pressure on the femoral nerves.[12] Injury has also been sustained in anticoagulated patients undergoing surgery owing to compression of the nerve from a hematoma in one of the surrounding muscles.[15] Hematomas occurring near the femoral triangle can result in flaccid paralysis of the quadriceps, loss of knee jerk, and loss of sensation extending from the anterior and medial aspect of the thigh traveling down along the medial side of the leg and foot with extension into the big toe.[12] In hip surgery, lateral and anterolateral approaches to the joint call for particular caution with respect to the femoral nerve.[15] Iatrogenic injury to the saphenous nerve is most closely associated with total stripping of the great saphenous vein owing to its close proximity to the vessel below the level of the knee.[15] Injury to the saphenous nerve can also be a result of improper placement of braces or stirrups during operations for positioning of the patient.[12] Femoral nerve injury following surgery can manifest itself as the patient falling when attempting to stand up postoperatively.[15] Any patient experiencing falls along with a loss in sensation over pertinent regions of the leg following surgery near the femoral nerve should be monitored and have femoral nerve injury ruled out.[15] Traumatic injuries including acute stretching of the femoral nerve during forced extension of the lower limb and fractures of the pubis can cause damage or even transection of the femoral nerve. Other injuries to the femoral nerve in the absence of trauma include spreading inflammatory reactions from benign or malignant masses (e.g., renal or appendix abscesses) and effects of radiation to the pelvis in patients with ovarian or uterine malignancies.[12]

If a patient exhibits symptoms of femoral nerve injury, the surgeon must consider motor and sensory deficits when determining where the injury is located, and therefore the manner of approach to the nerve and whether a graft is necessary.[5] If a femoral nerve is injured proximally, a midline abdominal incision is preferred, allowing control and access to the vasculature as well as a clear view of the entire femoral plexus and the obturator nerve.[5] This consists of palpating and marking the anterior superior iliac spine, the symphysis pubis, and the femoral artery, and drawing a line to connect the first two structures listed.[23] A line should also be drawn to indicate the location of the femoral artery such that it intersects the previously drawn line.[23] Depending on the patient's body habitus, the incision should roughly follow the lines just drawn and should be commenced halfway between the vertical line and the anterior superior iliac spine and just distal to the oblique line.[23] The ilioinguinal nerve requires special attention during this opening.[22] Medially, the incision should continue to the external abdominal oblique muscle and to the inguinal ligament on the anterior thigh.[23] Retraction of the peritoneum in a cranial and central direction should expose the fascia of the iliacus muscle.[23] After the psoas major muscle is identified and its fascia opened, the femoral nerve can be identified on the lateral border of the muscle; use of a nerve stimulator can help in the identification of its motor branches.[23] If the nerve injury is more distal, a direct approach is sometimes preferred as this allows the injury to be visualized optimally, and if the injury is close to the inguinal ligament, a "step cut" technique is recommended.[5] A nerve graft is often needed during femoral nerve surgery if there is a gap of more than 4 cm.[5] If the hip was flexed during surgical repair of the nerve, then to avoid injury such flexion should be maintained in a cast for approximately 3 weeks during convalescence.[5] Generally speaking, femoral nerve grafting produces good outcomes if the cause is iatrogenic.[5]

As with any other structure in the body, the femoral nerve and the lumbosacral plexus of which it is a part exhibit considerable variation in the general population.[3] Out of 18 specimens in one study, 5 did not exhibit a standard femoral nerve with contributions from L2 to L4 and forming at the level of L4–L5.[22] One study investigating iatrogenic injury to the nerve found that the most clinically relevant major variation was an altered position of the nerve at its entrance into the thigh: instead of being lateral to the femoral artery, it was between the femoral artery and vein.[7] However, many other minor variations of the nerve have been documented.[3] A study exclusively investigating variations of the femoral nerve revealed instances in which the nerve branched into two or three slips around the psoas major muscle fibers (these slips rejoined after bypassing the muscle and before passing under the inguinal ligament), or gave off only one anterior femoral cutaneous nerve instead of the anatomically normal two.[3] In this study, a surprising 88% of patients showed some kind of variation within the lumbosacral plexus overall, while 35.29% had a variation specifically in the femoral nerve.[3] As mentioned earlier, a slip in the psoas major muscle is not uncommon, and one study found its incidence as high as 2.2%.[3]

7.4 Conclusion

The femoral nerve is a prominent structure in the leg with fairly well-documented anatomical specifics down to the fascicular level and well-defined borders and landmarks; however, despite this anatomical knowledge, there is still disagreement about how to perform one of the most common procedures on the nerve. This should encourage all clinicians to seek a firmer grasp on the anatomy of the nerve and its possible variations in order to minimize the risk of iatrogenic injuries.

References

[1] Choy KW, Kogilavani S, Norshalizah M, et al. Topographical anatomy of the profunda femoris artery and the femoral nerve: normal and abnormal relationships. Clin Ter. 2013; 164(1):17–19

[2] Cho Sims G, Boothe E, Joodi R, Chhabra A. 3D MR neurography of the lumbosacral plexus: obtaining optimal images for selective longitudinal nerve depiction. AJNR Am J Neuroradiol. 2016; 37(11):2158–2162

[3] Anloague PA, Huijbregts P. Anatomical variations of the lumbar plexus: a descriptive anatomy study with proposed clinical implications. J Manual Manip Ther. 2009; 17(4):e107–e114

[4] Pećina MM, Nemanić JK, Markieitz AD. Tunnel Syndromes: Peripheral Nerve Compression Syndromes. 2nd ed. Boca Raton, FL: CRC Press; 1997:173–175

[5] Van Beek AL. Peripheral nerve injuries of the lower extremity. In: Omer GE, Spinner M, Van Beek AL, eds. Management of Peripheral Nerve Problems. 2nd ed. Philadelphia, PA: W.B. Saunders Company; 1998:58–59

[6] Gustafson KJ, Pinault GC, Neville JJ, et al. Fascicular anatomy of human femoral nerve: implications for neural prostheses using nerve cuff electrodes. J Rehabil Res Dev. 2009; 46(7):973–984

[7] Moore AE, Stringer MD. Iatrogenic femoral nerve injury: a systematic review. Surg Radiol Anat. 2011; 33(8):649–658

[8] Farny J, Drolet P, Girard M. Anatomy of the posterior approach to the lumbar plexus block. Can J Anaesth. 1994; 41(6):480–485

[9] Vloka JD, Hadzić A, Drobnik L, Ernest A, Reiss W, Thys DM. Anatomical landmarks for femoral nerve block: a comparison of four needle insertion sites. Anesth Analg. 1999; 89(6):1467–1470

[10] Orebaugh SL. The femoral nerve and its relationship to the lateral circumflex femoral artery. Anesth Analg. 2006; 102(6):1859–1862

[11] Lonchena TK, McFadden K, Orebaugh SL. Correlation of ultrasound appearance, gross anatomy, and histology of the femoral nerve at the femoral triangle. Surg Radiol Anat. 2016; 38(1):115–122

[12] Sauderland SS. Nerves and Nerve Injuries. 2nd ed. Edinburgh: Churchill Livingston; 1978:999–1009

[13] Aizawa Y. On the organization of the plexus lumbalis. I. On the recognition of the three-layered divisions and the systematic description of the branches of the human femoral nerve. Okajimas Folia Anat Jpn. 1992; 69(1):35–74

[14] Ritter JW. Femoral nerve "sheath" for inguinal paravascular lumbar plexus block is not found in human cadavers. J Clin Anesth. 1995; 7(6):470–473

[15] Mirjalili SA. Anatomy of the lumbar plexus. In: Tubbs RS, Rizk E, Shoja MM, Loukas M, Barbaro N, Spinner RJ, eds. Nerves and Nerve Injuries. Vol. 1. San Diego, CA: Elsevier; 2015:614–617

[16] Muhly WT, Orebaugh SL. Ultrasound evaluation of the anatomy of the vessels in relation to the femoral nerve at the femoral crease. Surg Radiol Anat. 2011; 33(6):491–494

[17] Mürtz P, Kaschner M, Lakghomi A, et al. Diffusion-weighted MR neurography of the brachial and lumbosacral plexus: 3.0 T versus 1.5 T imaging. Eur J Radiol. 2015; 84(4):696–702

[18] Rodrigues de Souza R, Gama EF, El-Razi Neto S, Maldonado D. Effects of metabolic syndrome on the ultrastructure of the femoral nerve in aging rats. Histol Histopathol. 2015; 30(10):1185–1192

[19] Vázquez MT, Murillo J, Maranillo E, Parkin IG, Sanudo J. Femoral nerve entrapment: a new insight. Clin Anat. 2007; 20(2):175–179

[20] Spratt JD, Logan BM, Abrahams PH. Variant slips of psoas and iliacus muscles, with splitting of the femoral nerve. Clin Anat. 1996; 9(6):401–404

[21] Azuelos A, Corò L, Alexandre A. Femoral nerve entrapment. Acta Neurochir Suppl (Wien). 2005; 92:61–62

[22] Davis TT, Bae HW, Mok JM, Rasouli A, Delamarter RB. Lumbar plexus anatomy within the psoas muscle: implications for the transpsoas lateral approach to the L4-L5 disc. J Bone Joint Surg Am. 2011; 93(16):1482–1487

[23] Pirela-Cruz MA. Surgical exposures of the peripheral nerves in the extremities. In: Omer GE, Spinner M, Van Beek AL, eds. Management of Peripheral Nerve Problems. 2nd ed. Philadelphia, PA: W.B. Saunders Company; 1998:197–198

8 Obturator Nerve

Michael Montalbano, Joy M. H. Wang

Abstract

The branches of the lumbar plexus are encountered in various invasive procedures. Therefore, a thorough knowledge of each of its branches is important to the clinician who performs such procedures. This chapter reviews the clinical anatomy of the obturator nerve. It is hoped that a better understanding of this nerve and its distribution will decrease patient morbidity.

Keywords: anatomy, posterior abdominal wall, nerves, complications, surgery

8.1 Embryology in General

As the embryo develops, neuronal axons follow the routes laid down by growth cones toward their target end points, distal to the neuronal soma. Continuous with the growth cones, these developing axons enter Schwann's cell tubes during migration. The growth cones consist of a triad: a peripheral zone made of actin within the filopodia and internally associated with microtubules; a central zone that provides for axon elongation with bundled microtubules; and a transitional zone that allows for traction between the central and peripheral zones.[1] Microtubules are crucial for development, providing two pathways for the growth cone to navigate forward. First, microtubules join in the peripheral zone to form an anchor that influences growth toward the adhesion. Second, microtubules can merge toward the growth of new axonal bodies, within the space provided by actin bundles. Eventually, the peripheral nerves congregate and form fascicles. Each fascicle is enveloped by a two-layer cellular mass that covers the mature nerve trunk. Its outer layer is composed of Schwann's cells that help proliferate axons, while the inner layer is composed of connective tissue components such as mesenchymal progenitor cells.[1]

This process of peripheral nerve elongation has been described in the 12th week of gestation in humans. Between the 14th and 16th weeks of pregnancy, Schwann's cells begin the process of myelination. Once formed, peripheral nerves consist of a triad of connective parts, namely endoneurium, perineurium, and epineurium. The endoneurium is the innermost neural layer, composed of two layers of collagen, directly supporting the individual nerve fiber. The perineurium, sandwiched between the endoneurium and epineurium, is formed by tight junctions that function to maintain ion concentrations required for neural function. As nerve fibers form clusters with surrounding connective tissue, they are labeled a "bundle." This bundle is wrapped again by a larger perineurium and then finally by the epineurium, the outermost layer of connective tissue that provides structural support.[1]

8.2 Spinal Cord Origin and Function

The obturator nerve (▶ Fig. 8.1 and ▶ Fig. 8.2) is derived from the second to fourth ventral rami, sharing the same roots as the femoral nerve. Its largest and smallest contributors are typically from L3 and L2, respectively.[2,3,4,5] Its main functions are to supply motor function to the major adductor muscles of the lower limb (obturator externus, adductor brevis, adductor longus, adductor magnus, gracilis, and, at times, pectineus) and the cutaneous sensation of the medial thigh. Through communicating fibers, it can also contribute to articular innervation of the knee and cutaneous sensation of a small area of the medial leg.

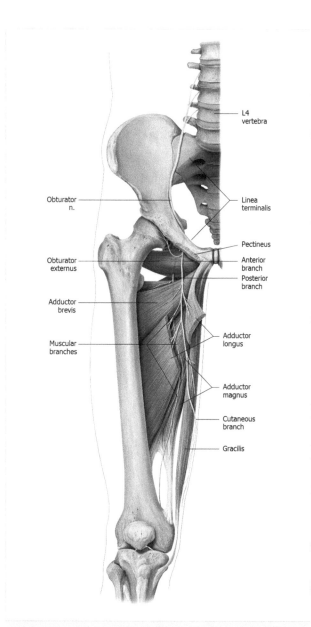

Fig. 8.1 Schematic drawing of the course of the obturator nerve. (Reproduced with permission from Gilroy AM, MacPherson BR, Ross LM, Schuenke M, Schulte E, Schumacher U. Atlas of Anatomy. 2nd ed. New York, NY: Thieme Medical Publishers; 2012. Illustration by Karl Wesker.)

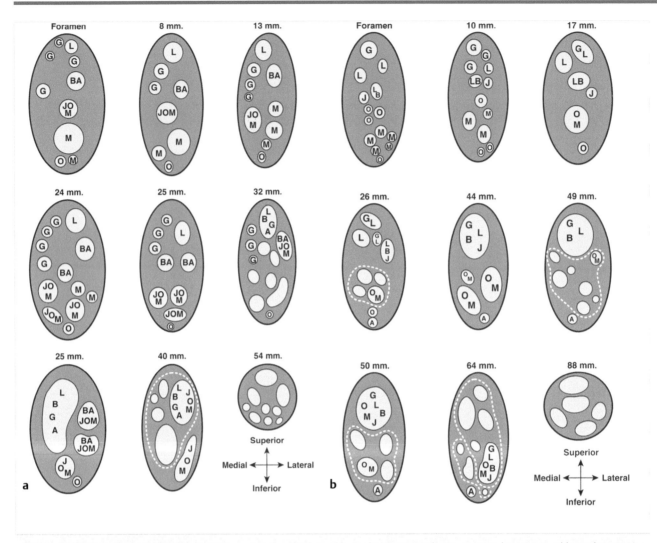

Fig. 8.2 (a, b) Internal topography of the obturator nerve. A, arterial; B, adductor brevis; G, gracilis-cutaneous; J, hip joint; L, adductor longus; M, adductor magnus; O, obturator externus.

8.3 Anatomy

Following its exit from the spinal cord, the obturator nerve runs a complex pathway deep within the pelvis. It descends medially along the posterior wall, just lateral to the lumbar vertebral column, and posterior to the psoas major muscle. It passes the sacroiliac joint, posterior to the common iliac artery and lateral to the internal iliac vessels. As it reaches the pelvic inlet, it travels anteriorly and slightly inferiorly, adjacent to the medial side of the pelvic wall, following the arcuate line, just superior to the obturator internus muscle. Throughout this course, the nerve is enveloped in the subperitoneal cellular tissue of the region, flattening and enlarging the nerve.[6] In this trajectory, it reaches the obturator canal, a small opening within the superior aspect of the larger, obturator foramen. The obturator foramen is mostly covered by the obturator membrane, apart from the opening of the canal, located 2.7 cm lateral and 1.7 cm inferior to the pubic tubercle.[7] The canal is bordered by the obturator sulcus of the pubic bone superiorly, and the internal and external obturator muscles inferiorly, with the obturator membrane forming the floor of

the tunnel.[8] Branching off from the internal iliac vessels, the obturator artery and vein travel just inferior to the nerve along the pelvic wall and through the obturator canal to exit the pelvis.[6]

As the nerve exits the obturator canal, it splits immediately into an anterior and posterior branch. Leaving the obturator canal, the anterior branch supplies the hip joint via the articular branch and branches a "twig" to the accessory obturator nerve, if that nerve is present.[4] The anterior division continues and then descends within a flat plane on the anterior surface of the obturator externus and adductor brevis muscles, deep to the pectineus and adductor longus muscles.[4,9] Within this pathway, it supplies the adductor longus and gracilis muscles, and at times the adductor brevis and pectineus muscles.[1,5] As it continues to the inferior border of the adductor longus, an arterial branch is supplied to the femoral artery, and a cutaneous branch communicates with the medial cutaneous nerve of the thigh and the saphenous nerve, forming the subsartorial nerve plexus; this plexus provides cutaneous sensation to the medial thigh.[1,2,5] Occasionally, this "subsartorial" cutaneous branch can continue on to provide sensation to the medial leg.[3,4]

The posterior branch of the obturator nerve pierces the anterior surface of the obturator externus muscle and then descends posterior to the adductor brevis muscle and anterior to the adductor magnus muscle. Within this pathway, the nerve divides into branches to supply the obturator externus, adductor magnus, and adductor brevis muscles. Typically, articular filaments are also sent to the knee joint, either by entering the adductor magnus distally or by passing via the adductor hiatus to the posterior knee, with the femoral artery. Within the popliteal fossa, the nerve descends with the popliteal artery and then pierces the oblique posterior ligament, thus providing sensory innervation to the cruciate ligaments and synovial membrane.[2,4,5,10]

8.4 Variations in Topography

Many variations can occur as the obturator nerve distinguishes itself from its lumbar roots. The obturator nerve can have additional roots from the first or fifth lumbar nerve. More specifically, the obturator nerve can arise in a "high" or "prefixed" form from L1–L4 or more rarely L1–L3. It can also arise in a "low" or "postfixed" form from L2–L5. In its typical form, the branch arising from the third lumbar nerve is the largest, while that arising from the second is often very small and may not contribute in some variations.[1,2,5]

Among the variations, changes in route are possible. The branch from the main nerve trunk to the obturator externus muscle can pass to the lateral instead of the usual medial side.[1] The articular branch to the hip has been seen to leave the main branch and run independently to the hip joint before passing the obturator foramen; its origin has also been seen to be the posterior, rather than the anterior, branch.[4,5]

The distribution of the obturator nerve branches can also vary. The nerve sometimes gives a branch to the pectineus or obturator internus.[5] The anterior cutaneous branch can be absent, in which case the cutaneous sensation of the medial thigh is supplied by the femoral nerve.[1] Similarly, when the anterior branch is missing, the posterior branch will innervate the adductor brevis and obturator externus.[2] Overall, multiple branches have been reported to the following structures: obturator internus, obturator artery, pectineus, and periosteum of pubis pelvic surface.[5] As well, when the communicating cutaneous nerve from the obturator is large, it can continue on from the subsartorial plexus, pierce the deep fascia lata at the knee, and communicate with the saphenous nerve to provide cutaneous sensation for the medial leg.[2,3,5] In this variation, the medial cutaneous nerve of the thigh is typically small and ends within the subsartorial plexus after providing a few cutaneous filaments.[2]

A final variation includes the presence of an accessory obturator nerve. Its prevalence has been reported to be approximately 8 to 9%[5,8]; however, numbers as high as 17 and 30% have also been reported.[5,11] If this is present, it is usually small and arises from the ventral rami of the third and fourth lumbar nerve roots; however, combinations of single to triple nerve roots ranging between L2 and L5 have been seen.[1,5] After leaving the nerve roots, it typically descends just anterior (often adherent) to the main obturator trunk, medial to the psoas major muscle, and then traverses the superior pubic ramus.[4,11] The nerve then descends within the psoas sheath and under Poupart's ligament (inguinal ligament), to run posterior to the pectineus.[4,5,11] In this path, it provides branches that may innervate one or more of the following: deep pectineus, hip joint, anterior branch of obturator, and adductor longus.[2,4,11] If only one branch is present, it typically innervates the deep pectineus and the hip joint, in lieu of the femoral branch.[1]

8.5 Intraneural Topography

The intraneural topography (▶ Fig. 8.2) of the obturator has been documented by examining the cross-sectional composition of the nerve in sections proximal to, at, and distal to the obturator foramen. Proximal to the foramen, the nerve divides into superior, intermediate, and inferior groups, based on cross-sectional areas. The superior group consists of bundles from the gracilis, cutaneous fibers, adductor longus, and adductor brevis muscles. The intermediate group consists of bundles from the obturator externus muscle and hip-joint fibers. The inferior group consists of bundles from the adductor magnus, obturator externus, and obturator vessels. In the proximal half of the pelvic section, toward the sacroiliac joint, the superior and inferior groups are intermingled in plexus formations. Conversely, as the nerve courses toward the distal half of the pelvis, the superior bundle is rarely engaged in plexus formation with the inferior group.

At the obturator foramen, the fibers for the gracilis, adductor longus, and adductor brevis lie toward the anteromedial portion of the bundle, while the fibers to obturator externus and adductor magnus are in a posterolateral position. Distal to the foramen, the obturator nerve courses through most of its muscles as bundles ranging from one to eight funiculi.

It appears that moving distally from the nerve roots, the aforementioned "superior group" of the obturator nerve largely corresponds to fibers that run along the anteromedial portion of the nerve when it reaches the foramen, and becomes the anterior branch when distal to the foramen. On the other hand, the aforementioned "intermediate" and "inferior group" within the pelvis largely correspond to fibers that run along the posterolateral portion of the nerve when it reaches the foramen, and become the posterior branch when distal to the foramen.

The average percentage cross-sectional area of the obturator nerve occupied within the funiculi has been measured at the foramen, midway along the lateral pelvic wall, and at the level of the sacroiliac joint and found to be 41, 49, and 52%, respectively.[5]

8.6 Pathology

Because of its deep anatomy, the most common cause of obturator pathology is compression. Some common sites of compression include: within the obturator canal near the vascular bundle of obturator vessels; in the fibromuscular canal anterior to the obturator membrane but posterior to the obturator externus; in the muscular tunnel where the posterior division separates the obturator externus; within the fascia located deep to the pectineus and adductor brevis muscles, but superficial to the obturator externus; and the proximal third of the adductor magnus.[12] Interestingly, the female reproductive anatomy can predispose women to obturator pathologies. In parturition, the fetal head can compress the obturator nerve against the pelvic wall, causing "obstetrical palsy."[8] Similarly, pelvic masses such as obturator hernias and ovarian tumors can also produce the same signs and symptoms.[5] Other compressive etiologies include bone osteophytes, obturator artery aneurysms, and retroperitoneal lesions.[2,8]

In addition to compression, due to the proximity of surrounding pelvic structures, their disease processes can affect the nerve. For example, as the obturator runs toward the obturator canal, it runs under or near the sigmoid colon. Cases of carcinoma of the large intestine and other pathologic growths in the pelvis must be kept in mind as differentials. Infection in the pelvis has been seen to follow the posterior branch into the thigh. Furthermore, the articular branch to the hip and filaments sent to the sacroiliac joint can be involved in joint pathology.[4]

Isolated mononeuropathy of the obturator nerve is rare. For example, in pathologies secondary to direct trauma, patients are more likely to present with complex comorbidities, as a pelvic fracture severe enough to cause lesion to the obturator nerve will likely also injure other structures such as spinal nerves, the lumbosacral plexus, and other peripheral leg nerves.[13] As well, labral tears of the hip can lead to acetabular labral cysts that not only impinge on the obturator nerve but also injure other nerves near the hip joint, such as the femoral and posterior sciatic nerves.[14,15]

There are reports of idiopathic obturator neuropathy, but there has been no significant evidence for true entrapment in anatomical variations such as a narrow obturator foramen. While obturator palsy has been reported in newborns, this is thought not to be congenital but secondary to a prolonged abnormal leg position in utero that overstretches the obturator nerve, with recovery usually within 2 weeks.[5,13,16] In cases of obturator hernia, compression of the obturator nerve causing pain referred to the hip, medial thigh, and knee is labeled the "Howship–Romberg sign."[2] This sign should not be confused with the "obturator sign," which is used to describe irritation of the obturator internus muscle, typically caused by appendicitis. Isolated lesions of the obturator nerve are extremely rare, but may occasionally occur as a result of direct trauma (sometimes during parturition) or in anterior dislocations of the hip. The nerve may also be damaged by an obturator hernia, or be involved together with the femoral nerve in retroperitoneal lesions that occur close to the origins of the lumbar plexus. A more distal nerve entrapment syndrome causing chronic medial thigh pain has been described in athletes with large adductor muscles.

There are several iatrogenic etiologies behind obturator neuropathy including hip arthroplasty, abdominal surgery, plastic surgery, forceps delivery, compression from retractor or surgical cement placement, and hematoma secondary to femoral venipuncture while anticoagulated.[15] Following hip arthroplasty, nerves close to the obturator foramen can be injured if methyl methacrylate escapes inferiorly from the acetabulum and exerts pressure on the obturator nerve near the superior ramus of the pubis.[5] The nerve can also be accidentally cut during radical pelvic resections for cancer. The nerve can also be accidentally cut during radical pelvic resections for cancer. Obturator paralysis has also been noted postoperatively in patients positioned on operating tables with the thighs acutely flexed, i.e., lithotomy position, to such an extent that the nerve leaves the bony obturator foramen.[5] However, iatrogenic injury more commonly involves the sciatic and femoral nerves.[13]

Iatrogenic complications, when they occur, need not be limited to neuropathy. For instance, the tension-free vaginal tape technique has been implicated in significant vascular and bowel injuries, in addition to obturator neuropathy.[12]

Musculoskeletal variations have also been shown to cause obturator nerve disturbances. Athletes with large adductor muscles can develop chronic medial thigh pain secondary to distal entrapment of the nerve.[2] They can also develop chronic groin pain due to chronic denervation of the adductor muscles.[10] Conversely, atrophied or weak adductors can lead to snapping hip syndrome.[17]

8.7 Imaging and Diagnostics

Ultrasound can be useful for exploring the nerve segments of the lower limb. The obturator nerve is best visualized by having the patient positioned with the leg straight and in a slight external rotation. However, the deep anatomical course underlying this region and the requisite patient positioning limit the usefulness of this imaging modality since only six nerves can be imaged in the hip, namely the lateral femoral cutaneous, femoral, sciatic, obturator, superior and inferior gluteal, and pudendal nerves.[18]

The best-established confirmation of obturator nerve lesions is finding electromyogram (EMG) abnormalities in the hip adductors. In such cases, the EMG of the adductor brevis, adductor longus, and gracilis muscles shows high-amplitude, long-duration, complex motor unit potentials and longer fibrillation potentials, corresponding to denervation and atrophy of these muscles.[10] These EMG findings can help differentiate obturator nerve deficits from similar pathologies such as lumbar and diabetic.[7] Alternatively, on T2 magnetic resonance imaging (MRI), an increased signal intensity in the medial thigh indicates that the muscles are undergoing denervation or atrophy with fatty infiltration. Specifically, the imaging signals that correspond to obturator neuropathy are more focal, more proximal, and spare the obturator externus.[9,15]

8.8 Surgical Interventions

There are several treatments for patients with obturator neuropathy. Most cases will use a combination of conservative management, physical therapy, and nonsteroidal anti-inflammatory drugs (NSAIDs) for analgesia. For many, a return to regular activity is expected within 6 weeks.[10] Surgical intervention may be required in cases with identifiable pelvic pathology, or when pain or weakness proves resistant to conservative management.[10] Percutaneous radiofrequency lesioning is a form of treatment used to alleviate refractory pain; however, it does have several complications including neuritis, neuroma formation, sensory loss, loss of motor function, and transient hematoma formation if patient is on anticoagulation.[19] Cryoanalgesia is another useful analgesic treatment modality but it carries the risk of deafferentation pain.[20] Alternatively, percutaneous thermocoagulation is a procedure used to denature proteins in the peripheral nerves, thus providing pain relief. While this method provides a longer duration of analgesia, it also entails a greater risk of inducing loss of motor function, neuroma formation, neuritis, and postprocedural neuroinflammation.[21]

Regional blockade is a key intervention for various neuropathies. Appropriate use of obturator nerve blocks has been associated with reduced consumption of NSAIDs and sustained pain relief for up to several months. For patients undergoing transurethral bladder tumor resection, there is a greater than 50% incidence of adductor muscle spasm postsurgery.[22] Obturator nerve blocks can be of great help to these patients by providing analgesia and managing spasticity for the pelvis and thigh.[7] As well, obturator nerve blocks can be modified for various applications. In patients with refractory, progressive hip displacement who have reached the maximum dose of botulinum toxin treatment, obturator nerve blocks using ethyl alcohol has been demonstrated as an alternate remedy.[23] In patients requiring general anesthesia, an obturator nerve block with spinal analgesia can be used.[24] Despite the utility of nerve blockades, some risks are involved. Incomplete nerve blocks can lead to bladder wall perforation or dissemination of a tumor secondary to thigh adductor muscle contractions.[18] The obturator nerve also has the highest failure rate of blockade among the triad of nerves involved in a three-in-one nerve block.[18] However, as techniques advance, the risks and difficulties involved with this procedure will undoubtedly decrease. In an anatomical study, a vertical obturator blocking technique landmarking only by palpation has been shown to have a high degree of accuracy (93.75%).[25]

In certain presentations, surgery may be unavoidable. A patient presenting with neuropathy secondary to arthroplasty might have a nerve encased in cement. Such patients should be observed carefully, with surgical exploration to follow if the symptoms fail to resolve. In cases of neuropathy resulting from pelvic trauma or intraoperative laceration, the patient could require nerve repair and grafting. For cases of progressive symptoms with unidentified causes, surgical exploration of the obturator canal should be conducted in search of a hernia or other tissue, e.g., endometriosis.[13]

Denervation or phenol injections are two other alternatives to treat adductor contractures, particularly when nerve blockage is unfeasible.[5] Denervation has been used constructively to avoid adductor contractures in paraplegic patients, and to avoid intraoperative complications during transurethral resection due to obturator nerve irritation.[26] Furthermore, studies suggest that the obturator nerve can serve as a potential nerve donor or graft site for various procedures. Surgical applications of the obturator nerve in facial reanimation procedures have been shown to be feasible.[27] In femoral nerve neurotization, the obturator nerve has been successfully used as a distal donor nerve. Autografting of motor nerves from the obturator to pudendal has also been done.[28] One technique particularly useful for high-level femoral nerve lesions is to transfer the anterior branch of the obturator nerve, which has been shown to successfully return power to at least two quadriceps femoris muscles.[29] However, this procedure involves neurorrhaphy within the pelvis, which complicates the procedure. Attempts at neurorrhaphy near the muscle to decrease recovery time have also been tried.[30]

References

[1] Tubbs RS, Rizk E, Shoja MM, Loukas M, Barbaro N, Spinner RJ. Nerves and Nerve Injuries, Volume 1: History, Embryology, Anatomy, Imaging, and Diagnostics. Cambridge, MA: Academic Press; 2015

[2] Standring S. Gray's Anatomy: The Anatomical Basis of Clinical Practice. 41st ed. London: Elsevier; 2016

[3] Thane GD. Quain's Elements of Anatomy, Volume 3, Part 2: The Nerves. 10th ed. London: Longmans, Green, and Co.; 1895

[4] Schaeffer JP. Morris' Human Anatomy: A Complete Systematic Treatise. 11th ed. New York, NY: McGraw-Hill Book Company, Inc.; 1953

[5] Sunderland S. Nerves and Neve Injuries. 2nd ed. London: Churchill Livingstone; 1978

[6] Cruveilhier J. The Anatomy of the Human Body. New York, NY: Harper & Brothers; 1844

[7] Jo SY, Chang JC, Bae HG, Oh JS, Heo J, Hwang JC. A morphometric study of the obturator nerve around the obturator foramen. J Korean Neurosurg Soc. 2016; 59(3):282–286

[8] Pecina MM, Krmptoc-Nemanic J, Markiewitz AD. Tunnel Syndromes: Peripheral Nerve Compression Syndromes. 2nd ed. Boca Raton, FL: CRC Press; 1997

[9] Martinoli C, Miguel-Perez M, Padua L, Gandolfo N, Zicca A, Tagliafico A. Imaging of neuropathies about the hip. Eur J Radiol. 2013; 82(1):17–26

[10] Tipton JS. Obturator neuropathy. Curr Rev Musculoskelet Med. 2008; 1(3–4): 234–237

[11] Henry AK. Extensile Exposure. 2nd ed. London: Churchill Livingstone; 1973

[12] Kumka M. Critical sites of entrapment of the posterior division of the obturator nerve: anatomical considerations. J Can Chiropr Assoc. 2010; 54(1):33–42

[13] Stewart JD. Focal Peripheral Neuropathies. 3rd ed. Philadelphia, PA: LWW; 2000

[14] Kim SH, Seok H, Lee SY, Park SW. Acetabular paralabral cyst as a rare cause of obturator neuropathy: a case report. Ann Rehabil Med. 2014; 38(3):427–432

[15] Yukata K, Arai K, Yoshizumi Y, Tamano K, Imada K, Nakaima N. Obturator neuropathy caused by an acetabular labral cyst: MRI findings. AJR Am J Roentgenol. 2005; 184(3) Suppl:S112–S114

[16] Tubbs RS, Sheetz J, Salter G, Oakes WJ. Accessory obturator nerves with bilateral pseudoganglia in man. Ann Anat. 2003; 185(6):571–572

[17] Oh J, Kang M, Park J, Lee JI. A possible cause of snapping hip: intrapartum obturator neuropathy. Am J Phys Med Rehabil. 2014; 93(6):551

[18] Soong J, Schafhalter-Zoppoth I, Gray AT. Sonographic imaging of the obturator nerve for regional block. Reg Anesth Pain Med. 2007; 32(2):146–151

[19] Chaiban G, Paradis T, Atallah J. Use of ultrasound and fluoroscopy guidance in percutaneous radiofrequency lesioning of the sensory branches of the femoral and obturator nerves. Pain Pract. 2014; 14(4):343–345

[20] Rigaud J, Labat JJ, Riant T, Hamel O, Bouchot O, Robert R. Treatment of obturator neuralgia with laparoscopic neurolysis. J Urol. 2008; 179(2):590–594, discussion 594–595

[21] Yavuz F, Yasar E, Ali Taskaynatan M, Goktepe AS, Tan AK. Nerve block of articular branches of the obturator and femoral nerves for the treatment of hip joint pain. J Back Musculoskeletal Rehabil. 2013; 26(1):79–83

[22] Tekgül ZT, Divrik RT, Turan M, Konyalioğlu E, Şimşek E, Gönüllü M. Impact of obturator nerve block on the short-term recurrence of superficial bladder tumors on the lateral wall. Urol J. 2014; 11(1):1248–1252

[23] Park ES, Rha DW, Lee WC, Sim EG. The effect of obturator nerve block on hip lateralization in low functioning children with spastic cerebral palsy. Yonsei Med J. 2014; 55(1):191–196

[24] Khorrami M, Hadi M, Javid A, et al. A comparison between blind and nerve stimulation guided obturator nerve block in transurethral resection of bladder tumor. J Endourol. 2012; 26(10):1319–1322

[25] Feigl GC, Ulz H, Pixner T, Dolcet C, Likar R, Sandner-Kiesling A. Anatomical investigation of a new vertical obturator nerve block technique. Ann Anat. 2013; 195(1):82–87

[26] Kendir S, Akkaya T, Comert A, et al. The location of the obturator nerve: a three-dimensional description of the obturator canal. Surg Radiol Anat. 2008; 30(6):495–501

[27] Rozen S, Rodriguez-Lorenzo A, Audolfsson T, Wong C, Cheng A. Obturator nerve anatomy and relevance to one-stage facial reanimation: limitations of a retroperitoneal approach. Plast Reconstr Surg. 2013; 131(5):1057–1064

[28] Houdek MT, Wagner ER, Wyles CC, Moran SL. Anatomical feasibility of the anterior obturator nerve transfer to restore bowel and bladder function. Microsurgery. 2014; 34(6):459–463

[29] Tung TH, Chao A, Moore AM. Obturator nerve transfer for femoral nerve reconstruction: anatomic study and clinical application. Plast Reconstr Surg. 2012; 130(5):1066–1074

[30] Goubier JN, Teboul F, Yeo S. Transfer of two motor branches of the anterior obturator nerve to the motor portion of the femoral nerve: an anatomical feasibility study. Microsurgery. 2012; 32(6):463–465

9 Furcal Nerve

Naomi Ojumah

Abstract

The branches of the lumbar plexus are frequently encountered in various invasive procedures. Therefore, a thorough knowledge of each of its branches is important to the clinician who performs such procedures. This chapter reviews the clinical anatomy and associated pathologies of the furcal nerve. Variations in the furcal nerve could contribute to atypical presentations of lumbar radiculopathy. It is hoped that a better understanding of this nerve and its distribution will decrease patient morbidity.

Keywords: lumbosacral radicular syndromes, lumbosacral trunk, lumbar plexus, sacral plexus

9.1 Introduction

The lumbosacral plexus has had less attention than the brachial plexus probably due to there being less injuries to it.[1] The lumbar plexus is often formed by a contribution from the 12th thoracic nerve, the first three lumbar ventral rami, and the greater part of the fourth lumbar ventral ramus. The lumbosacral plexus is formed by the remaining small part of the fourth lumbar nerve and the fifth lumbar nerve (lumbosacral trunk)[2] and the upper sacral nerves.[3] Various types of lumbosacral nerve root anomalies have been described in the literature. The existing classifications of nerve root abnormalities consider convergence, intradural or extradural anastomosis, and division.[4,5]

The furcal nerve has been variably defined, but many consider it the nerve that enters into the formation of both the lumbar and sacral plexuses, usually as a result of a nerve dividing, or forking, between the two plexuses[6,7,8,9] serving as a link between the two plexuses (▸ Fig. 9.1)[1]—for example, a part of the L4 ventral ramus that joins with L5 ventral ramus to form the lumbosacral trunk. Some, however, have described the furcal nerve as a separate nerve traveling alongside the L4 nerve root in the intervertebral foramen, having separate anterior and posterior root fibers and its own dorsal root ganglion, and thus indicating that it is its own independent nerve root. It has also been found to have fibers contributing to neighboring nerves— 26% to the femoral nerve, 18% to the obturator nerve, and 16% to the lumbosacral trunk.[10] Schaeffer[8] has specifically described the furcal nerve as "when the fourth nerve enters into the formation of both lumbar and sacral plexuses, it may be called the furcal nerve, but this name is also applied to any of the nerves that enter into the formation of both plexuses, so there may be one or more furcal nerves." Others have defined the furcal nerve simply as the entire ventral ramus of the L4 spinal nerve.

9.2 Variations of the Furcal Nerve

The different deviations are thought to be a result of a deviation from the normal fetal development during the first four weeks of life.[1] Kikuchi et al performed cadaveric dissections including coronal and sagittal sectioning of the lumbosacral region in order to better delineate the anatomy of the furcal nerve. The furcal nerve was found in up to 93% of their dissections and mainly as L4. The furcal nerve has been referred to as the boundary root.[10] However, although most furcal nerves arise at the L4 level, they can occur at any level from L1 to S1.[5,7,8,9,11] When the furcal nerve arises cranial to L4, the lumbar plexus is termed prefixed; a more caudal emergence is termed postfixed.[6,7,8,9,11] In Bardeen and Elting's findings, 42.3% were found to be normal, 36% prefixed, and 21.5% postfixed.[12] Several other variations of the furcal nerve have also been described. The furcal nerve may consist of L3 and L4 in some cases, and other times, it may consist of L4 and L5. These "doubled" furcal nerves have an incidence of 0.8% (L3 and L4 more common than L4 and L5).[3,13] At times, the L4 branch to the sacral plexus is missing, leaving L5 as the sole furcal nerve or boundary root. Interestingly, in rhesus monkeys, as a rule there are seven lumbar vertebrae and the L5 ventral ramus is usually the furcal nerve.[14]

Kikuchi et al further classified the anatomical variations of the furcal nerve into six types (A through F) on the basis of the level at which they arose: A, two furcal nerves at the L3 and L4 root levels; B, one furcal nerve at the cephalad side of the L4 root; C, one furcal nerve root at the L4 level following the same course as the proper L4; D, two furcal nerves at the cephalad side of the L4 root; E, two furcal nerves at L4 and L5 roots, respectively; and F, a furcal nerve at the cephalad side of the L5 nerve root.[10] Earlier reports suggested the prevalence of extra connections to be as high as 20%, although the 20% was in patients with radicular symptoms and not in cadavers.[5,15,16]

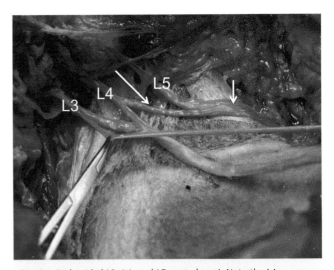

Fig. 9.1 Right-sided L3, L4, and L5 ventral rami. Note the L4 contribution (*left arrow*) to the L5 ventral ramus forming the lumbosacral trunk (*right arrow*) that continues distally to interconnect with upper sacral ventral rami and thus forming the lumbosacral trunk. The obturator nerve is being retracted laterally. Lateral to the obturator nerve, the large femoral nerve is seen. Depending on the author, the L4 ventral ramus or the connection (*left arrow*) to the L5 ventral ramus could be termed the furcal nerve in this specimen.

9.3 Clinical Significance of the Furcal Nerve

These variations described above create several controversies including the atypical sciatica presentation and discrepancy between clinical presentation and imaging, and interestingly, there are few reports regarding the detailed anatomy of the furcal nerve with respect to its involvement in different clinical conditions such as lumbosacral radicular symptoms.[15,17,18] For patients with radiculopathy, a selective spinal nerve root block approach is used and the choice of what root is usually determined by the clinical presentation and imaging identification of nerve root compression. L5 or S1 radiculopathy usually presents as pain below the knee up to the foot, and L2–L4 radiculopathy is perceived as pain projecting to the knee, thigh, or groin. L4 radiculopathy also typically involves the medial leg. However, in a subset of patients, the clinical picture is confusing and there are a number of reasons for this, variable furcal nerve contribution being one of them.[10,19] In a study by Bartynski et al, L4 injection provoked typical gluteal, hip, or posterior thigh pain (sciatica) in 5 out of 32 patients, consistent with a prominent furcal nerve contribution to the sacral plexus, with 3 of these patients with pain projecting to the ankle or foot.[19] Clinical suspicion and awareness plus a thorough magnetic resonance imaging (MRI) examination can be useful in identifying this subset of patients.[3] With an increased prevalence of posterolateral approaches to the spine, surgeons must pay attention to the various presentations of a furcal nerve so as to avoid nerve injury. It is also important to be able to recognize patients with atypical sciatica as those patients may have a furcal nerve with a conjoined nerve root. A thorough understanding of anatomical variations and insight into the anomalies of the lumbosacral plexus reduces the incidence of failed back surgery and enhances surgical success.

9.4 Conclusion

Since nerve variations can present in a nonclassical and confusing fashion, preoperative diagnosis of these variations is essential for explaining atypical clinical presentations and selecting a safe and effective surgical treatment. If a single lesion at a single level results in radiculopathy in the distribution of two separate nerve roots, the furcal nerve could be involved.

References

[1] Matejčík V. Anatomical variations of lumbosacral plexus. Surg Radiol Anat. 2010; 32(4):409–414

[2] Gray H. 1918. Anatomy of the Human Body. Available at: http://www.bartleby.com/107/212.html

[3] Harshavardhana NS, Dabke HV. The furcal nerve revisited. Orthop Rev (Pavia). 2014; 6(3):5428

[4] Chotigavanich C, Sawangnatra S. Anomalies of the lumbosacral nerve roots. An anatomic investigation. Clin Orthop Relat Res. 1992(278):46–50

[5] Haijiao W, Koti M, Smith FW, Wardlaw D. Diagnosis of lumbosacral nerve root anomalies by magnetic resonance imaging. J Spinal Disord. 2001; 14(2):143–149

[6] Clemente CD. Gray's Anatomy of the Human Body. 30th ed. Philadelphia, PA: Lea & Febiger; 1985:1225–1235

[7] Hollinshead WH. Anatomy for Surgeons, Vol 3. New York, NY: Harper and Row; 1964:597–605

[8] Schaeffer JP. Morris' Human Anatomy: A Complete Systemic Treatise. Philadelphia, PA: The Blakiston Company; 1946

[9] Standring S. Gray's Anatomy. 39th ed. Philadelphia, PA: Elsevier; 2005

[10] Kikuchi S, Hasue M, Nishiyama K, Ito T. Anatomic features of the furcal nerve and its clinical significance. Spine. 1986; 11(10):1002–1007

[11] Romanes GJ. Cunningham's Textbook of Anatomy. 12th ed. Oxford: Oxford University Press; 1981

[12] Bardeen CR, Elting AW. A statistical study of the variations in the formation and position of the lumbosacral plexus in man. Anat Anz. 1901; 19(1):124–209

[13] Bergman RA, Thompson SA, Afifi AA, Saadeh F. Compendium of Human Anatomic Variation. Nervous System. Baltimore, MD: Urban and Schwarzenberg; 1988:143–146

[14] Paterson AM. The origin and distribution of the nerves to the lower limb. J Anat Physiol. 1894; 28(Pt 2):169–193

[15] d'Avella D, Mingrino S. Microsurgical anatomy of lumbosacral spinal roots. J Neurosurg. 1979; 51(6):819–823

[16] Maiuri F, Gambardella A. Anomalies of the lumbosacral nerve roots. Neurol Res. 1989; 11(3):130–135

[17] Kikuchi S, Hasue M, Nishiyama K, Ito T. Anatomic and clinical studies of radicular symptoms. Spine. 1984; 9(1):23–30

[18] Parke WW, Watanabe R. Lumbosacral intersegmental epispinal axons and ectopic ventral nerve rootlets. J Neurosurg. 1987; 67(2):269–277

[19] Bartynski WS, Kang MD, Rothfus WE. Adjacent double-nerve root contributions in unilateral lumbar radiculopathy. AJNR Am J Neuroradiol. 2010; 31(2):327–333

10 Accessory Obturator Nerve

Matthew Protas, R. Shane Tubbs

Abstract

The branches of the lumbar plexus are frequently encountered in various invasive procedures. Therefore, a thorough knowledge of each of its branches is important to the clinician who performs such procedures. This chapter reviews the clinical anatomy and associated pathologies of the accessory obturator nerve. Variations of this nerve could contribute to atypical presentations of lumbar radiculopathy. It is hoped that a better understanding of this nerve and its distribution will decrease patient morbidity.

Keywords: accessory obturator nerve, anterior internal crural nerve, lumbar plexus variations, obturator nerve variation, psoas muscle

10.1 Introduction

The accessory obturator nerve (AON) was first reported in 1672 by Isbrand van Diemerbroeck,[1] who stated that it was found in roughly one in every three persons and originated from the third and fourth lumbar nerves (▶ Fig. 10.1 and ▶ Fig. 10.2).[1] Not until 1794 was it described in depth by Schmidt. Since its discovery, it has been termed the anterior internal crural nerve, accessory nerve of the internal crural nerve, and the nerve of the coxofemoral articulation.[2] Some have proposed that the AON should be named the accessory femoral nerve owing to its typical derivation from the posterior part of the anterior division of L3 and L4, its function, and its anatomical course over the pubic ramus.[3]

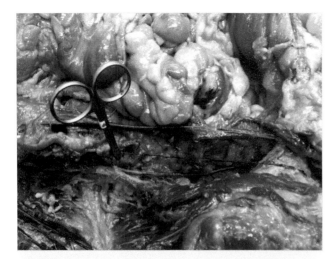

Fig. 10.1 Cadaveric example of a right-sided accessory obturator nerve. The small threadlike nerve above the scissors is the accessory obturator nerve. Note its course over the pubis. More deeply below the scissors, the obturator nerve is seen coursing out the obturator foramen.

10.2 Origin

When present, the AON arises from L3 or more commonly L3 and L4 between the roots of the femoral and obturator nerves. It can also arise from L2, L3, and L4; or L2 and L3; or from the obturator nerve directly.[4,5] Katritsis et al found it was formed by roots from the anterior primary divisions of L3 and L4 (63.6%) or L2, L3, and L4 (10.6%), or L2 and L3 (7.6%), or L3 (6.1%), or from the trunk of the obturator nerve (12.1%).[6] Ellis reported one case in which the AON arose from the trunk of the obturator nerve.[7] Quain et al described the obturator nerve as originating in association with the anterior crural nerve in two cases.[8]

10.3 Anatomy

The prevalence of the AON has consistently been reported as ranging from 10 to 30%.[9,10,11] Population samples in individual studies have been too small for reliable estimates of the overall prevalence of the AON. Most studies of it have failed to record gender or unilateral bias. Sim and Webb and Akkaya et al reported a greater prevalence in females and of left-sided AON, but these results could have been misleading owing to the low numbers of specimens.[12,13] The largest study by Katritsis et al, which examined 1,000 plexuses, revealed no gender difference in the prevalence of an AON in the lumbar plexus, but there was still a left-sided dominance in unilateral cases. This suggests a lack of association between side dominance and gender.

The AON branching from the trunk of the obturator nerve (12.1%)[6] is incompatible with the proposal that it be termed the accessory femoral nerve. Misidentification of the AON can lead to surgical complications such as those in a case reported by Jirsch and Chalk,[14] which demonstrated the importance of these variations in surgical practice. In this case, the AON was thought to be the obturator nerve, which led to the obturator nerve being injured during elective laparoscopic tubal occlusion. Techniques such as magnetic resonance imaging (MRI) and intraoperative nerve stimulation can be used to locate it.[12]

10.4 Course

In 100% of the plexuses examined that had an AON, Katritsis et al found that it passed 2 to 3 cm anterolateral to the obturator nerve and medial to the psoas major toward the obturator foramen, but instead of passing through the canal, it passed over the superior pubic ramus, staying medial to the psoas muscle. Woodburne described the AON as passing directly over the pubic ramus under the femoral vein. Once it crosses the pubic ramus, the nerve descends dorsally to the pectineus muscle, where it typically divides into three branches: one entering the anterior hip joint, one entering the dorsomedial aspect of the pectineus muscle, and one passing medially to anastomose with the anterior branch of the obturator nerve.[11,15] In a rare

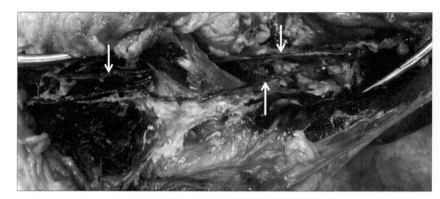

Fig. 10.2 Cadaveric example of a left-sided accessory obturator nerve (lower arrow). The psoas major is retracted laterally to show the obturator nerve (upper arrows). In this specimen, the accessory obturator nerve crosses over the pubis to join the anterior branch of the obturator nerve.

case reported by Rohini et al, the AON emerged on the medial side of the psoas major, entered the femoral triangle, divided into the three typical terminal branches, and passed superficially to the pectineus muscle instead of deep to it.[16]

10.5 Variations

Katritsis et al studied 1,000 plexuses (132 with AON) and found that 36.4% of AONs had variant origins. Although most of these variations were not drastically different, it is important to recognize that the AON can derive from the trunk of the obturator nerve or the anterior crural nerve.[8] Multiple variations of the three terminal divisions have been reported. Katritsis et al saw that after supplying the pectineus, the AON branched off behind the pectineus muscle and supplied the anterior branch (14.3%), posterior branch (4.65%), or trunk of the obturator nerve (6.1%), or the femoral nerve (2.3%). Woodburne also reported that a single branch supplying the adductor longus is not uncommon, along with other additional branches. A very common variation of the AON makes it the sole innervation of the pectineus muscle rather than the typical dual innervation with the femoral nerve.[11] Quain et al described a small cutaneous branch that supplies the inner thigh and upper proximal inner leg. Allen and Shakespeare reported a similar finding of the AON anastomosing with the obturator nerve and supplying cutaneous innervation to the skin of the inner thigh.[17] In one case reported by Tubbs et al, a pseudoganglion was found in association with an AON.[18]

10.6 Landmarks

Akkaya et al reported that the AON had a mean distance of 1.6 cm from the femoral nerve, and was 2.0 cm superior and 2.0 cm anterior to the upper wall of the external opening of the obturator canal, 4.0 cm from the pubic tubercle, and 4.6 cm from the median plane. Although no measurements of the AON have been reported, it is described as "smaller than the usual obturator nerve."[8,11,19]

In view of the close proximity of the lateral femoral cutaneous nerve to the AON in the pelvis, it is important to be able to distinguish them. The lateral femoral cutaneous nerve is formed from the posterior division of L2 and L3.[20] It passes laterally to the psoas muscle instead of medially as the AON does.

10.7 Embryology

There are conflicting accounts of the embryological origin of the AON. According to the original hypothesis of its derivation, the AON arises from a splitting of the obturator nerve caused by the developing obturator foramen.[11,■] The fact that the pubis develops around the obturator nerve, enclosing it in the obturator foramen, threw doubt on this proposal.[11,21] Howell also asserted that when the pubis develops around the obturator nerve, it separates it from the AON. Yasar et al[22] reported an AON in 4 of 20 lumbar plexuses in 10 fetuses between gestational ages 24 and 28 weeks. Woodburne described the pectineus as a "border muscle" in embryological development. This is because it is located between the muscles typically innervated by the obturator and femoral nerves; it is located in the anterior thigh but its function is similar to that of an adductor medial thigh muscle. The development of this muscle and its innervation further questions whether the AON and its innervation of this border muscle more closely represent the femoral or the obturator nerve. The AON innervates the pectineus on its dorsomedial aspect, while the femoral branch that arises distally to the inguinal ligament turns medially, travels dorsal to the femoral vessels, and finally innervates the muscle on the ventrolateral aspect.[11] With this in mind, the arguments for naming the AON "the accessory femoral nerve" are called into question by the similar way in which the pectineus is innervated. Bolk described the femoral innervation as frequently being an independent branch and very loosely associated with the femoral nerve.[23] However, Woodburne proposed that the innervation might differ because the dorsomedial obturator portion of the pectineus muscle was phylogenetically separated from the ventrolateral femoral portion. This questions whether the phylogenetic separation of the pectineus muscle might be responsible for the embryological development of the AON. In a 14-mm embryo, a distinct branch of the femoral nerve was found to innervate the pectineus.[11,24] Leche suggested that in some mammals there is an obturator intermedius muscle in addition to the obturator externus during development.[25] He proposed that this obturator intermedius becomes associated with the pectineus muscle, leading to dual innervation by both the femoral nerve and the AON. Grafenberg described a 6-week-old human embryo in which the muscles of the anterior and medial thigh developed from a single primordial muscle,[26] which was innervated by both the femoral and obturator nerves. Uneven splitting of this primordial muscle could account for the changes in innervation leading to the development of the AON. Visual evidence for this was suggested in a study by Bardeen, who believed that a mass associated with the embryonic external obturator and pectineus muscles was the area where the obturator nerve would innervate.[24] Further support is provided by its course and location on the dorsal aspect of the pectineus muscle after crossing the pelvic brim and before splitting into its terminal branches. The proposal that the AON first formed because of a phylogenic separation is supported by its atypical path over the pubic ramus (which is the known path for innervation of the anterior thigh muscles) instead of through the obturator canal.

10.8 Clinical Implications

Akkaya et al reported that an AON could negatively affect the clinical efficacy of an obturator nerve block. They stated that if the patient had an AON, it too might need to be blocked. AON blockage can be recommended for thigh surgeries, treatment of pain, and diagnosis of hip joint pain.[16] Akkaya et al showed that in 12 cadavers the AON was located a mean distance of 4 cm lateral to the pubic tubercle, which should be used as a guide for AON block. Positioning for such a block should be 2 cm lateral and caudal to the pubic tubercle. The needle should then be rotated 30 degrees lateral and inserted toward the superior edge of the superior pubic ramus.[12] Failure to block the obturator nerve completely along with the AON during transurethral bladder surgery can lead to life-threatening hemorrhage owing to the proximity of the overextended bladder to an accessory obturator artery.[27,28] However, Akata et al were unsure whether it was inadequate anesthesia or lack of direct targeting of the AON that caused the life-threatening hemorrhage. Akkaya et al argued that the best way to prevent injury is to plan for the presence of the AON regardless of the situation to ensure proper obturator nerve blockage.

References

[1] Swanson LW. Neuroanatomical Terminology: A Lexicon of Classical Origins and Historical Foundations. New York, NY: Oxford University Press; 2015:29

[2] Cruveilhier J. The Anatomy of the Human Body. 1st ed. New York, NY: Harper & Brothers; 1844

[3] McMinn RMH. Last's Anatomy: Regional and Applied. 9th ed. Marrickville, New South Wales: Elsevier; 2003:397

[4] Bergman RA, Thompson SA, Afifi AK. Catalogue of Human Variations. Baltimore, MD: Urban & Schwarzenberg; 1984:158–161

[5] Bergman RA, Thompson SA, Afifi AA, Saadeh F. Compendium of Human Anatomical Variations. Baltimore, MD: Urban and Schwarzenburg; 1988:143–148

[6] Katritsis E, Anagnostopoulou S, Papadopoulos N. Anatomical observations on the accessory obturator nerve (based on 1000 specimens). Anat Anz. 1980; 148(5):440–445

[7] Ellis G. Demonstrations of Anatomy. London: Smith Elder and Company. 1887; 11:543, 631.

[8] Quain J, Sharpey W, Thomson A, Cleland JG. Quain's Elements of Anatomy. 7th ed. London: Walton and Maberly; 1867:663–664

[9] Hollinshead WH. Anatomy for Surgeons, Vol 2: The Thorax, Abdomen and Pelvis. London: Cassell & Co. 1956:636–638

[10] Lennon RL, Horlocker TT. Mayo Clinic Analgesic Pathway: Peripheral Nerve Blockade for Major Orthopedic Surgery and Procedural Training Manual. Boca Raton, FL: CRC Press; 2006:6

[11] Woodburne RT. The accessory obturator nerve and the innervation of the pectineus muscle. Anat Rec. 1960; 136:367–369

[12] Sim IW, Webb T. Anatomy and anaesthesia of the lumbar somatic plexus. Anaesth Intensive Care. 2004; 32(2):178–187

[13] Akkaya T, Comert A, Kendir S, et al. Detailed anatomy of accessory obturator nerve blockade. Minerva Anestesiol. 2008; 74(4):119–122

[14] Jirsch JD, Chalk CH. Obturator neuropathy complicating elective laparoscopic tubal occlusion. Muscle Nerve. 2007; 36(1):104–106

[15] Standring S. Gray's Anatomy. 40th ed. London: Churchill Livingstone; 2008:1069–1081

[16] Rohini M, Yogesh AS, Banerjee C, Goyal M. Variant accessory obturator nerve? A case report and embryological review. J Med Health Sci. 2012; 1:7–9

[17] Allen H, Shakespeare EO. A System of Human Anatomy: Bones and Joints. 2nd ed. Philadelphia, PA: H. C. Lea's Son & Company; 1883:566

[18] Tubbs RS, Sheetz J, Salter G, Oakes WJ. Accessory obturator nerves with bilateral pseudoganglia in man. Ann Anat. 2003; 185(6):571–572

[19] Gray H. Anatomy, Descriptive and Surgical. 1st ed. Philadelphia, PA: Blanchard and Lea; 1867:582

[20] Anloague PA, Huijbregts P. Anatomical variations of the lumbar plexus: a descriptive anatomy study with proposed clinical implications. J Manual Manip Ther. 2009; 17(4):e107–e114

[21] Howell AB. The phylogenetic arrangement of the muscular system. Anat Rec. 1936; 66:295–316

[22] Yasar S, Kaya S, Temiz C, Tehli O, Kural C, Izci Y. Morphological structure and variations of lumbar plexus in human fetuses. Clin Anat. 2014; 27(3):383–388

[23] Bolk L. Beziehungenzwischen Skelett, Muskulatur und Nerven der Extremitaten. Mowh. Jb. 1894; 21:241–277

[24] Bardeen CR. Development and variation of the nerves and the musculature of the inferior extremity and of the neighboring regions of the trunk in man. Am J Anat. 1906; 6:259–390

[25] Leche W. Muskulatur. Saugethiere: Mammalia. In: Bronn's Klassen und Ordnungen des Thierreichs. 1900. Leipzig: Thiel.

[26] Grafenberg E. Die Entwickelung der Menschlichen Beckenmuskulatur. Anat Hefte 1904; 23:431–493

[27] Akata T, Murakami J, Yoshinaga A. Life-threatening haemorrhage following obturator artery injury during transurethral bladder surgery: a sequel of an unsuccessful obturator nerve block. Acta Anaesthesiol Scand. 1999; 43(7); 784–788

[28] Atanassoff PG, Weiss BM, Brull SJ. Lidocaine plasma levels following two techniques of obturator nerve block. J Clin Anesth. 1996; 8(7):535–539

11 Variations of the Lumbar Plexus

Nihal Apaydin, Michele Davis

Abstract

The nerves of the body are often varied in their course and composition from person to person and from side to side in the same individual. The lumbar plexus is no exception. Therefore, a good understanding of the variant anatomy seen in the lumbar plexus is important to the clinician and student of anatomy. Herein, the more common anatomical variations of the lumbar plexus and its branches are discussed.

Keywords: anatomy, anomaly, variant, morphology, surgery, imaging

11.1 Introduction

Variations in the formation and distribution of the lumbosacral plexus and its branches have been the subject of several investigations. One of the first detailed descriptions of the anatomy of the lumbosacral plexus was provided by the French anatomist and pathologist Cruveilhier in 1844.[1] The classical definitions and common classifications were formulated during the late 1800s and early 1900s. Eisler studied variations in the lumbosacral plexus extensively, paying particular attention to the thickness and the number of different spinal nerves entering the formation or its individual branches; and Paterson defined the separation of the nerves into dorsal and ventral groups, documenting the ordinary pattern of formation of the lumbosacral plexus.[2,3] He also introduced the term "nervus furcalis." Sherrington introduced the terms "prefixed" and "postfixed" for cases in which the plexus originated more superiorly (rostrally) for prefixed or more inferiorly (caudally) for postfixed plexuses than the more usual pattern.[4] Bardeen and Elting used the terms "proximal" and "distal" in much the same way as Sherrington used "prefixed" and "postfixed."[5] They suggested that the distal limit of the lumbar plexus is less definite than the proximal one and portions of more distal lumbar nerves join with the sacral nerves to form the sacral plexus. They also concluded that race, sex, and side of the body have little or no relationship to variations in the lumbosacral plexus. Severeano in 1904 studied 50 bodies bilaterally and classified the formation of the lumbar plexus into three types: ordinary (formation normale), prefixed (formation supérieure), and postfixed (formation inférieure).[6]

The descriptions in the current literature and the variations identified in case reports are based mainly on these early publications. Variations in the formation of the lumbosacral plexus have long been a source of diagnostic confusion, aside from atypical clinical and electromyographic findings. It is also important to know that muscle innervation can change independently of the number of the roots entering the plexus because the connections between the plexus roots vary.

The lumbosacral plexus provides the nerve supply to the pelvis and lower limb, in addition to the autonomic supply to the pelvic organs. It is formed by the union of the anterior primary divisions of the lumbar, sacral, and coccygeal nerves. For convenience of description and because of the differences in position and course of some of the nerves arising from it, it is subdivided into four parts: lumbar, sacral, pudendal, and coccygeal. It must be remembered that these plexuses overlap and that there are no definite lines of demarcation between their origins and distributions. Also, the distribution of the nerves in the limbs is not typically segmental and is interrupted by the overlapping of the areas of distribution.[7,8,9,10,11]

11.2 Lumbar Plexus

The lumbar plexus is located in the posterior abdominal wall, in front of the transverse processes of the lumbar vertebrae and deep inside or posterior to the psoas major muscle (▶ Fig. 11.1). Variations in the position of the plexus are usually accompanied by variations in the vertebral column itself. While the origin of the various branches of the lumbar plexus varies according to whether the plexus is prefixed, ordinary, or postfixed, it is typically by the union of the anterior rami of the first three lumbar nerves and usually a part of the fourth lumbar nerve, and it projects laterally and caudally from the intervertebral foramina. A communicating branch from T12, also known as the subcostal nerve, often joins the first lumbar nerve. The range of variations in the formation of the lumbar plexus is summarized in ▶ Table 11.1.[7,8,9,10,11]

The lumbosacral plexus is usually bilaterally asymmetric. In its usual form, the L2–L4 ventral rami first bifurcate into anterior and posterior primary divisions. The L1 nerve splits into cranial and caudal branches after receiving a contribution from T12. The cranial branch is thicker and bifurcates into the

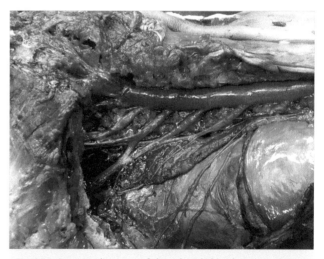

Fig. 11.1 Posterior dissection of the right-sided lumbar plexus following a hemilaminectomy and exposure of the lumbar dura mater. The thecal sac has been filled with saline and the lower ribs, posterior sacrum, and upper iliac crest have been removed. To the right, the lower right diaphragm is seen with overlying parietal pleura. The psoas major muscle is seen anterior to the major components of the lumbar plexus, which, in this specimen, has a "normal" composition.

Table 11.1 Range of variation of the lumbar plexus[5]

Nerve	Prefixed plexus (high form)	Usual pattern	Postfixed plexus (low form)
Lateral femoral cutaneous	L1, L2	L2, L3	L3, L4
Femoral	T12, L4	L1, L4	L1, L5
Obturator	L1, L4	L2, L3	L2, L5
Furcal	L3, L4	L4	L4, L5

iliohypogastric and ilioinguinal nerves; the former is also formed by the subcostal nerve in individuals where this nerve contributes to the lumbar plexus. The caudal branch of the L1 nerve unites with the anterior division of L2 to form the genito-femoral nerve. The anterior divisions of the L2–L4 roots form the obturator nerve. The posterior divisions of L2 and L3 further split into two. The thinner branches unite to form the lateral femoral cutaneous nerve; the thicker ones, together with a contribution from the posterior division of L4, join to create the femoral nerve. The psoas major and quadratus lumborum are innervated by the T12 and L1 nerves and the L2–L4 anterior primary divisions.[7,8,9,10,11,12] The anterior division of L4 is commonly divided between the lumbar and sacral plexuses, hence it is called the furcal (meaning forked) nerve.[3] Fibers from the anterior division of L4 join the anterior division of L5 and create the lumbosacral trunk to join the sacral plexus. Eisler found the furcal nerve to be formed by L5 in 19 out of 22 variations noted in the formation of the lumbar plexus; in only two cases was it formed by L3. The proportion of L4 contributing to the sacral plexus is also variable. The common formation of the lumbar plexus is the manner of division of this nerve: in a postfixed plexus, it contributes all or most of its fibers to the lumbar plexus, while in a prefixed one it contributes few or none. More rarely, an appreciable part of the 12th thoracic or a part of the 5th lumbar nerve participates in the formation of prefixed and postfixed plexuses, respectively.[7,8,9,12]

Matejcík reported the variations of the lumbosacral plexus in 50 cadavers and found the prefixed type in 19 cases and postfixed in 5, the rest being the ordinary form. He also reported that the T12 and L1 roots are thicker in the prefixed type. In this type, the L4 root contributes more significantly to the sacral plexus and the S3 and S4 roots are absent. If the L4 root does not contribute to the sacral plexus or contributes only minimally, the L5 root is also thinner, S1–S3 are thicker, and S4 is also present. As expected, in the postfixed type, the L5 root is the largest contributor to the sacral plexus. These variations at the level of neural root formation are reported to be the most common variations of the lumbosacral plexus.[13] Mine Erbil et al described a rare variation: occurrence of the prefixed type on one side and the postfixed type on the other.[14]

The lumbosacral trunk, either a single trunk formed by the union of L4 and L5 or two parallel but nonunited trunks, also appears medial to the psoas muscle, usually within the pelvis itself, on the anterior surface of the sacrum. It lies medial and posterior to the obturator nerve and is usually not visible from the abdomen, since it is covered first by the psoas muscle and then by the hypogastric vessels. The iliolumbar artery typically passes between the lumbosacral trunk and the obturator

nerve.[7] Urbanowicz studied the connections between the lumbar and sacral plexuses bilaterally in 122 subjects.[15] The plexuses were joined by a single nervus furcalis in 91.8% of subjects and by a doubled one in 0.8%. The single furcal nerve was formed by the abdominal nerve L4 in 80% and L5 in 7.7%. The doubled furcal nerve arose from L3 and L4 in 0.4% of cases and from L4 and L5 in 0.4%. Usually, the major part of the furcal nerve arising from L4 went to the lumbar plexus, and from L5 to the sacral plexus. In 7.4% of cases, no connection between the plexuses could be found.[15] In a series of 20 fetal specimens, Yasar et al observed a single furcal nerve, which originated only from the L4 spinal nerve.[16] A sixth lumbar nerve that contributes to the sacral plexus has been described.[17]

11.3 Branches of the Lumbar Plexus

11.3.1 Iliohypogastric Nerve

The iliohypogastric nerve usually originates from the ventral ramus of the L1 spinal nerve. It emerges from the upper lateral border of the psoas major, crossing obliquely behind the lower renal pole and in front of the quadratus lumborum. Above the iliac crest, it enters the posterior part of the transversus abdominis. Between the transversus abdominis and internal oblique, it divides into lateral and anterior cutaneous branches. The lateral cutaneous branch runs through the internal and external oblique above the iliac crest, a little behind the iliac branch of the T12 spinal nerve. It is distributed to the posterolateral gluteal skin. The anterior cutaneous branch runs between the internal oblique and transversus abdominis and innervates both muscles. It runs through the internal oblique approximately 2 cm medial to the anterior superior iliac spine (ASIS) and through the external oblique aponeurosis approximately 3 cm above the superficial inguinal ring, and is then distributed to the suprapubic skin supplying sensory branches. The iliohypogastric nerve usually gives communicating branches to the subcostal and ilioinguinal nerves.[10,11] The iliac branch of the iliohypogastric nerve can be absent, replaced by the lateral cutaneous branch of the 12th thoracic nerve. The hypogastric branch can supply the pyramidalis muscle and be joined with the 12th thoracic nerve. The iliohypogastric nerve is sometimes derived from the 12th thoracic nerve and can also receive a root from the 11th.[7,8,9] Anloague and Huijbregts demonstrated the absence of the iliohypogastric nerve in 20.6% of the lumbar plexuses they investigated.[18] Sometimes its anterior branch is replaced by the ilioinguinal nerve just before the former exits from the external inguinal ring.[19]

11.3.2 Ilioinguinal Nerve

The ilioinguinal nerve is usually smaller than the iliohypogastric nerve and arises with it from the first lumbar ventral ramus. It emerges from the lateral border of the psoas major, with or just inferior to the iliohypogastric nerve. It passes obliquely across the quadratus lumborum and the upper part of the iliacus and enters the transversus abdominis near the anterior end of the iliac crest. Here, it sometimes connects with the iliohypogastric nerve. It pierces the internal oblique lower than the iliohypogastric, supplies it, and then traverses the inguinal canal below the spermatic cord. Sometimes it passes deep to the inguinal ligament.[19] It emerges with the cord from the superficial inguinal ring and supplies the proximal medial skin of the thigh and the skin over the root of the penis and upper part of the scrotum in males. In females, it innervates the skin covering the mons pubis and the adjoining labium majus. The ilioinguinal and iliohypogastric nerves are reciprocal in size. The ilioinguinal is occasionally very small and ends by joining the iliohypogastric, a branch of which then takes its place.[10,11]

This nerve can be small, terminating near the iliac crest by joining the iliohypogastric nerve, as they exit through the psoas major muscle. In this case, the iliohypogastric nerve sends branches to replace the absent terminal part of the ilioinguinal nerve. The ilioinguinal nerve can be entirely absent, its distribution being taken over by the genital branch of the genitofemoral nerve; the iliohypogastric nerve supplies its territory. The ilioinguinal nerve can also be replaced by either the genital (more commonly) or femoral branches of the genitofemoral nerve. The ilioinguinal can provide a lateral cutaneous or iliac branch to supply the skin in the region of the ASIS. It can partially or completely replace the genital branch of the genitofemoral nerve or the lateral femoral cutaneous nerve. It sometimes arises from L2 instead of L1. Sometimes it gives a communicating branch to the lateral femoral cutaneous nerve. If such a branch is present, it pierces the external oblique aponeurosis near the ASIS and joins the nerve in that vicinity.[7,8,9,19]

The ilioinguinal and iliohypogastric nerves sometimes arise as a common trunk, usually separating between the transversus and internal oblique muscles. The ilioinguinal nerve can be derived from the last thoracic nerve (T12), from a loop between the L2 and L3 nerves, or even from the L2 and L3 nerves directly. It can also supply branches to the rectus abdominis muscle. In a study of 200 cadavers, the ilioinguinal nerve was reported to arise from the lumbar plexus in 72.5% and by a common trunk with the iliohypogastric nerve in 25%; it was absent in 2.5%. It was formed from one root in 92.5% and from two roots in about 5% of cases. In 86%, it carried fibers from one spinal nerve (primarily from L1), and in 11% from two (T12–L1; L1–L2; or L2–L3). Within the inguinal canal, the nerve usually lies ventral to the spermatic cord (60% of cases) but it can lie posterior the cord or within it. It usually leaves the superficial inguinal ring medially but sometimes through its lateral aspect. In some cases, the nerve runs outside the inguinal ring.[7,8,9,19]

11.3.3 Genitofemoral Nerve

The genitofemoral nerve is formed within the substance of the psoas major, originating from the L1 and L2 ventral rami. It descends obliquely through the muscle to emerge on its anterior border, opposite the third or fourth lumbar vertebra. It then descends beneath the peritoneum on the psoas major, crosses obliquely behind the ureter, and divides above the inguinal ligament into genital and femoral branches; it often divides close to its origin, in which case its branches emerge separately from the psoas major. The genital branch innervates the genital area. It crosses the lower part of the external iliac artery, entering the inguinal canal by the deep ring. It supplies the cremaster and the skin of the scrotum in males. In females, it accompanies the round ligament and ends in the skin of the

mons pubis and labium majus. The femoral branch provides sensory innervation of the medial upper thigh and the skin over the femoral vessels. It descends lateral to the external iliac artery, passing behind the inguinal ligament. It then enters the femoral sheath lateral to the femoral artery. It pierces the anterior layer of the femoral sheath and fascia lata and supplies the skin anterior to the upper part of the femoral triangle. It connects with the femoral intermediate cutaneous nerve and supplies the femoral artery.[10,11]

Some authors consider this to be the most variable nerve of the lumbar plexus. Its genital and femoral branches can arise separately from the lumbar plexus. Either of them can be derived entirely from the L1 or L2 nerves. It occasionally arises from L3. The genital branch sometimes receives fibers from the T12 nerve. The genitofemoral or either of its branches (genital or femoral) can be absent. In such cases, the ilioinguinal nerve replaces the genital branch while the lateral cutaneous or the anterior femoral nerve replaces the femoral branch. The branches of the genitofemoral can replace the ilioinguinal nerve or communicate with it. The genital branch can bypass the deep inguinal ring, running superficial to it in the aponeurosis of the external abdominal oblique muscle. The femoral branch can replace or join the lateral or middle cutaneous nerve. Occasionally, the femoral branch has an extensive cutaneous distribution to the upper two-thirds of the thigh. The genital branch can supply the lower fibers of the internal oblique and transversalis muscles. Occasionally, the nerve divides within the substance of the psoas muscle and its terminal branches emerge separately from the anterior surface of that muscle. In a study of 200 cadavers, the genitofemoral nerve arose as a single trunk in 80% and as two separate branches (genital and femoral) in 20%. The single trunk can arise from L1, L2, or L3. The two separate trunks can arise from L1, L2 or L1, L2, and L3. In the present study, L2 contributed to the nerve in all cases but L3 in only 0.75%. The level of division into terminal branches is also highly variable.[7,8,9,19] Anloague and Huijbregts demonstrated variations of the genitofemoral nerve in 47.1% of the cases they dissected.[18] The most common variation included a split of this nerve into genital and femoral branches within the substance of the psoas muscle (26.5%). In 20.6%, this bifurcation occurred at the upper rather than middle portion of the anterior surface of the psoas. Sim and Webb also found that the nerve divided into genital and femoral branches prior to emergence from the psoas major in only 5 of 60 plexuses (8.3%).[33]

11.3.4 Lateral Femoral Cutaneous Nerve

This is an exclusively sensory nerve. Several variations in its formation, course, and branches have been reported. In its usual form, it arises from posterior divisions of L2 and L3, but it can arise in a "high form" (prefixed) from L1 and L2 or in a "low form" (postfixed) from L3 and L4. It can also arise from the femoral nerve or as an independent branch of the lumbar plexus. It emerges from the lateral border of the psoas major and crosses the iliacus obliquely toward the ASIS, parallel to the iliac crest. It supplies sensory fibers to the parietal peritoneum in the iliac fossa. The right nerve passes posterolateral to the cecum, separated from it by the fascia iliaca and peritoneum. The left nerve passes behind the lower part of the descending colon. It supplies the parietal peritoneum in the iliac fossa. Both nerves pass behind or through the inguinal ligament approximately 1 cm medial to the ASIS and anterior to, or through, the sartorius into the thigh. The nerve can be absent on one side and be replaced by a branch of the anterior femoral cutaneous nerve or by the ilioinguinal nerve.[8,9] Carai et al reported that the lateral femoral cutaneous nerve could not be found in 13 (8.8%) of 148 patients who received surgical intervention for meralgia paresthetica.[20] The nerve usually passes behind or through the inguinal ligament, variably medial to the ASIS (commonly 1 cm) and anterior or posterior to or through the sartorius into the thigh. It can pass beneath the inguinal ligament at a point midway between the ASIS and the femoral artery. It is sometimes associated with the anterior femoral cutaneous nerve until it passes distal to the inguinal ligament.[8,9] Then it divides into anterior and posterior branches. The anterior branch becomes superficial approximately 10 cm distal to the ASIS and supplies the skin of the anterior and lateral thigh as far as the knee. It contributes to the formation of the peripatellar plexus, connecting with the cutaneous branches of the anterior division of the femoral nerve and the infrapatellar branch of the saphenous nerve. The posterior branch pierces the fascia lata higher than the anterior branch, and divides to supply the skin on the lateral surface from the greater trochanter to about mid-distance along the thigh. It can also supply the gluteal skin. In some cases, the posterior branch emerges from beneath the inguinal ligament about 5 cm medial to the ASIS and can be replaced by a branch of the genitofemoral nerve.[8,9] Anloague and Huijbregts demonstrated variation in the lateral femoral cutaneous nerve in 17.6% of the cases they dissected.[18] In its variant form, it arose either from the L1 and L2 nerve roots or solely from L2. Another variation included a bifurcation of the lateral femoral nerve within the pelvic cavity prior to its exit near the ASIS. Such bifurcations normally occur after the nerve exits the pelvis.[18]

de Ridder et al reported that in 24 of the 200 cadavers they dissected the lateral femoral cutaneous nerve arose from L1 and L2, and even solely from L2 and L3.[21] Sim and Webb reported that in 22 of 60 plexuses (36.7%), the lateral femoral cutaneous nerve arose from the first two lumbar nerves. The nerve arose solely from the L2 ventral ramus in only one plexus (1.7%), and in six plexuses (10%) it derived directly from the femoral nerve, making for a total of 48.3% variations for this nerve. Mine Erbil et al reported a patient where the right lateral femoral cutaneous nerve was derived from the anterior divisions of the L2 and L3 nerve roots.[14] Webber classified the neural contribution to the lateral femoral cutaneous nerve into eight distinct patterns in 50 plexuses they examined.[6] Grothaus et al found that it bifurcated into additional branches before crossing the inguinal ligament in 27.6% of 29 cadavers.[22] Carai et al also reported early nerve bifurcation in 37.8% of 148 cases.[20] Mine Erbil et al reported similar bifurcations of this nerve into either two or three branches in 2 of 56 plexuses (3.5%).[14] Rosenberger et al found that in 23% of 53 cadavers, the lateral femoral cutaneous nerve gave rise to two branches.[23] Anatomical variations of the nerve were found in about 25% of the patient population in a study by de Ridder et al.[21] Kosiyatrakul et al examined its location in relation to the ASIS and the iliac crest in 96 cadaveric specimens and revealed that 18.8% passed lateral to the ASIS.[24] Dimitropoulos et al demonstrated that the nerve was absent under the inguinal ligament in one

patient; instead, it was found crossing the iliac crest at a distance of 2 cm laterally to the ASIS.[25] Mischkowski et al described a case of a lateral femoral cutaneous nerve that crossed at a distance less than 5 mm superolaterally from the most anterior point of the anterior superior iliac spine.[26] Erbil et al observed two variations in the 28 cadavers they examined.[27] In one of these specimens, the ventral rami of the S1–S2 spinal nerves were united and then divided into four branches, the obturator, femoral and two lateral femoral cutaneous nerves. In the other case, they noted three lateral femoral cutaneous nerves, all piercing the psoas major muscle anterolaterally. Two of these nerves were united by a communicating branch anterior to the iliacus muscle.[27]

11.3.5 Femoral Nerve

This is a motor and sensory nerve derived from the posterior divisions of the ventral rami of the L2–L4 spinal nerves. It is located lateral to the psoas muscle, in the cleavage between the psoas and iliacus. In its course to the thigh, the femoral nerve can pierce the iliacus. It is covered by the iliac fascia, which separates it from the major vessels. Here, it gives off branches that supply the iliacus and pectineus and sends sensory fibers to the femoral artery. Posterior to the inguinal ligament, it lies lateral to the femoral artery and is separated from it by part of the psoas major. Under the inguinal ligament, the femoral nerve lies lateral to the femoral artery and vein (VAN from medial to lateral). However, it has also been reported to enter the thigh between the femoral artery and vein. It has anterior and posterior divisions. The anterior division has two sensory branches that supply the anteromedial thigh and two muscular branches that supply the sartorius and pectineus muscles. The posterior division has one sensory branch, the saphenous nerve, and muscular branches to the quadriceps. The muscular branch to the rectus femoris also supplies the hip joint, while the muscular branches to the three vasti muscles also supply the knee joint.[10,11]

In *Gray's Anatomy*, the femoral nerve is described as having three main divisions: nerve to the pectineus, anterior division, and posterior division.[11] The anterior division gives the intermediate and medial cutaneous nerves of the thigh and the nerve to the sartorius. The posterior division gives the saphenous nerve and muscular branches to the quadriceps femoris. There are also unnamed vascular branches, which travel along the femoral artery and its branches.

Anloague and Huijbregts demonstrated variations of the femoral nerve in 35.3% of the lumbar plexuses they investigated.[18] In those cases, the nerve divided into two and sometimes three separate slips within the mid-substance of the psoas major. Spratt et al reported that 3 out of 136 plexuses (2.2%) contained a variant slip of the iliacus and psoas major muscles that split the femoral nerve.[28] In a case report, Jelev et al noted similar variations of the iliacus and psoas muscles splitting the femoral nerve.[29]

The anterior cutaneous branch can arise from the beginning of the femoral nerve or directly from the lumbar plexus. It can partly or completely replace the femoral branch of the genitofemoral nerve. The posterior branch of the medial cutaneous nerve is sometimes very small or absent, in which case the obturator or saphenous nerves provide its usual area of supply.

The saphenous nerve can end at the knee and be replaced in the leg by a branch of the tibial nerve. The patellar branch of the saphenous nerve can arise from the nerve to the vastus medialis. The saphenous sometimes provides the medial dorsal digital nerve to the great toe. Branches from the femoral nerve to the tensor fasciae latae and adductor longus have also been reported. A branch was also found passing behind the femoral artery and vein, joining an accessory obturator nerve and supplying part of the obturator muscle. The portion of the nerve arising from L4 can run a separate course. Leaving the pelvis with the superior gluteal nerve, it can pass under the fascia lata to supply the rectus femoris and vastus lateralis.[8,9]

The intermediate cutaneous nerve of the thigh has a separate origin from the lumbar plexus. This nerve sometimes arises from the lumbar plexus or from the beginning of the femoral nerve and partially or totally replaces the femoral branch of the genitofemoral nerve.[19]

Saphenous Nerve

This is a sensory nerve that originates from the posterior division of the femoral nerve (L3–L4) in the inguinal region. It is the largest and longest cutaneous branch of the femoral nerve. It descends lateral to the femoral artery in the femoral triangle and enters the adductor canal, where it crosses in front of the artery to lie medial to it. At the distal end of the canal, it leaves the artery and emerges through the aponeurotic covering of the vastoadductor membrane with the saphenous branch of the descending genicular artery. As it leaves the adductor canal, it gives off an infrapatellar branch that contributes to the peripatellar plexus. It then pierces the fascia lata between the tendons of the sartorius and gracilis, becoming subcutaneous to supply the prepatellar skin. It descends along the medial tibial border with the long saphenous vein. It passes in front of the medial malleolus in the ankle before terminating around the base of the first metatarsal on the medial side of the foot. It divides distally into a branch that continues along the tibia to the ankle and one that passes anterior to the ankle to supply the skin on the medial side of the foot, often as far as the first metatarsophalangeal joint. It can connect with the medial branch of the superficial fibular nerve.[8,9,10,11]

11.3.6 Obturator Nerve

The obturator is the nerve of the medial compartment of the thigh. It arises from the anterior divisions of the second to fourth lumbar ventral rami. It can have additional roots from the first or fifth lumbar nerve. It can arise in a "high form" from L1, L2, L3, and L4 (very rarely from L1, L2, and L3), or in a "low form" from L2, L3, L4, and L5. In its usual form, the branch from the third is the largest, while that from the second is often very small. The second lumbar nerve does not always contribute to it. The obturator descends through the psoas major and emerges from its medial border at the pelvic brim running down between this muscle and the lumbar vertebral column. It crosses the sacroiliac joint behind the common iliac artery and lateral to the internal iliac vessels, running along the lateral pelvic wall medial to the obturator internus, anterosuperior to the obturator vessels. It can run in a bony canal prior to entering the obturator foramen.[30] Tubbs et al reported this nerve to

appear at a mean distance of 5 cm inferior to the supracristal plane on a vertical line through the ASIS and having a mean distance of 3 cm lateral to the midline.[31] It enters the thigh through the upper part of the obturator foramen. Near the foramen, it divides into anterior and posterior branches, which are separated at first by part of the obturator externus and more distally by the adductor brevis. One study found that the nerve divided within the pelvis in 23.22%, in the obturator canal in 51.78%, and in the thigh in 25%.[18] The branch from the main trunk of the nerve to the obturator externus muscle can pass to the lateral (instead of the medial) side of the obturator nerve. It gives articular branches to the hip and knee and can supply the skin on the medial thigh and leg. The anterior sensory branch is frequently missing, and in those cases the femoral nerve also supplies the medial thigh. The highly variable distribution of the cutaneous branch of the obturator nerve has contributed to the confusion about how much of the medial thigh and the knee the obturator nerve innervates. Branches to the following structures have also been reported: the obturator internus and pectineus muscles, obturator artery, and periosteum of the pelvic surface of pubis.[8,9,10,11] Locher et al noted substantial anatomical variation in the location of the branches, which were not all the same in the cadaveric specimens they dissected.[32]

The anterior branch of the obturator leaves the pelvis anterior to the obturator externus and descends in front of the adductor brevis, deep to the pectineus and adductor longus. It can pass posterior to the adductor brevis muscle. The anterior branch innervates the gracilis, adductor brevis and adductor longus, and sometimes the pectineus. It can communicate with the accessory obturator nerve (when this nerve is present). It also gives articular branches to the hip joint. Sometimes it supplies the skin of the medial side of the thigh. It can communicate with the medial cutaneous and saphenous branches of the femoral nerve to form the subsartorial plexus. The contribution of the obturator nerve to this plexus is highly variable. When its communicating branch is large and reaches the leg, the posterior branch of the medial cutaneous nerve is small. Occasionally, the communicating branch to the medial femoral cutaneous and saphenous branches continues as a cutaneous branch to the thigh and leg. When this occurs, the nerve emerges from the distal border of the adductor longus to descend along the posterior margin of the sartorius to the knee. Here, it pierces the deep fascia and connects with the saphenous nerve to supply the skin on the medial side of the leg.

The posterior branch of the obturator nerve has a short trajectory. It usually pierces the obturator externus anteriorly and passes beneath the adductor brevis to the front of the adductor magnus. It can also pass posterior to the adductor brevis muscle. The posterior branch gives branches to the obturator externus, adductor magnus, and adductor brevis when the latter is not supplied by the anterior division. It gives branches to the knee joint and popliteal artery.

11.3.7 Accessory Obturator Nerve

An accessory obturator nerve has a reported incidence of 30, 29 (of 120 cases), 11, 8, and 3%.[2,6,7,33] In contrast, Tubbs et al reported finding not a single accessory obturator nerve in 22 plexuses.[31] When present, it arises from the L3 or more commonly the L3 and L4 nerves between the roots of the femoral and obturator nerves. It can also arise from L2, L3, and L4; or L2, L3; or only L3; or from the obturator nerve.[8,9] In a series of 1,000 specimens from 500 embalmed adult human cadavers, the accessory obturator nerve was present in 13.2% (13.3% of the males and 12.9% of the females) with predominance on the left side of the body.[34] Sim and Webb also noted that it occurred more frequently on the left side and in females.[33] Katritsis et al found it to be formed by roots from the anterior primary divisions of L3 and L4 (63.6%) or L2, L3, and L4 (10.6%), or L2 and L3 (7.6%), or L3 (6.1%), or from the trunk of the obturator nerve (12.1%).[34]

The accessory obturator nerve usually courses medial and posterior to the obturator nerve and is usually not visible from the abdomen, since it is covered first by the psoas muscle and then by the hypogastric vessels. It courses with the obturator nerve to the level of the brim of the pelvis but is sometimes closely related to the femoral nerve. However, instead of passing through the obturator foramen like the obturator nerve, it descends along the medial border of the psoas muscle, crosses over the superior ramus of the pubic bone, passes beneath the pectineus, and terminates in three branches, which are also variable. These terminal branches usually replace the femoral branch to the pectineus and supply the muscle and the hip joint. It can also give branches to the adductor muscles by rejoining the obturator nerve. However, sometimes these only supply the pectineus or make a significant contribution to the innervation of the adductor muscles.[7,8,9]

References

[1] Cruveilhier J. The Anatomy of the Human Body. New York, NY: Harper & Brothers; 1844

[2] Eisler P. Der Plexus lumbosacralis des Menschen. Berlin: Halle; 1892

[3] Paterson AM. The origin and distribution of nerves to the lower limb. J Anat Physiol. 1893; 28(Pt 1):84–95

[4] Sherrington CS. Notes on the arrangement of some motor fibers in the lumbo-sacral plexus. J Physiol. 1892; 13(6):621–772, 17

[5] Bardeen CR, Elting AW. A statistical study of the variations in the formation and position of the lumbosacral plexus in man. Anat Anz. 1901; 19:124–128, 209–232

[6] Webber RH. Some variations in the lumbar plexus of nerves in man. Acta Anat (Basel). 1961; 44:336–345

[7] Hollinshead WH. Anatomy for Surgeons, Vol. 2: The Thorax, Abdomen and Pelvis. London: Cassell & Co. Ltd.; 1956:636–638

[8] Bergman RA, Thompson SA, Afifi AK, Saddeh FA. Compendium of Human Anatomical Variations. Baltimore, MD: Urban & Schwarzenburg; 1988;143–148

[9] Bergman RA, Thompson SA, Afifi AK. Catalogue of Human Variations. Baltimore: Urban & Schwarzenberg 1984;158–161

[10] Williams A. Pelvic girdle and lower limb. In: Standring S, ed. Gray's Anatomy. 39th ed. New York, NY: Elsevier; 2005;1456–1499

[11] Mahadevan V. Pelvic girdle and lower limb. In: Standring S, ed. Gray's Anatomy. 40th ed. New York, NY: Elsevier; 2008;1327–1429

[12] Urbanowicz Z, Zaluska S. Formation of the lumbar plexus in man and macaca. Folia Morphol (Warsaw). 1969; 28:256–271

[13] Matejcík V. Anatomical variations of lumbosacral plexus. Surg Radiol Anat. 2010; 32(4):409–414

[14] Mine Erbil K, Onderoğlu S, Başar R. Unusual branching in lumbar plexus. Case report. Folia Morphol (Warsz). 1998; 57(4):377–381

[15] Urbanowicz Z. Connections between the lumbar and the sacral plexus in man. Folia Morphol (Warsz). 1981; 40(3):271–279

[16] Yasar S, Kaya S, Temiz C, Tehli O, Kural C, Izci Y. Morphological structure and variations of lumbar plexus in human fetuses. Clin Anat. 2014; 27(3):383–388

[17] Lane WA. Some variations in the human skeleton. J Anat Physiol. 1886; 20(Pt 3):388–404

[18] Anloague PA, Huijbregts P. Anatomical variations of the lumbar plexus: a descriptive anatomy study with proposed clinical implications. J Manual Manip Ther. 2009; 17(4):e107–e114

[19] Aasar YH. Anatomical Anomalies. Cairo: Fouad I University Press; 1947;92–101

[20] Carai A, Fenu G, Sechi E, Crotti FM, Montella A. Anatomical variability of the lateral femoral cutaneous nerve: findings from a surgical series. Clin Anat. 2009; 22(3):365–370

[21] de Ridder VA, de Lange S, Popta JV. Anatomical variations of the lateral femoral cutaneous nerve and the consequences for surgery. J Orthop Trauma. 1999; 13(3):207–211

[22] Grothaus MC, Holt M, Mekhail AO, Ebraheim NA, Yeasting RA. Lateral femoral cutaneous nerve: an anatomic study. Clin Orthop Relat Res. 2005(437):164–168

[23] Rosenberger RJ, Loeweneck H, Meyer G. The cutaneous nerves encountered during laparoscopic repair of inguinal hernia: new anatomical findings for the surgeon. Surg Endosc. 2000; 14(8):731–735

[24] Kosiyatrakul A, Nuansalee N, Luenam S, Koonchornboon T, Prachaporn S. The anatomical variation of the lateral femoral cutaneous nerve in relation to the anterior superior iliac spine and the iliac crest. Musculoskelet Surg. 2010; 94(1):17–20

[25] Dimitropoulos G, Schaepkens van Riempst J, Schertenleib P. Anatomical variation of the lateral femoral cutaneous nerve: a case report and review of the literature. J Plast Reconstr Aesthet Surg. 2011; 64(7):961–962

[26] Mischkowski RA, Selbach I, Neugebauer J, Koebke J, Zöller JE. Lateral femoral cutaneous nerve and iliac crest bone grafts–anatomical and clinical considerations. Int J Oral Maxillofac Surg. 2006; 35(4):366–372

[27] Erbil KM, Sargon FM, Sen F, et al. Examination of the variations of lateral femoral cutaneous nerves: report of two cases. Anat Sci Int. 2002; 77(4):247–249

[28] Spratt JD, Logan BM, Abrahams PH. Variant slips of psoas and iliacus muscles, with splitting of the femoral nerve. Clin Anat. 1996; 9(6):401–404

[29] Jelev L, Shivarov V, Surchev L. Bilateral variations of the psoas major and the iliacus muscles and presence of an undescribed variant muscle–accessory iliopsoas muscle. Ann Anat. 2005; 187(3):281–286

[30] Varricchio P, Pinhal-Enfield G, Melovitz-Vasan C, Vasan N. Uncommon course of obturator nerve through an osseous tunnel: clinical relevance. IJAV. 2013; 6:133–135

[31] Tubbs RS, Salter EG, Wellons JC, III, Blount JP, Oakes WJ. Anatomical landmarks for the lumbar plexus on the posterior abdominal wall. J Neurosurg Spine. 2005; 2(3):335–338

[32] Locher S, Burmeister H, Böhlen T, et al. Radiological anatomy of the obturator nerve and its articular branches: basis to develop a method of radiofrequency denervation for hip joint pain. Pain Med. 2008; 9(3):291–298

[33] Sim IW, Webb T. Anatomy and anaesthesia of the lumbar somatic plexus. Anaesth Intensive Care. 2004; 32(2):178–187

[34] Katritsis E, Anagnostopoulou S, Papadopoulos N. Anatomical observations on the accessory obturator nerve (based on 1000 specimens). Anat Anz. 1980; 148(5):440–445

12 High-Resolution Magnetic Resonance Neurography of the Lumbar Plexus

Claudia Cejas, Diego Leonardo Pineda Ordóñez, Inés Tatiana Escobar Buitrago, Mercedes Serra, Fabio Barroso

Abstract

The lumbar plexus may be involved in various disorders of the peripheral nerves. Magnetic resonance neurography (MRN) is a recent addition to the diagnostic tool set for assessing the lumbar plexus and peripheral nerves. It provides anatomical detail of the plexus components, showing enlargement and/or abnormal signal when affected by disease. MRN is particularly useful for assessing focal lesions due to neoplasia, infiltration, and inflammatory diseases, and for defining the extent and degree of nerve injury after trauma. Additionally, it is increasingly being used to characterize polyneuropathies. This chapter reviews the imaging of the lumbar plexus and its branches. A better understanding of the nerve roots and their distribution may contribute to decrease the procedure-related morbidity.

Keywords: lumbar plexus, neuropathies, magnetic resonance, neurography, anatomy, posterior abdominal wall, nerves, complications, surgery

12.1 Introduction

Magnetic resonance neurography (MRN) is a recent addition to the set of tools for the assessment of the lumbar plexus (LP) and peripheral nerves. The objective of this chapter is to review state-of-the-art MRN imaging techniques used to characterize disorders affecting the LP.

With the current techniques, MRN allows the examiner to distinguish mononeuropathies from polyneuropathies or tumors from inflammatory disease; to establish the exact location of a lesion; to quantify degrees of nerve injury related to trauma; and to localize nerve entrapment.

12.2 Anatomy

The LP is formed by the ventral rami arising between L1 and L4, in some cases with a small contribution from T12. The anterior divisions of these roots form anterior nerve branches including the iliohypogastric and ilioinguinal nerves (L1), the genitofemoral nerve (L1–L2), and the obturator nerve (L2–L4). The posterior divisions form posterior nerve branches, as the femoral nerve (L2–L4) and the lateral femoral cutaneous nerve (L2–L3, occasionally L4) (▶ Fig. 12.1).

Iliohypogastric, ilioinguinal, and genitofemoral nerves supply sensory innervation to the lower abdomen, genitals, and inner thigh. The lateral femoral cutaneous nerve does supplies the anterolateral thigh. The femoral and obturator nerves, on the other hand, provide motor innervation to pelvic and anterior and medial thigh muscles.[1,2,3]

12.3 Lumbar Plexus Evaluation Protocol

For magnetic resonance imaging (MRI) studies of the LP, 3.0-tesla scanners are ideal since they provide better signal-to-noise ratio and contrast resolution, essentials for assessing the complexity of this structure.[4] Sequences for lumbosacral plexus study include T1- and T2-weighted images with and without fat suppression, and diffusion-weighted imaging (DWI). For homogeneous fat–water separation, special 2, 3, or multipoint Dixon protocols are used, such as IDEAL (Iterative Decomposition of water and fat with Echo Asymmetry and Least squares estimation) developed by Reeder for General Electric (GE) Healthcare.[48] Other options include Dixon TSE developed by Siemens Healthcare, or mDixon developed by Philips Healthcare. Fat suppression techniques such as short tau inversion recovery (STIR) or spectral adiabatic inversion recovery (SPAIR) are also used.[5] Special volumetric acquisitions with high spatial resolution can be applied, such as CUBE developed by GE Healthcare, SPACE (Sampling Perfection with Application Optimized Contrast) developed by Siemens Healthcare, or VISTA

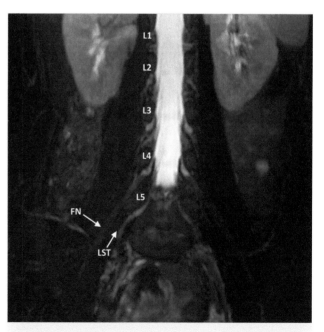

Fig. 12.1 Coronal IDEAL T2-weighted image with fat suppression. MIP reconstruction identifying L1 to L4 roots, forming the lumbar plexus and the femoral nerve (FN); the figure also shows the L5 root and lumbosacral trunk.

(Volume Isotropic Turbo spin echo Acquisition) developed by Philips Healthcare.

Volumetric sequences may be visualized through multiplanar reformations (MPRs), curved planar reformations, and maximum intensity projections (MIP). It allows one to follow the nerve across the organ and compares either size or signal intensity with the normal side in order to discriminate normal anatomy from pathology.[6]

T1-weighted images are optimal for anatomical assessment, allowing perineural fat to be adequately outlined; if needed, fat suppression and intravenous contrast can be used to identify perineural enhancement. On fat-suppressed T2-weighted images, the contrast between background and water signal of the perineurium allows excellent MPR and MIP reconstructions along the nerve course, demonstrating changes in thickness or signal intensity that could be even measured.[7] DWIs with different b values are also useful for assessing nerves, allowing extensive MIP reconstructions without vessels overlapping. DWI is also valuable for studying tumors with a high degree of cellularity. Muscles affected by denervation may show hyperintensity in fat suppressed T2-weighted images during the acute phases due to edema, and hyperintensity in T1-weighted images during chronic phases because of fatty infiltration.[8]

12.4 Pathological Conditions Affecting the Lumbar Plexus

LP could be involved in various disorders of the peripheral nerves. ▶ Table 12.1 lists the categories of peripheral nerve disorders that manifest with abnormalities in LP MRN.

12.4.1 Lumbar Plexopathies

Trauma and Entrapment

Effects of direct trauma over the LP are rare due to the protective effect of the pelvic rim. Lumbar plexopathies caused by penetrating injuries, or root avulsions resulting from traffic accidents, are more common.[9]

Traumatic injury of the sciatic nerve may occur during surgery over or in the proximities of the gluteal muscles.

LP entrapment is frequent in serious spine osteoarthritis, and when it is associated with scoliosis may cause radicular compression[3] (▶ Fig. 12.2).

Psoas muscle injuries such as hematomas or abscesses can generate LP or femoral nerve compression.[10]

On MRN, fusiform enlargement of the nerve with high signal intensity on T2-weighted images, effacement of the perineural fat, and contrast enhancement are the imaging features of the formation of neuroma. In addition, signal changes in paraspinal and limb muscles innervated by the affected root or nerve trunk are common signs of denervation.

Tumors

Intrinsic Tumors

The LP is a common site for the development of peripheral nerve sheath tumor (PNST). The most common neurogenic tumors are schwannomas and neurofibromas. There are three types of neurofibroma: localized, diffuse, and plexiform.[11,12]

In general terms, schwannomas are eccentric to the nerve and encapsulated within the perineurium. Neurofibromas can occur either sporadically or in the context of neurofibromatosis type 1 (NF1).

In PNST, MRN shows well-defined focal or fusiform masses. A dumbbell shape is typical for paraspinal lesions with neuroforaminal enlargement (▶ Fig. 12.3). Different classic imaging landmarks have also been described such as target nodule, contrast-enhancing tail, fascicular disarrangement of fibers, split perineural fat, and bag-of-worms appearance. It is almost impossible to distinguish between schwannomas and focal neurofibromas based solely in imaging features[11,13] (▶ Fig. 12.4).

Malignant peripheral nerve sheath tumors (MPNSTs) can occur in patients with NF1 or can develop de novo. Most MPNSTs are ill-defined masses larger than 5 cm in diameter and spread along large nerve trunks and may enlarge rapidly[14] (▶ Fig. 12.5).

Matsumine et al[15] described MRI characteristics that distinguish between benign and malignant PNSTs. Large size, irregular tumor shape, peripheral enhancement, perilesional edema, and presence of T1-hyperintense areas are important features of MPNSTs.

"Neurolymphomatosis" is a term used to describe infiltration of roots and peripheral nerves by lymphoma. It is a rare extranodal manifestation of both B-cell and T-cell non-Hodgkin lymphoma (90%) or leukemia (10%) (neuroleukemiosis).[16] The diagnosis is based on clinical presentation, presence of lymphoma cells in spinal fluid, and nodular enlargement of plexus, roots, and peripheral nerves.[17] On MRN, nodular enlargement of dorsal roots and an LP with varying enhancement after contrast administration may be seen.[18]

Table 12.1 Causes of lumbar plexopathies

Inflammatory disorders	Immune or vascular disorders	Neoplastic and infiltrative processes	Trauma or entrapment	Iatrogenic
Diabetes, sarcoidosis, amyloidosis, vasculitis	Guillain–Barré syndrome, chronic demyelinating polyneuropathy, multifocal mononeuropathy	• Intrinsic tumors: PNST, MPNST, perineurioma, neurolymphoma • Extrinsic tumors: perineural infiltration: prostate colorectal, gynecological cancers	Trauma, injury, retroperitoneal abscesses or hematomas, posttraumatic neuroma	Hip or pelvic surgery, radiation neuropathy

Abbreviations: MPNST, malignant peripheral nerve sheath tumor; PNST, peripheral nerve sheath tumor.

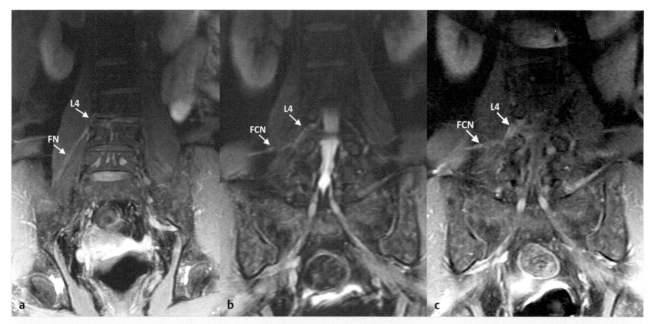

Fig. 12.2 Nerve entrapment. Fifty-eight-year-old woman with left lumbar scoliosis and degenerative changes at L3–L4 level. **(a, b)** Coronal fat-saturated proton density weighted image. Thickening and high signal intensity of L4 nerve root, femoral nerve (FN), and lateral femoral cutaneous nerve (LFCN) is identified (*arrows*). **(c)** Coronal fat-saturated T1-weighted image after intravenous contrast shows enhancement of the same nerves.

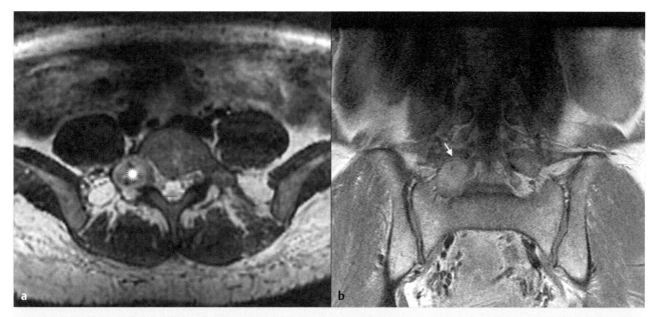

Fig. 12.3 Schwannoma. Fifty-year-old female patient. **(a)** Axial CUBE T2-weighted image. An expansive oval-shaped mass is identified in the right foramen at L5–S1 level (*asterisk*). **(b)** Coronal T1-weighted image after intravenous contrast shows L5 nerve root has expanded (*arrow*) surrounding the enhanced lesion.

Extrinsic Tumors

Perineural spread of malignancy in peripheral nerves is less common, but is known to occur in rectal, prostate, and cervix cancers. Dissemination of prostate adenocarcinoma is associated with advanced disease. However, it has been recently established that approximately 15% of cases have perineural spread at the initial presentation,[19] making it crucial to differentiate spread from radiation-induced neuropathy.

MRN is very useful for depicting perineural tumor involvement. In addition to high signal intensity on T2-weighted images, nodular enhancement is typically present in perineural tumor infiltration[20] (▶ Fig. 12.6).

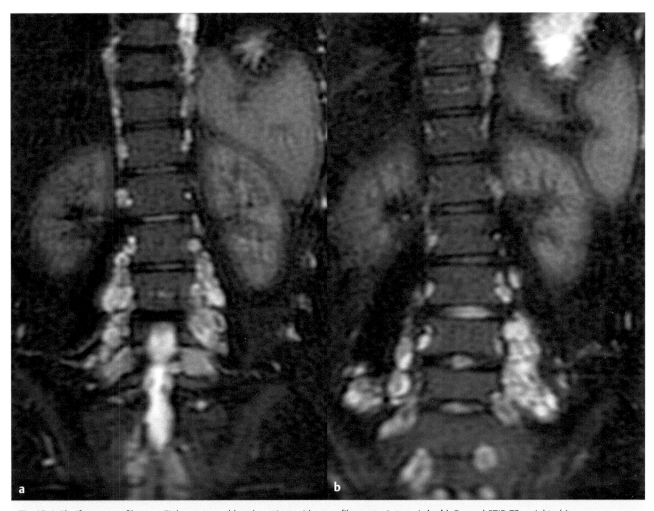

Fig. 12.4 Plexiform neurofibroma. Eighteen-year-old male patient with neurofibromatosis type I. **(a, b)** Coronal STIR T2-weighted images. Multilobulated and coalescent hyperintense masses are observed along the nerve roots and branches of the LP.

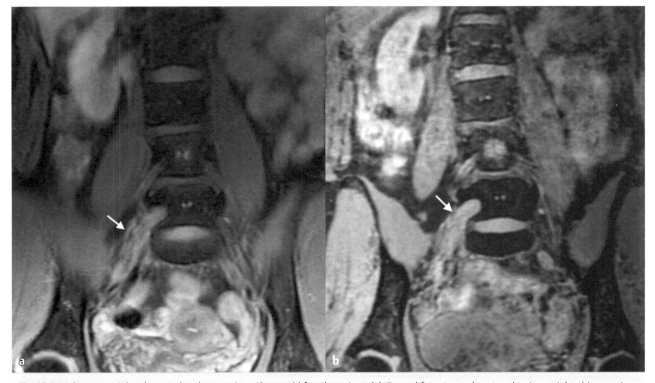

Fig. 12.5 Malignant peripheral nerve sheath tumor in a 40-year-old female patient. **(a)** Coronal fat-saturated proton density–weighted image. A heterogeneous hyperintense lesion is observed enlarging L5 nerve root (*arrow*). **(b)** Coronal IDEAL T1-weighted image with fat suppression and intravenous contrast administration. Lesion enhancement is observed (*arrow*).

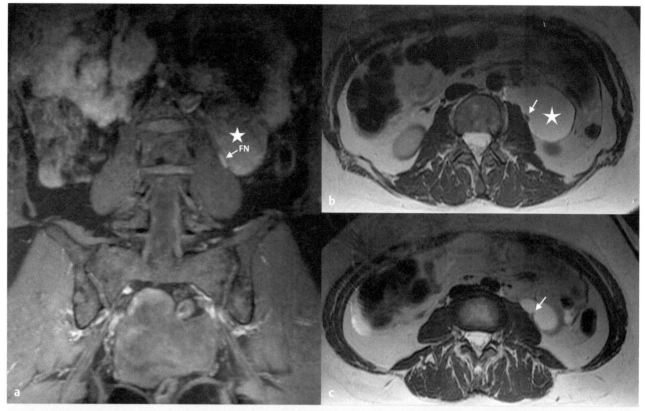

Fig. 12.6 Nerve entrapment by tumor. Forty-seven-year-old woman with lymphangioleiomyomatosis. MRI is performed due to left lumbar pain. Coronal IDEAL T1-weighted image with fat suppression **(a)** and axial T2-weighted images **(b, c)** show an oval-shaped lesion in the left retroperitoneum (*star*). The femoral nerve (FN) is thickened and hyperintense (*arrow*) on both sequences, entrapment between the lesion and the psoas muscle is evident.

Radiation Neuropathy

The LP is frequently exposed to radiation treatment in the setting of pelvic tumors such as prostate, colorectal, and gynecological tumors. When high doses of radiation are administrated, radiation-induced neuropathy can occur. Concurrent chemotherapy appears to potentiate radiation effects.[21]

On MRN, a pattern of fibrosis can be seen along affected nerves or roots, represented by low signal on both T1 and T2. Diffuse thickening and nerve enhancement can be durable.[22]

12.4.2 Lumbar Plexus Abnormalities in Peripheral Neuropathies

Diabetes

The clinical presentation of diabetic neuropathy (DPN) varies widely. It may start as symmetric length-dependent sensorimotor polyneuropathy, mononeuropathy, radiculopathy, multifocal mononeuropathy, autonomic neuropathy, or lumbosacral polyradiculoneuropathy.[22,23]

Pathology findings in DPN include ischemic nerve injury (multifocal fiber loss, focal perineural thickening and degeneration, microvessel neovascularization and injury neuroma) and perivascular inflammation (microvasculitis and hemosiderin-laden macrophages).[24]

On MRN, the most frequent finding in LP involvement is hyperintense abnormal signal from the proximal thigh muscles on T2-weighted images, reflecting acute or subacute denervation. Muscles innervated by femoral and obturator nerves are the most frequently affected[25] (► Fig. 12.7). In later stages, muscles may appear hyperintense signals on T1-weighted images as a consequence of fatty degeneration.[26]

Nerve abnormal findings include diffuse enlargement with an increased T2 signal, or contrast enhancement of the thoracic and lumbar roots. Nerves are less frequently affected individually.[27]

Guillain–Barré Syndrome

Guillain–Barré syndrome is an acute, rapidly progressive immune-mediated inflammatory polyradiculoneuropathy. Most common features are weakness, hyporeflexia, or areflexia. Clinical variants include: acute inflammatory demyelinating polyradiculoneuropathy, acute motor axonal neuropathy, acute motor sensory axonal neuropathy, and Miller Fisher's syndrome.[28]

Diagnosis is based on clinical findings. Cerebrospinal fluid analysis shows albumin-cytological dissociation. Nerve conduction studies most commonly show reduced velocities or conduction block in demyelinating forms, and reduced compound muscle action potential amplitude in axonal varieties of the disease.[29]

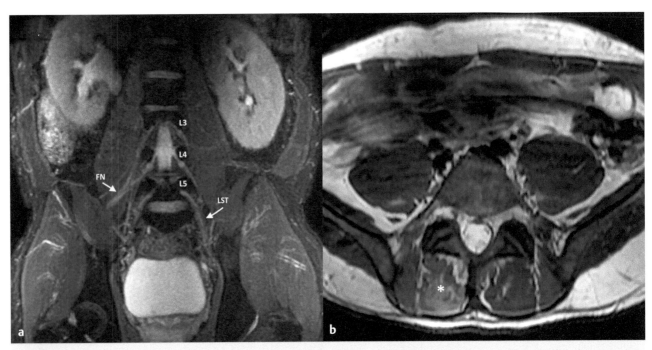

Fig. 12.7 Diabetic polyneuropathy in a 43-year-old male patient. **(a)** Coronal IDEAL T2-weighted image with fat suppression. Diffuse hyperintensity and thickening of right-sided L3 and L4 nerve roots, right femoral nerve, and left L5 nerve root are observed (*arrows*). Fascicular appearance and predominant involvement of the right femoral nerve (FN). **(b)** Axial T2-weighted image. Hyperintense signal of right-sided paravertebral muscles is observed at L5 as a sign of muscle edema and fatty infiltration, possibly related to denervation (*asterisk*). (Reproduced with permission from Cejas et al. [3])

The main MRI finding is thickening and contrast enhancement of spinal nerves, cauda equina, and conus medullaris, with more prominent contrast enhancement in the anterior roots.[30]

MRI can also be useful for predicting the clinical course of the disease. Coşkun et al[31] suggest that MRI follow-up on the third month or later can benefit the prediction of clinical recovery.

MRI helps rule out myelitis and compressive myelopathy when clinical diagnosis is uncertain.[32]

Chronic Inflammatory Demyelinating Polyneuropathy

Chronic inflammatory demyelinating polyneuropathy (CIDP) is an autoimmune demyelinating polyradiculoneuropathy with a wide range of clinical symptoms.[33] It includes a typical form characterized by symmetrical polyneuropathy involving both proximal and distal territories, an asymmetrical form known as multifocal acquired demyelinating sensory and motor neuropathy (Lewis-Sumner syndrome or MADSAM), and a demyelinating acquired distal symmetric polyneuropathy.[34]

Several reports have demonstrated enlargement of LP nerves in patients with CIDP.[35,36]

A typical CIDP case predominantly shows nerve hypertrophy, whereas MADSAM is characterized by multifocal fusiform peripheral nerve trunk hypertrophy.[37] MRN images show fusiform enlargement and thickening of nerve roots due to segmental demyelination, axonal degeneration, fiber loss, and reactive events (i.e., onion-bulb formation).[38]

In some cases, contrast enhancement of nerve sheaths has been reported, and this can persist even after therapy.[35]

In addition, hypertrophy of the cauda equina nerve roots can be seen in some cases[39] (▶ Fig. 12.8).

Hereditary Motor and Sensory Neuropathy or Charcot–Marie–Tooth Disease

Inherited peripheral neuropathies of the Charcot–Marie–Tooth (CMT) spectrum are the most common form of hereditary neuropathy.[40] The number of genetic abnormalities recognized as responsible for this clinical entity is steadily increasing. The most common is a chromosomal duplication of locus 17p11.2, containing the *PMP22* gene.[41] The next most common is a mutation in the gene encoding the GJ1B protein, also known as connexin, located on the X chromosome, followed by point mutations in the *PMP22* and *P0* genes. The total number of genetic abnormalities recognized as associated with CMT is close to 80.[42,43]

This group of disorders is characterized by childhood onset, although clinical presentation can occur at any age. Typical manifestations include distal muscle weakness and sensory loss, diminished or absent tendon reflexes, and foot deformities.[44]

Diagnosis has historically relied on clinical manifestations, family history, and electrophysiological measurements. A positive family history can indicate autosomal dominant, autosomal recessive, and X-linked patterns of inheritance. Electrophysiological assessment provides insight into the predominant pathological abnormality—demyelinating, axonal, or intermediate. Currently, definitive categorization of the disease requires molecular characterization of the genetic abnormality responsible.[45]

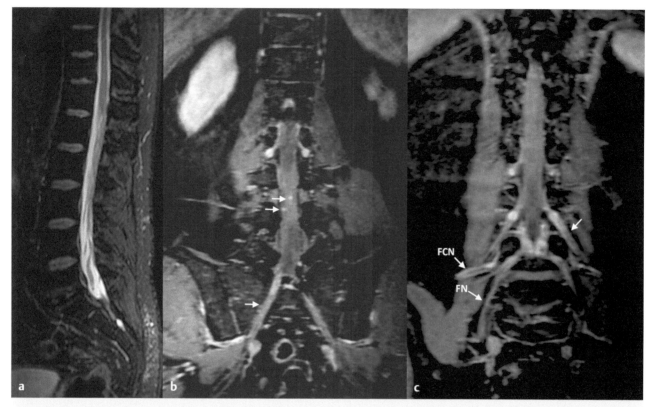

Fig. 12.8 Chronic inflammatory demyelinating polyneuropathy (CIDP) in a 54-year-old man. **(a)** Sagittal IDEAL T2-weighted image with fat suppression. Irregular thickening and disorganization of cauda equina nerve roots is observed. **(b, c)** Coronal IDEAL T1-weighted images with fat suppression. Nodular enhancement of cauda equina nerve roots (*top arrows* on **b**) as well as thickening and perineural enhancement of lumbosacral plexus nerves (*bottom arrow* on **b, c**).

Today, MRN is important for detecting abnormal patterns and establishing the exact location and extent of lesions. Ellegala et al[46] studied nine cases of different CMT varieties, reporting abnormal signal intensity on T1- and T2-weighted images. On T1-weighted images, nerve areas were larger with moderate fat infiltration, whereas on T2-weighted images the nerves appeared hyperintense.

References

[1] Soldatos T, Andreisek G, Thawait GK, et al. High-resolution 3-T MR neurography of the lumbosacral plexus. Radiographics. 2013; 33(4):967–987

[2] Delaney H, Bencardino J, Rosenberg ZS. Magnetic resonance neurography of the pelvis and lumbosacral plexus. Neuroimaging Clin N Am. 2014; 24(1): 127–150

[3] Cejas C, Escobar I, Serra M, Barroso F. High resolution neurography of the lumbosacral plexus on 3T magneteic resonance imaging. Radiologia. 2015; 57(1):22–34

[4] Chhabra A, Flammang A, Padua A, Jr, Carrino JA, Andreisek G. Magnetic resonance neurography: technical considerations. Neuroimaging Clin N Am. 2014; 24(1):67–78

[5] Del Grande F, Santini F, Herzka DA, et al. Fat-suppression techniques for 3-T MR imaging of the musculoskeletal system. Radiographics. 2014; 34(1):217–233

[6] Chhabra A, Lee PP, Bizzell C, Soldatos T. 3 Tesla MR neurography–technique, interpretation, and pitfalls. Skeletal Radiol. 2011; 40(10):1249–1260

[7] Freund W, Brinkmann A, Wagner F, et al. MR neurography with multiplanar reconstruction of 3D MRI datasets: an anatomical study and clinical applications. Neuroradiology. 2007; 49(4):335–341

[8] Yamabe E, Nakamura T, Oshio K, Kikuchi Y, Ikegami H, Toyama Y. Peripheral nerve injury: diagnosis with MR imaging of denervated skeletal muscle-experimental study in rats. Radiology. 2008; 247(2):409–417

[9] Sugimoto Y, Ito Y, Tomioka M, et al. Risk factors for lumbosacral plexus palsy related to pelvic fracture. Spine. 2010; 35(9):963–966

[10] Ailianou A, Fitsiori A, Syrogiannopoulou A, et al. Review of the principal extra spinal pathologies causing sciatica and new MRI approaches. Br J Radiol. 2012; 85(1014):672–681

[11] Kransdorf MJ. Benign soft-tissue tumors in a large referral population: distribution of specific diagnoses by age, sex, and location. AJR Am J Roentgenol. 1995; 164(2):395–402

[12] Prada CE, Rangwala FA, Martin LJ, et al. Pediatric plexiform neurofibromas: impact on morbidity and mortality in neurofibromatosis type 1. J Pediatr. 2012; 160(3):461–467

[13] Jee WH, Oh SN, McCauley T, et al. Extraaxial neurofibromas versus neurilemmomas: discrimination with MRI. AJR Am J Roentgenol. 2004; 183(3):629–633

[14] Kransdorf MJ. Malignant soft-tissue tumors in a large referral population: distribution of diagnoses by age, sex, and location. AJR Am J Roentgenol. 1995; 164(1):129–134

[15] Matsumine A, Kusuzaki K, Nakamura T, et al. Differentiation between neurofibromas and malignant peripheral nerve sheath tumors in neurofibromatosis 1 evaluated by MRI. J Cancer Res Clin Oncol. 2009; 135(7):891–900

[16] Grisariu S, Avni B, Batchelor TT, et al. International Primary CNS Lymphoma Collaborative Group. Neurolymphomatosis: an International Primary CNS Lymphoma Collaborative Group report. Blood. 2010; 115(24):5005–5011

[17] Baehring JM, Damek D, Martin EC, Betensky RA, Hochberg FH. Neurolymphomatosis. Neuro-oncol. 2003; 5(2):104–115

[18] Del Grande A, Sabatelli M, Luigetti M, et al. Primary multifocal lymphoma of peripheral nervous system: case report and review of the literature. Muscle Nerve. 2014; 50(6):1016–1022

[19] Hébert-Blouin MN, Amrami KK, Myers RP, Hanna AS, Spinner RJ. Adenocarcinoma of the prostate involving the lumbosacral plexus: MRI evidence to support direct perineural spread. Acta Neurochir (Wien). 2010; 152(9):1567–1576

[20] Crush AB, Howe BM, Spinner RJ, et al. Malignant involvement of the peripheral nervous system in patients with cancer: multimodality imaging and pathologic correlation. Radiographics. 2014; 34(7):1987–2007

[21] Said G, Krarup C. Diagnosis of brachial and lumbosacral plexus lesions. In: Aminoff MJ, Boller F, Swaab DF, eds. Peripheral Nerve Disorders: Handbook of Clinical Neurology. London: Elsevier; 2013:115-293

[22] Tesfaye S, Boulton AJ, Dyck PJ, et al. Toronto Diabetic Neuropathy Expert Group. Diabetic neuropathies: update on definitions, diagnostic criteria, estimation of severity, and treatments. Diabetes Care. 2010; 33(10):2285–2293

[23] Dyck PJB. Radiculoplexus neuropathies: diabetic and nondiabetic varieties. In: Dyck PJ, Thomas PK, eds. Peripheral Neuropathy. Vol. 2. 4th ed. Philadelphia, PA: Elsevier; 2005:1993–2015

[24] Gwathmey KG, Burns TM, Collins MP, Dyck PJ. Vasculitic neuropathies. Lancet Neurol. 2014; 13(1):67–82

[25] Poliachik SL, Friedman SD, Carter GT, Parnell SE, Shaw DW. Skeletal muscle edema in muscular dystrophy: clinical and diagnostic implications. Phys Med Rehabil Clin N Am. 2012; 23(1):107–122, xi

[26] Wattjes MP, Kley RA, Fischer D. Neuromuscular imaging in inherited muscle diseases. Eur Radiol. 2010; 20(10):2447–2460

[27] Massie R, Mauermann ML, Staff NP, et al. Diabetic cervical radiculoplexus neuropathy: a distinct syndrome expanding the spectrum of diabetic radiculoplexus neuropathies. Brain. 2012; 135(Pt 10):3074–3088

[28] Ropper AH. The Guillain-Barré syndrome. N Engl J Med. 1992; 326(17):1130–1136

[29] Asbury AK. Diagnostic considerations in Guillain-Barré syndrome. Ann Neurol. 1981; 9 Suppl:1–5

[30] Wilmshurst JM, Thomas NH, Robinson RO, Bingham JB, Pohl KR. Lower limb and back pain in Guillain-Barré syndrome and associated contrast enhancement in MRI of the cauda equina. Acta Paediatr. 2001; 90(6):691–694

[31] Coşkun A, Kumandaş S, Paç A, Karahan OI, Guleç M, Baykara M. Childhood Guillain-Barré syndrome. MR imaging in diagnosis and follow-up. Acta Radiol. 2003; 44(2):230–235

[32] Kumar S. Guillain-Barré syndrome. Spinal MR findings. J Pediatr Neuroradiol. 2014; 3(3):153–154

[33] Dyck PJ, Pineda A, Swanson C, Low P, Windebank A, Daube J. The Mayo Clinic experience with plasma exchange in chronic inflammatory-demyelinating polyneuropathy (CIDP). Prog Clin Biol Res. 1982; 106:197–204

[34] Van den Bergh PY, Hadden RD, Bouche P, et al. European Federation of Neurological Societies, Peripheral Nerve Society. European Federation of Neurological Societies/Peripheral Nerve Society guideline on management of chronic inflammatory demyelinating polyradiculoneuropathy: report of a joint task force of the European Federation of Neurological Societies and the Peripheral Nerve Society - first revision. Eur J Neurol. 2010; 17(3):356–363

[35] Adachi Y, Sato N, Okamoto T, et al. Brachial and lumbar plexuses in chronic inflammatory demyelinating polyradiculoneuropathy: MRI assessment including apparent diffusion coefficient. Neuroradiology. 2011; 53:3–11

[36] Shibuya K, Sugiyama A, Ito S, et al. Reconstruction magnetic resonance neurography in chronic inflammatory demyelinating polyneuropathy. Ann Neurol. 2015; 77(2):333–337

[37] Tazawa K, Matsuda M, Yoshida T, et al. Spinal nerve root hypertrophy on MRI: clinical significance in the diagnosis of chronic inflammatory demyelinating polyradiculoneuropathy. Intern Med. 2008; 47(23):2019–2024

[38] Ginsberg L, Platts AD, Thomas PK. Chronic inflammatory demyelinating polyneuropathy mimicking a lumbar spinal stenosis syndrome. J Neurol Neurosurg Psychiatry. 1995; 59(2):189–191

[39] Ishida K, Wada Y, Tsunemi T, Kanda T, Mizusawa H. Marked hypertrophy of the cauda equina in a patient with chronic inflammatory demyelinating polyradiculoneuropathy presenting as lumbar stenosis. J Neurol. 2005; 252(2):239–240

[40] Skre H. Genetic and clinical aspects of Charcot-Marie-Tooth's disease. Clin Genet. 1974; 6(2):98–118

[41] Raeymaekers P, Timmerman V, Nelis E, et al. The HMSN Collaborative Research Group. Duplication in chromosome 17p11.2 in Charcot-Marie-Tooth neuropathy type 1a (CMT 1a). Neuromuscul Disord. 1991; 1(2):93–97

[42] Chance PF, Fischbeck KH. Molecular genetics of Charcot-Marie-Tooth disease and related neuropathies. Hum Mol Genet. 1994; 3(Spec No):1503–1507

[43] Klein CJ, Duan X, Shy ME. Inherited neuropathies: clinical overview and update. Muscle Nerve. 2013; 48(4):604–622

[44] Krajewski KM, Lewis RA, Fuerst DR, et al. Neurological dysfunction and axonal degeneration in Charcot-Marie-Tooth disease type 1A. Brain. 2000; 123 (Pt 7):1516–1527

[45] Ionasescu VV. Charcot-Marie-Tooth neuropathies: from clinical description to molecular genetics. Muscle Nerve. 1995; 18(3):267–275

[46] Ellegala DB, Monteith SJ, Haynor D, Bird TD, Goodkin R, Kliot M. Characterization of genetically defined types of Charcot-Marie-Tooth neuropathies by using magnetic resonance neurography. J Neurosurg. 2005; 102(2):242–245

[47] Reeder SB, Pineda AR, Wen Z, et al. Iterative decomposition of water and fat with echo asymmetry and least-squares estimation (IDEAL): application with fast spin-echo imaging. Magn Reson Med. 2005; 54:636–644

[48] Grayev A, Reeder S, Hanna A. Use of Chemical Shift Encoded Magnetic Resonance Imaging (CSE-MRI) for high resolution fat-suppressed imaging of the brachial and lumbosacral plexuses. European Journal of Radiology. 2016; 85 (6):199–207

13 Lesions Involving the Lumbar Plexus

Arun Gunasekaran, Noojan Kazemi

Abstract

The lumbar plexus and its branches can be affected by various pathologies. Therefore, a thorough knowledge of not only the surgical anatomy of the lumbar plexus but also how these can be involved with disease is important to the clinician. This chapter reviews various pathological entities that can involve the lumbar plexus and its branches. It is hoped that a better understanding of these pathologies will improve patient outcomes from their treatment and decrease morbidity.

Keywords: lumbar plexus pathology, plexus lesions, posterior abdominal wall, nerves, complications, surgery

13.1 Introduction

The lumbar plexus, formed by the ventral primary rami of the L1–L4 nerve roots, provides innervation to the muscles of the lower extremity and pelvic girdle. The route taken by the roots of the lumbar plexus—exiting the spinal column lateral to the intervertebral foramen and piercing the psoas major, where the plexus itself is formed—makes these nerves vulnerable to many pathologies. These include neoplasms such as peripheral nerve sheath tumors, infections, neuropathic degeneration, and hematological, iatrogenic, and traumatic complications. This chapter will describe a number of these pathologies arising in and adjacent to the lumbar plexus and will address potential treatment options.

13.2 Anatomy

The lumbar plexus, composed of the ventral rami of the L1–L4 spinal nerve roots, travels into and is formed within the body of the psoas major muscle, coalescing to produce several prominent nerves. The obturator nerve (L2–L4) exits from the medial aspect of the psoas major and travels caudally, innervating the adductor muscles housed in the medial compartment of the thigh. The femoral nerve (L2–L4) emerges from the lateral aspect of the psoas major roughly at the level of the L4–L5 intervertebral disc and courses caudally in the groove between the psoas major and iliacus muscle, providing innervation to the latter as well as the muscles of the anterior compartment of the thigh, such as the sartorius and the quadriceps femoris.

The lumbosacral trunk (L4–L5) lies deep to the obturator nerve and joins the sacral plexus in the pelvis, forming the lumbosacral plexus. Although it is not technically part of the lumbar plexus proper, the lumbosacral trunk cannot be ignored, both because of its contribution from the L4 and L5 nerve roots and because of its proximity to the lumbar plexus. Two smaller nerves, the ilioinguinal (L1) and the iliohypogastric (L1), enter the abdominal cavity dorsal to the medial arcuate ligament and pass along the ventral surface of the quadratus lumborum muscle, eventually innervating the abdominal muscles and skin of the inguinal area. The genitofemoral nerve (L1–L2) perforates the ventral surface of the psoas major at the level of the L4 vertebra and travels caudally on its surface, splitting near its distal end into the genital branch, which supplies the cremaster muscle, and the femoral branch, which supplies the skin inferomedial to the inguinal ligament. Finally, the lateral cutaneous nerve of the thigh (L2–L3) courses inferolaterally on the ventral aspect of the iliacus muscle, eventually entering the thigh medial to the anterior superior iliac spine, supplying the skin on the ventrolateral surface of the thigh.[1]

13.3 Lesions of the Lumbar Plexus

Lesions involving the lumbar plexus include those arising from the plexus itself and those originating from adjacent structures (e.g., psoas muscle abscesses). These lesions can include compressive pathology such as neoplasms or can be non-compressive. Examples of the latter include neuropathy, infection, iatrogenic injury, and trauma.

13.3.1 Tumors

Schwannoma

Schwannomas are a subclass of peripheral nerve sheath tumors that arise from the myelin-producing cells of the peripheral nervous system. Owing to their neural crest origin, they stain positively for S-100 immunohistochemically—an important diagnostic factor used for the histological differentiation of these tumors. Schwannomas also stain strongly with calretinin but weakly for CD34.[2] They can be classified into those that occur sporadically (which are much more common) and those arising in conjunction with an underlying inherited condition, such as familial schwannomatosis and neurofibromatosis type II (NF-2).[3]

Schwannomas are most commonly found in the head and neck region (e.g., bilateral vestibular schwannomas in NF-2), but they can also arise from the peripheral nerves of the mediastinum and the periphery and, less commonly, the nerves of the pelvis.[4,5]

Rarely, these tumors have been reported to arise from within the body of the psoas major from the sheath of one of the nerves of the lumbar plexus, such as a femoral or obturator nerve.[6,7,8,9] Although rare, these retroperitoneal schwannomas can grow large, possibly causing symptoms consistent with compression of the adjacent structures (e.g., urinary obstruction and hydroureteronephrosis).[4] Furthermore, patients with these lesions can present with chronic pelvic and abdominal pain.[6,10] These tumors also present initially with pain that becomes worse with movement or with weight-bearing exercise, often progressing to neuropathic symptoms from the affected nerve itself (e.g., the femoral nerve). These symptoms can include paresthesia and neuralgia on the affected side as well as weakness of the muscles innervated by the nerves.[11] Lesions can be treated conservatively through surveillance, or removed when symptoms develop.

Familial Schwannomatosis

Familial schwannomatosis is extremely rare, characterized by multiple schwannomas in the absence of acoustic neuromas (▶ Fig. 13.1, ▶ Fig. 13.2, ▶ Fig. 13.3, ▶ Fig. 13.4).[12,13] Genetically, individuals with familial schwannomatosis have mutations distinct from those found in NF-2, namely a novel germline mutation in SMARCB1.[13] Patients frequently present with symptoms similar to those of individuals with benign schwannomas, such as pelvic and abdominal pain, and occasionally neuropathic symptoms. Suspicion for this condition should be raised if there are multiple lesions without the (bilateral) vestibular schwannomas characteristically seen with NF-2. Magnetic resonance imaging (MRI) is frequently used to visualize the schwannomas, while surgical resection is the preferred method of treatment, although chronic pain is frequently reported even after surgical resection.[12]

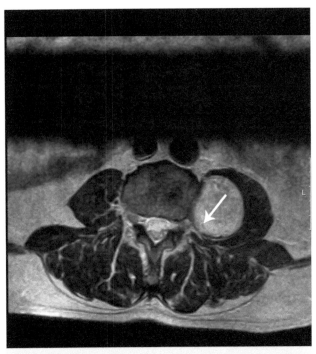

Fig. 13.1 A 65-year-old man with a background of familial schwannomatosis presenting with left intrapsoas schwannoma arising from a branch of the lumbar plexus. T2-weighted contrast enhancing MRI reveals the mass (*arrow*).

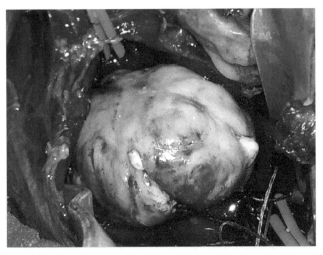

Fig. 13.2 Intraoperative photo of mass in patient as seen in Fig. 13.1.

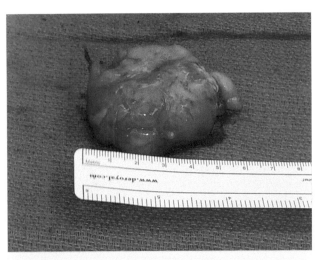

Fig. 13.3 Resected mass from Fig. 13.2.

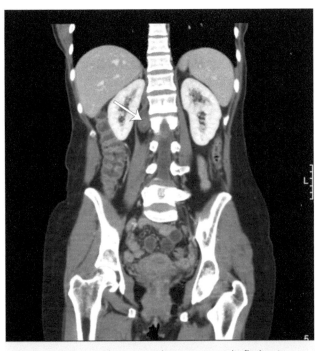

Fig. 13.4 A 50-year-old woman with progressive right flank pain. Coronal plane CT illustrating right intra-psoas major mass medial to the kidney (Note mass at *arrow*).

Neurofibroma

Neurofibromas, like schwannomas, are tumors that arise from the peripheral nerve sheath (▶ Fig. 13.5, ▶ Fig. 13.6, ▶ Fig. 13.7, ▶ Fig. 13.8, ▶ Fig. 13.9). Like schwannomas, they also arise from the neural crest, so they too stain for S-100 immunohistochemically.[2] Unlike schwannomas, however, they test positive for CD34 because they contain increased and varied intracellular material. On the other hand, they stain poorly for calretinin, a marker that is strongly positive in schwannomas.[2,14] While most neurofibromas are frequently discovered as isolated tumors, they can also be associated with the autosomal dominant disorder neurofibromatosis type I (NF-1).[14,15] They can occur in the head and neck (so-called diffuse neurofibromas) and in association with major nerve trunks, as in the case of plexiform neurofibromas.

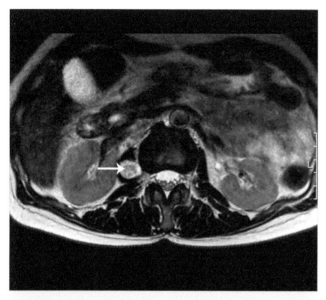

Fig. 13.5 Preoperative, T2-weighted, axial MRI with contrast of adult female presenting with right flank pain.

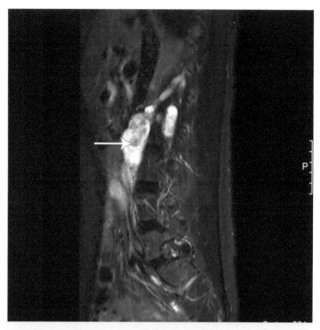

Fig. 13.6 Preoperative, sagittal MRI with contrast.

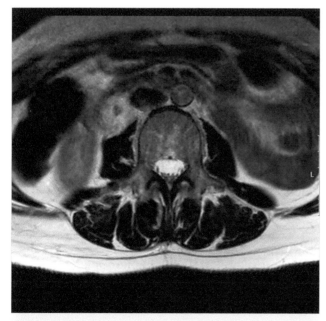

Fig. 13.7 Postoperative, axial, T2-weighted MRI of patient seen in Fig. 13.5, and diagnosis of L2 neurofibroma.

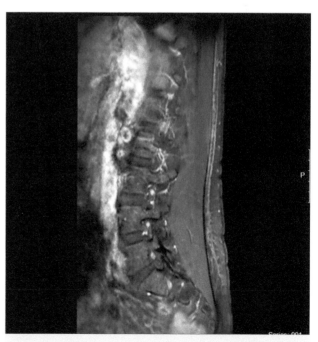

Fig. 13.8 Sagittal, contrasted, postoperative MRI of Fig. 13.6.

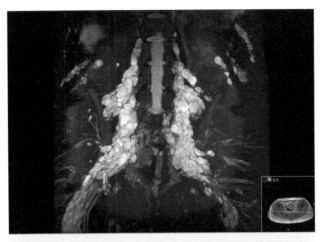

Fig. 13.9 A 24-year-old woman presenting with abdominal pain and bilateral sciatica. MRI neurography demonstrated multiple lesions along the branches of the lumbar plexus and bilateral sciatic nerves, consistent with neurofibromatosis type 1 (NF-1).

In patients with NF-1, there are several reports of neurofibromas arising within the body of the psoas muscle, affecting the lumbar plexus, and those arising from the lumbosacral plexus in the pelvis.[16,17] Owing to the size and location of neurofibromas within the pelvis and retroperitoneal space, symptoms can vary, but are similar in presentation to those of schwannomas (discussed above). These include nonspecific symptoms such as abdominal pain and more specific ones such compressive neuropathy of the lumbar plexus (most commonly the femoral nerve), and corresponding sequelae of weakness of the lower extremities with diminished reflexes and sensation.[18]

While a thorough medical and family history can often point toward a diagnosis of neurofibroma, imaging modalities remain essential for detecting these lesions. They are often detected incidentally by computed tomography (CT), but when they are suspected, more advanced imaging modalities such as MRI are needed to visualize soft tissue and bony involvement.[19,20,21,22,23,24] Additionally, individuals with substantial lumbosacral plexus involvement can show abnormalities on electromyography (EMG) of the anterior and medial compartment muscles.

Retroperitoneal plexiform neurofibromas characteristically appear as hypodense lesions in the retroperitoneal space on CT imaging, lacking symmetry. As with schwannomas, an increase in size in a relatively short time is worrying because it suggests potential malignancy.[25] Treatment, as with schwannomas, is either continued surveillance or definitive surgical resection as appropriate.

Malignant Peripheral Nerve Sheath Tumors (MPNST)

MPNSTs can arise from plexiform neurofibromas (most commonly associated with NF-1) or secondarily due to radiation exposure.[26,27,28,29] These malignant tumors are frequently found in the trunk and distal appendages, and are often associated with major nerve trunks such as the lumbar plexus.[28,30,31] Diagnosis usually depends on biopsy, but imaging modalities such as positron emission tomography (PET) can be used to differentiate benign neurofibromas from MPNSTs[28,32,33] Treatment is

often multifaceted and involves surgical resection or chemotherapy for nonresectable tumors.[28,32,34]

Lymphoma

While very rare, lymphoma can also arise directly within the plexus, leading to a plexopathy, or can spread via direct compression from an enlarged lymph node.[35] Spreading from the nodes, the disease can involve the muscle (e.g., psoas or iliacus).[36] The symptomatology of these lesions will depend on the severity of involvement. Imaging (such as MRI with contrast) can be used to diagnose such lesions. Treatment often includes a diagnostic biopsy and nonoperative management such as chemotherapy.

Other Malignant Tumors

Malignant tumors of three possible origins have been reported within the lumbar plexus. First, a primary tumor can spread from its original adjacent location and involve the plexus.[37] Second, tumors can metastasize to the tissue surrounding the plexus. Third, they can metastasize directly to the plexus itself. These tumors include gastrointestinal, colorectal, and genitourinary carcinomas as well as a wide range of sarcomas.[38] Although the grade and cell of origin of tumors can differ, pain has been reported as a most consistent symptom.[38,39] Imaging findings of these malignant lesions are not always pathognomonic. While MRI is better at visualizing nerve and soft tissue involvement, CT is extremely useful for assessing osseous involvement. Even with contrast, these lesions can have a nonspecific appearance and cannot easily be distinguished from other pathologies in the region.[40] Treatments are often multimodal and include radiation, chemotherapy, or surgery, although newer agents such as monoclonal antibodies have been used for specific conditions (e.g., giant cell tumors). Other lesions that arise in the region can include primary bone tumors such as sarcomas or chordomas.

13.3.2 Infection

Lumbar plexus pathologies can also arise from infection by organisms such as *Staphylococcus aureus*, *Escherichia coli*, *Mycobacterium tuberculosis* (TB), and a number of other less common etiologies. Compressive neuropathy of the lumbar plexus and its branches can result from infections of the psoas because the plexus is embedded within the psoas muscle. Infections of the psoas muscle can be primary or secondary. If secondary, they are frequently due to spread from the gastrointestinal or genitourinary systems, the colorectal area, or the spine. In fact, discitis osteomyelitis of the lumbar vertebrae is a potent cause of psoas muscle abscesses with lumbar plexus involvement and subsequent compression. The two most common etiologies of primary infection of the psoas muscle are *S. aureus* and *E. coli*, which are also the two most common infectious agents in the United States,[41] while TB remains the most common cause worldwide.

Staphylococcus aureus and Escherichia coli

S. aureus is a gram-positive coccus, a frequent asymptomatic colonizer of human body surfaces. While many etiologies can cause psoas abscess formation (the pathogenesis of which is suspected to be related to hematological spread), the most common cause of primary psoas abscesses is *S. aureus*.[42,43]

Classical physical symptoms of a psoas abscess, whether caused by *S. aureus* or *E. coli*, are fever, pain radiating to the flank (most common) and thigh, and pain upon movement of the psoas muscle (i.e., hip movement).[44,45] However, patients can also present with more generalized symptoms such as a nausea, vomiting, and fatigue. Upon physical examination, specific signs can include a physical mass that is palpable in the region of the psoas muscle, or extreme pain upon flexion of the hip.

Laboratory values are frequently consistent with those of acute infection, including elevated CRP, ESR, and leukocytosis.[45] Imaging modalities such as intravenous contrast-enhanced CT scans of the abdomen and pelvis are particularly useful for visualizing these abscesses. Following initial visualization, MRI can be used to visualize soft tissue and hence local involvement.[20,21,45,46,47] Definitive microbiological diagnosis involves obtaining a biopsy via needle aspiration or by surgery. For an uncomplicated abscess, percutaneous drainage with placement of a pigtail catheter is the preferred treatment option, along with long-term antibiotic therapy.

Other common causes of lumbar plexopathy are discitis and osteomyelitis. Bacteria can seed the intervertebral disc via hematogenous spread and then radiate outward into the vertebrae.[48] Infection can also spread from contiguous structures (e.g., aorta or bowel) into the disc space and bony structures.[49] Once an infection is established, it can spread into the adjacent soft tissue structures including the retroperitoneal space and psoas muscle, producing an abscess or posteriorly causing an epidural abscess compressing the spinal cord or cauda equina.[50] The most common cause of discitis–osteomyelitis and subsequent abscess formation is *S. aureus*, while other etiological agents include *Pseudomonas* spp., *Candida* spp., group A and B *Streptococcus* spp., and *Brucella* spp.[51,52] Patients with discitis-osteomyelitis frequently present with pain and fever, along with pain upon palpation of the overlying infection. As expected, they also have leukocytosis and elevated CRP and ESR values. Diagnosis is established once again by positive cultures obtained via needle biopsy or from surgical drainage of the abscess. Treatment is long-term antibiotic therapy or surgical debridement and fixation if conservative treatment has failed or symptoms have dramatically worsened with neurological deficits.

Tuberculosis (TB)

While the infectious agents discussed above are frequently the cause of psoas muscle infection and discitis–osteomyelitis leading to lumbar plexopathy in the United States, *M. tuberculosis* continues to be the main cause of it worldwide.[41] *M. tuberculosis* is an acid-fast bacterium that causes tuberculosis, which manifests as a pulmonary tract infection in the vast majority of cases. However, in approximately 10%, there is widespread extrapulmonary involvement including lymph nodes, cardiac pleura, spinal column (Pott's disease), central nervous system, and the abdomen and pelvis.[53]

TB infection of the lumbar plexus, while not common in the United States, is frequently cited in the literature. Nonspecific symptoms of TB infection include weight loss and night sweats.

Presentations of TB tend to be significantly less specific than *S. aureus* infections. In individuals with suspected psoas muscle abscess, a positive acid-fast lung smear is diagnostic of infection.[54] As with other infiltrative lesions, abscesses caused by TB can lead to lumbar plexopathy with ensuing neurological symptoms. A large abscess can be detected on CT[19,20,22,23,24] while MRI can be used to visualize soft tissue, nerve, and bony involvement in great detail.[20,21,46]

Other

Other less common causes of psoas muscle abscess and subsequent lumbar plexopathy are *Klebsiella pneumonia*, especially in patients with diabetes. These infections can be accompanied by gas formation at the site of infection, which is linked with a high mortality rate (80%).[55] There are rare reports of abscess due to *Streptococcus pneumoniae*, *Streptococcus moniliformis*, and *Nocardia* spp.[56,57,58] Additionally, *Salmonella* spp. and *Candida* spp. have been described as causes of psoas abscesses and subsequent lumbar plexopathy, although these are exceedingly rare.[43,59,60] As above, definitive diagnosis is obtained using needle biopsy of the lesion, with treatment frequently including percutaneous drainage and long-term antibiotic therapy.

13.4 Neuropathy And Plexopathy

Lumbar plexopathy can also arise due to idiopathic or autoimmune-mediated degenerative changes. Chronic inflammatory demyelinating polyneuropathy (CIDP) is one immune-mediated cause of lumbar plexus degeneration leading to neuropathy. Neuralgic amyotrophy, a rapidly progressing degenerative condition, can often present with mixed lumbar plexus and sacral plexus symptoms, with pain being reported in the distribution of both plexuses. Unlike neurogenic plexopathies of the brachial plexus, involvement of the lumbar and sacral plexuses are often reported as progressive in nature, with an initial acute pain course followed by months or occasionally years of diminished strength in the affected muscles.[61]

Another common cause of lumbar plexopathy is diabetes mellitus (DM), called diabetic amyotrophy, which is thought to be caused by an accumulation of transient microvascular ischemic events sustained over a long period. Owing to the size and distribution of the femoral and obturator nerves in relation to the others within the plexus, these two are most commonly affected, and so in consequence are the muscles within their distribution. These include atrophy and weakness of the anterior and medial muscle compartments of the thigh, with the patellar reflex frequently absent.[61]

13.5 Hematoma

The rich vascular supply around the lumbar plexus makes ischemia rather unlikely, but also makes the plexus particularly susceptible to compression due to hemorrhage. Hematomas in the area can have etiological beginnings in many places, such as retroperitoneal hemorrhage (to be discussed below, under iatrogenic pathologies[62]) and hematomas directly within the psoas and iliacus muscles, including those iatrogenically created through bleeds.[63,64,65] Ruptured aneurysms in and around the distribution of the internal iliac artery have also been reported to compress the lumbar plexus, leading to deficits.[61]

Hematomas of the psoas and iliacus muscles can cause lumbar plexopathy, especially in individuals on anticoagulation therapy who fall or sustain trauma. These patients are more susceptible to rupturing of retroperitoneal blood vessels, especially those in the body of the psoas muscle, forming an iliopsoas hematoma. Bleeding within the body of the muscle can compress the lumbar plexus, most commonly affecting the femoral and obturator nerves, and can lead to initial symptoms of moderate to severe pain with pain upon extension of the hip.[66,67] (The larger a hematoma becomes, the more likely it is to compress the femoral nerve *and* the rest of the plexus; smaller hematomas tend to be limited to femoral nerve compression.[64,66]) The preferred imaging modality for initial visualization of the hematoma is CT, while MRI is preferred for visualizing bony and nerve involvement.[19,20,21,22,23,24,46] Therapeutic options include observation, reversal of anticoagulation, needle aspiration or placement of an in-situ drain to assist with evacuation of the degraded blood products.

13.6 Trauma

Traumatic causes of lumbar plexus injuries are very rare because the plexus is well protected. The most common causes of traumatic injury to the lumbar plexus involve motor vehicle and motorcycle accidents.[68] Individuals with post-MVA/motorcycle-related lumbar plexus injuries are usually found to have varied degrees of functional deficit in both the femoral and obturator nerves, leading to weakness in the iliopsoas and quadriceps muscles. Additionally, pelvic fractures secondary to high speed trauma can cause lumbar or sacral plexopathy.[66] While often demanding surgical intervention, they are frequently treated with conservative therapy. Unfortunately, because high-speed traumatic injuries frequently involve many organs, lumbar or sacral plexopathy can go undetected unless an additional investigation is conducted such as EMG, nerve conduction study (NCS), or advanced imaging such as MRI neurography.

13.7 Iatrogenic

A frequent cause of iatrogenic retroperitoneal hemorrhage is a pre-operative lumbar plexus block in the setting of anticoagulation therapy.[61,69,70] Symptoms include an inability to move muscles innervated by the lumbar plexus, but the deficits are most easily noticed in the distribution of the femoral nerve and present as inability or weakness in knee extension and hip flexion, and potentially sensory loss in the anterior thigh.

Another common and novel mode of iatrogenic injury to the lumbar plexus is during lateral trans-psoas lumbar interbody fusion (LLIF). (▶ Fig. 13.10) This technique is considered a minimally invasive alternative to the traditional posterior (PLIF) or anterior lumbar interbody fusion surgery (ALIF). A recent study found that roughly 23.8% of those undergoing LLIF reported post-operative plexopathies while only 15.8% of ALIF patients, 7.8% of PLIF patients, and 2% of TLIF patients reported the same symptoms.[71] Additional studies have demonstrated the benefit of continuous intraoperative EMG to monitor the integrity of the nerves of the lumbar plexus during the lateral approach to

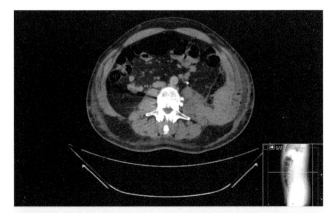

Fig. 13.10 A 69-year-old man presenting with left psoas and retroperitoneal hematoma following an L2/L3 lateral transpsoas lumbar interbody fusion procedure.

the lumbar spine.[72] Common symptoms following a lateral transpsoas procedure such as LLIF include anterior thigh numbness and hip flexion weakness, though the other branches of the lumbar plexus can also be injured during the approach. It is suggested that the etiology of injury is related to the retraction time of the psoas muscle as opposed to the placement of a tube through which LLIF is typically performed.[73]

A post-operative complication of abdominal surgeries known as an arterial pseudoaneurysm can expand to a size large enough to compress the lumbosacral plexus. Aortic dissection can also compress the plexus via a similar mechanism, leading to weakness or focal motor deficits of the muscles involved.[74]

13.8 Miscellaneous

Other causes of lumbar plexopathy are rare and are therefore infrequently reported in the literature. Endometriosis of the lumbar plexus has been reported sporadically, leading to neurological deficits associated with the nerve affected. Imaging modalities such as MRI have been useful in visualizing these lesions.[75,76] Patients with extramedullary hematopoiesis due to profound anemia (e.g., B-thalassemia major) have been reported to have compression of the plexus because of hematopoietic proliferation.[76,77] Lastly, piriformis syndrome can also cause compression of the sciatic nerve, the major branch of the lumbosacral plexus, leading to symptoms expected with nerve compression.[76,78]

13.9 Conclusion

The importance of the lumbar plexus in providing innervation to the cutaneous and motor supply to the lower limb cannot be overemphasized. Despite its close and "protective" proximity to the psoas muscle, it is vulnerable to several common pathologies with potentially devastating consequences for lower extremity neurological function.

Hopefully, a better understanding of the nature of these pathologies, as described above, will minimize iatrogenic injuries and improve the overall treatment of these important and potentially devastating lesions.

References

[1] Moore KL, Agur AMR, Dalley AF. Essential Clinical Anatomy. 4th ed. Baltimore, MD: Lippincott Williams and Wilkins; 2011

[2] Fine SW, McClain SA, Li M. Immunohistochemical staining for calretinin is useful for differentiating schwannomas from neurofibromas. Am J Clin Pathol. 2004; 122(4):552–559

[3] Hanemann CO, Evans DG. News on the genetics, epidemiology, medical care and translational research of Schwannomas. J Neurol. 2006; 253(12):1533–1541

[4] Jindal T, Mukherjee S, Kamal MR, et al. Cystic schwannoma of the pelvis. Ann R Coll Surg Engl. 2013; 95(1):e1–e2

[5] Liu DS, Brazenor G, Chu P, Danne P. Lumbar plexus schwannoma causing recurrent syncope. J Clin Neurosci. 2012; 19(11):1594–1596

[6] Dawley B. A retroperitoneal femoral nerve schwannoma as a cause of chronic pelvic pain. J Minim Invasive Gynecol. 2008; 15(4):491–493

[7] Kanta M, Petera J, Ehler E, et al. Malignant schwannoma of the obturator nerve. Bratisl Lek Listy (Tlacene Vyd). 2013; 114(10):584–586

[8] Mansukhani SA, Butala RR, Shetty SH, Khedekar RG. Sciatic nerve schwannoma: a case report. J Orthop Surg (Hong Kong). 2015; 23(2):259–261

[9] Muramatsu K, Ihara K, Yoshida Y, Taguchi T. Intramuscular schwannoma arising from the psoas major muscle. Clin Neurol Neurosurg. 2008; 110(5):532–533

[10] D'Silva KJ, Dwivedi AJ, Barnwell JM. Schwannoma of the psoas major muscle presenting with abdominal and back pain. Dig Dis Sci. 2003; 48(8):1619–1621

[11] Hsu YC, Shih YY, Gao HW, Huang GS. Intramuscular schwannoma arising from the psoas muscle presenting with femoral nerve neuropathy. South Med J. 2010; 103(5):477–479

[12] Merker VL, Esparza S, Smith MJ, Stemmer-Rachamimov A, Plotkin SR. Clinical features of schwannomatosis: a retrospective analysis of 87 patients. Oncologist. 2012; 17(10):1317–1322

[13] Sestini R, Bacci C, Provenzano A, Genuardi M, Papi L. Evidence of a four-hit mechanism involving SMARCB1 and NF2 in schwannomatosis-associated schwannomas. Hum Mutat. 2008; 29(2):227–231

[14] Rodriguez FJ, Folpe AL, Giannini C, Perry A. Pathology of peripheral nerve sheath tumors: diagnostic overview and update on selected diagnostic problems. Acta Neuropathol. 2012; 123(3):295–319

[15] Muir D, Neubauer D, Lim IT, Yachnis AT, Wallace MR. Tumorigenic properties of neurofibromin-deficient neurofibroma Schwann cells. Am J Pathol. 2001; 158(2):501–513

[16] Kalra N, Vijayanadh O, Lal A, Khandelwal N, Mukherjee KK, Suri S. Retroperitoneal plexiform neurofibroma mimicking psoas abscesses. Australas Radiol. 2005; 49(4):330–332

[17] Tavakkoli H, Asadi M, Mahzouni P, Foroozmehr A. Ulcerative colitis and neurofibromatosis type 1 with bilateral psoas muscle neurofibromas: a case report. J Res Med Sci. 2009; 14(4):261–265

[18] Shafir M, Holland JF, Cohen B, Aufses AH, Jr. Radical retroperitoneal tumor surgery with resection of the psoas major muscle. Cancer. 1985; 56(4):929–933

[19] Gruenwald I, Abrahamson J, Cohen O. Psoas abscess: case report and review of the literature. J Urol. 1992; 147(6):1624–1626

[20] Mallick IH, Thoufeeq MH, Rajendran TP. Iliopsoas abscesses. Postgrad Med J. 2004; 80(946):459–462

[21] Mückley T, Schütz T, Kirschner M, Potulski M, Hofmann G, Bühren V. Psoas abscess: the spine as a primary source of infection. Spine. 2003; 28(6):E106–E113

[22] Navarro López V, Ramos JM, Meseguer V, et al. GTI-SEMI Group. Microbiology and outcome of iliopsoas abscess in 124 patients. Medicine (Baltimore). 2009; 88(2):120–130

[23] Takada T, Terada K, Kajiwara H, Ohira Y. Limitations of using imaging diagnosis for psoas abscess in its early stage. Intern Med. 2015; 54(20):2589–2593

[24] Zissin R, Gayer G, Kots E, Werner M, Shapiro-Feinberg M, Hertz M. Iliopsoas abscess: a report of 24 patients diagnosed by CT. Abdom Imaging. 2001; 26(5):533–539

[25] Wechsler RJ, Nino-Murcia M. Computed tomography of ilio-psoas muscle tumors. Comput Radiol. 1984; 8(4):229–235

[26] Baehring JM, Betensky RA, Batchelor TT. Malignant peripheral nerve sheath tumor: the clinical spectrum and outcome of treatment. Neurology. 2003; 61(5):696–698

[27] Ducatman BS, Scheithauer BW, Piepgras DG, Reiman HM, Ilstrup DM. Malignant peripheral nerve sheath tumors. A clinicopathologic study of 120 cases. Cancer. 1986; 57(10):2006–2021

[28] Kim DH, Murovic JA, Tiel RL, Moes G, Kline DG. A series of 397 peripheral neural sheath tumors: 30-year experience at Louisiana State University Health Sciences Center. J Neurosurg. 2005; 102(2):246–255

[29] Perrin RG, Guha A. Malignant peripheral nerve sheath tumors. Neurosurg Clin N Am. 2004; 15(2):203–216

[30] Patel TD, Shaigany K, Fang CH, Park RC, Baredes S, Eloy JA. Comparative analysis of head and neck and non-head and neck malignant peripheral nerve sheath tumors. Otolaryngol Head Neck Surg. 2016; 154(1):113–120

[31] Stucky CC, Johnson KN, Gray RJ, et al. Malignant peripheral nerve sheath tumors (MPNST): the Mayo Clinic experience. Ann Surg Oncol. 2012; 19(3):878–885

[32] Bhattacharyya AK, Perrin R, Guha A. Peripheral nerve tumors: management strategies and molecular insights. J Neurooncol. 2004; 69(1–3):335–349

[33] Brahmi M, Thiesse P, Ranchere D, et al. Diagnostic accuracy of PET/CT-guided percutaneous biopsies for malignant peripheral nerve sheath tumors in neurofibromatosis type 1 patients. PLoS One. 2015; 10(10):e0138386

[34] Porter DE, Prasad V, Foster L, Dall GF, Birch R, Grimer RJ. Survival in malignant peripheral nerve sheath tumours: a comparison between sporadic and neurofibromatosis type 1-associated tumours. Sarcoma. 2009; 2009:756395

[35] Roncaroli F, Poppi M, Riccioni L, Frank F. Primary non-Hodgkin's lymphoma of the sciatic nerve followed by localization in the central nervous system: case report and review of the literature. Neurosurgery. 1997; 40(3):618–621, discussion 621–622

[36] Muttarak M, Peh WC. CT of unusual iliopsoas compartment lesions. Radiographics. 2000; 20(Spec No):S53–S66

[37] Benyahya E, Etaouil N, Janani S, et al. Sciatica as the first manifestation of a leiomyosarcoma of the buttock. Rev Rhum Engl Ed. 1997; 64(2):135–137

[38] Taylor BV, Kimmel DW, Krecke KN, Cascino TL. Magnetic resonance imaging in cancer-related lumbosacral plexopathy. Mayo Clin Proc. 1997; 72(9):823–829

[39] Jaeckle KA. Nerve plexus metastases. Neurol Clin. 1991; 9(4):857–866

[40] Even-Sapir E, Parag Y, Lerman H, et al. Detection of recurrence in patients with rectal cancer: PET/CT after abdominoperineal or anterior resection. Radiology. 2004; 232(3):815–822

[41] Maker VK, Guzman-Arrieta ED. Retroperitoneum and Great Vessels of the Abdomen in Cognitive Pearls in General Surgery. New York, NY: Spring Sciences; 2014:473

[42] Franco-Paredes C, Blumberg HM. Psoas muscle abscess caused by Mycobacterium tuberculosis and Staphylococcus aureus: case report and review. Am J Med Sci. 2001; 321(6):415–417

[43] Lin MF, Lau YJ, Hu BS, Shi ZY, Lin YH. Pyogenic psoas abscess: analysis of 27 cases. J Microbiol Immunol Infect. 1999; 32(4):261–268

[44] Chern CH, Hu SC, Kao WF, Tsai J, Yen D, Lee CH. Psoas abscess: making an early diagnosis in the ED. Am J Emerg Med. 1997; 15(1):83–88

[45] Tomich EB, Della-Giustina D. Bilateral psoas abscess in the emergency department. West J Emerg Med. 2009; 10(4):288–291

[46] Lee JK, Glazer HS. Psoas muscle disorders: MR imaging. Radiology. 1986; 160(3):683–687

[47] Lee YT, Lee CM, Su SC, Liu CP, Wang TE. Psoas abscess: a 10 year review. J Microbiol Immunol Infect. 1999; 32(1):40–46

[48] Berbari EF, Kanj SS, Kowalski TJ, et al. Infectious Diseases Society of America. 2015 Infectious Diseases Society of America (IDSA) Clinical Practice Guidelines for the diagnosis and treatment of native vertebral osteomyelitis in adults. Clin Infect Dis. 2015; 61(6):e26–e46

[49] McHenry MC, Easley KA, Locker GA. Vertebral osteomyelitis: long-term outcome for 253 patients from 7 Cleveland-area hospitals. Clin Infect Dis. 2002; 34(10):1342–1350

[50] Park KH, Cho OH, Jung M, et al. Clinical characteristics and outcomes of hematogenous vertebral osteomyelitis caused by gram-negative bacteria. J Infect. 2014; 69(1):42–50

[51] Lew DP, Waldvogel FA. Osteomyelitis. Lancet. 2004; 364(9431):369–379

[52] Nolla JM, Ariza J, Gómez-Vaquero C, et al. Spontaneous pyogenic vertebral osteomyelitis in nondrug users. Semin Arthritis Rheum. 2002; 31(4):271–278

[53] Golden MP, Vikram HR. Extrapulmonary tuberculosis: an overview. Am Fam Physician. 2005; 72(9):1761–1768

[54] Stoeckli TC, Mackin GA, De Groote MA. Lumbosacral plexopathy in a patient with pulmonary tuberculosis. Clin Infect Dis. 2000; 30(1):226–227

[55] Chang CM, Ko WC, Lee HC, Chen YM, Chuang YC. Klebsiella pneumoniae psoas abscess: predominance in diabetic patients and grave prognosis in gas-forming cases. J Microbiol Immunol Infect. 2001; 34(3):201–206

[56] Dubois D, Robin F, Bouvier D, et al. Streptobacillus moniliformis as the causative agent in spondylodiscitis and psoas abscess after rooster scratches. J Clin Microbiol. 2008; 46(8):2820–2821

[57] Giladi M, Sada MJ, Spotkov J, Bayer AS. Pneumococcal psoas abscess: report of a case and review of the world literature. Isr J Med Sci. 1996; 32(9):771–774

[58] Palavutitotai N, Chongtrakoo P, Ngamskulrungroj P, Chayakulkeeree M. Nocardia beijingensis psoas abscess and subcutaneous phaeohyphomycosis caused by phaeoacremonium parasiticum in a renal transplant recipient: the first case report in Thailand. Southeast Asian J Trop Med Public Health. 2015; 46(6):1049–1054

[59] Aoyama M, Nemoto D, Matsumura T, Hitomi S. A fatal case of iliopsoas abscess caused by Salmonella enterica serovar Choleraesuis that heterogeneously formed mucoid colonies. J Infect Chemother. 2015; 21(5):395–397

[60] Heyd J, Meallem R, Schlesinger Y, et al. Clinical characteristics of patients with psoas abscess due to non-typhi Salmonella. Eur J Clin Microbiol Infect Dis. 2003; 22(12):770–773

[61] Preston DC, Shapiro BE. Electromyography and Neuromuscular Disorders: Clinical-Electrophysiologic Correlations. 3rd ed. London: Elsevier Saunders; 2013

[62] Emery S, Ochoa J. Lumbar plexus neuropathy resulting from retroperitoneal hemorrhage. Muscle Nerve. 1978; 1(4):330–334

[63] Aveline C, Bonnet F. Delayed retroperitoneal haematoma after failed lumbar plexus block. Br J Anaesth. 2004; 93(4):589–591

[64] Conesa X, Ares O, Seijas R. Massive psoas haematoma causing lumbar plexus palsy: a case report. J Orthop Surg (Hong Kong). 2012; 20(1):94–97

[65] Ginanneschi U, Capus L, Smrekar V, Dell'Antonio A, Fabiani P, Visintin A. [Partial paralysis of the right lumbar plexus caused by a traumatic hematoma of the ileo-psoas muscle]. Chir Ital. 1985; 37(2):165–173

[66] Aminoff MJ, Daroff RB. Encyclopedia of the Neurological Sciences. 1st ed. Amsterdam: Academic Press; 2003

[67] Ozçakar L, Sivri A, Aydinli M, Tavil Y. Lumbosacral plexopathy as the harbinger of a silent retroperitoneal hematoma. South Med J. 2003; 96(1):109–110

[68] Garozzo D, Zollino G, Ferraresi S. In lumbosacral plexus injuries can we identify indicators that predict spontaneous recovery or the need for surgical treatment? Results from a clinical study on 72 patients. J Brachial Plex Periph Nerve Inj. 2014; 9(1):1

[69] Kaymak B, Ozçakar L, Cetin A, Erol O, Akoğlu H. Bilateral lumbosacral plexopathy after femoral vein dialysis: synopsis of a case. Joint Bone Spine. 2004; 71 (4):347–348

[70] Klein SM, D'Ercole F, Greengrass RA, Warner DS. Enoxaparin associated with psoas hematoma and lumbar plexopathy after lumbar plexus block. Anesthesiology. 1997; 87(6):1576–1579

[71] Epstein NE. More nerve root injuries occur with minimally invasive lumbar surgery, especially extreme lateral interbody fusion: A review. Surg Neurol Int. 2016; 7 Suppl 3:S83–S95

[72] Bendersky M, Solá C, Muntadas J, et al. Monitoring lumbar plexus integrity in extreme lateral transpsoas approaches to the lumbar spine: a new protocol with anatomical bases. Eur Spine J. 2015; 24(5):1051–1057

[73] Uribe JS, Isaacs RE, Youssef JA, et al. SOLAS Degenerative Study Group. Can triggered electromyography monitoring throughout retraction predict postoperative symptomatic neuropraxia after XLIF? Results from a prospective multicenter trial. Eur Spine J. 2015; 24 Suppl 3:378–385

[74] Lefebvre V, Leduc JJ, Choteau PH. Painless ischaemic lumbosacral plexopathy and aortic dissection. J Neurol Neurosurg Psychiatry. 1995; 58(5):641

[75] Binkovitz LA, King BF, Ehman RL. Sciatic endometriosis: MR appearance. J Comput Assist Tomogr. 1991; 15(3):508–510

[76] Planner AC, Donaghy M, Moore NR. Causes of lumbosacral plexopathy. Clin Radiol. 2006; 61(12):987–995

[77] Carazo ER, Herrera RO, de Fuentes TM, Rull JP, Muñoz CM. Presacral extramedullary haematopoiesis with involvement of the sciatic nerve. Eur Radiol. 1999; 9(7):1404–1406

[78] Ozaki S, Hamabe T, Muro T. Piriformis syndrome resulting from an anomalous relationship between the sciatic nerve and piriformis muscle. Orthopedics. 1999; 22(8):771–772

14 Injury to the Lumbar Plexus Following Lateral Lumbar Spine Fusion Procedures

Peter Grunert, Joy M. H. Wang, R. Shane Tubbs

Abstract

Neurological deficits from lumbar plexus nerve injuries commonly occur in patients undergoing lateral approaches. However, it is not yet clear which structures are typically injured at each anatomical cross-section and by what mechanism they are injured. Knowledge of the complex plexus anatomy, specifically its mediolateral course, is critical in order to avoid approach-related injuries.

Keywords: transpsoas approach, spine surgery, iatrogenic injury, anatomy, nerves, lateral spine surgery

14.1 Introduction

The lateral transpsoas approach to the lumbar spine is increasingly being used to treat degenerative changes requiring fusion.[1] In contrast to conventional posterior spinal fusion techniques, this minimally invasive approach spares extensive posterior tissue dissection and resection for cage implantation and decreases operative time, blood loss, postoperative pain, and tissue trauma.[1] Although minimally invasive, this procedure has the approach-related risk to cause lumbar plexus nerve injuries secondary to the insertion and dilation of dilatators or retractors (▶ Fig. 14.1, ▶ Fig. 14.2, ▶ Fig. 14.3, ▶ Fig. 14.4). Plexus injuries are reported from 6 to 33%, often presenting as neuropathic pain and motor or sensory deficits.[1,2,3]

Several cadaveric anatomical studies on plexus nerve anatomy for lateral approaches have been published[4,5]; however, few have systematically documented the types of injury typically observed at each spinal level after such procedures. In the cadaveric study of Grunert et al, approximately 50% of all operated-upon segments had plexus nerve injuries occurring at segments L1–L4 and involving nerve roots as well as motor and sensory nerves.[6] In a similar cadaveric study, Banagan et al found direct nerve injuries from lateral approaches in 25% of operated segments.[7] The higher percentage in the former study could be explained as follows.

First, Banagan et al openly dissected the surface of the psoas major muscle. Then, under direct visualization, they inserted dilator tubes through the anterior third of the muscle in order to achieve an "ideal position."[7] Alternatively, Grunert et al used a standard operative technique, inserting tubes without direct visualization.[6] Second, the Banagan et al study only assessed segments L3–L5, whereas Grunert et al studied L1–L5.[6,7] In Grunert et al's study, most of the lumbar plexus nerve injuries observed were in the upper lumbar levels (L1–L3).[6] Thus, solely investigating levels L3–L5 could significantly underestimate the injury potential of these procedures.

Other groups have conducted cadaveric anatomy studies without performing transtubular procedures in order to locate safe zones or docking points. Benglis et al described a ventral migration of the lumbosacral plexus on the lumbar disc spaces from L2 to L5, indicating that the tubular docking point should be placed more anteriorly at more caudal levels.[5] Similar results were described by Moro et al and Uribe et al, who subdivided each vertebral segment into four quarters (zone I to zone IV) from the anterior to the posterior border of the vertebral body.[4,8] Although describing the relationship of the plexus nerves to the lateral vertebral body surface helps in determining ideal docking points, it oversimplifies the complex plexus anatomy, as the nerves run in both anteroposterior and mediolateral directions. As shown in the study by Grunert et al, injuries can occur throughout the entire trajectory of the lateral approach. Over 50% of the nerve injuries occurred either at the lateral aspect of the psoas major muscle, in the retroperitoneal space, within the outer abdominal muscles, or in the subcutaneous tissue of the abdominal wall, predominantly affecting the subcostal, ilioinguinal, iliohypogastric, and lateral femoral cutaneous nerves.[6] Dakwar et al described the anatomical course of the plexus nerves lateral to the psoas major muscle in great detail.[9] However, the surgically relevant question—for each lumbar level, at what anatomical location can these nerves be encountered and injured—has not been addressed.

To clarify where those nerves can be encountered, Grunert et al subdivided their approach into four mediolateral anatomical zones superficial to deep and medial to lateral: zone I, the psoas major muscle; zone II, the retroperitoneal fat tissue; zone III, the outer abdominal muscles; zone IV, the subcutaneous tissue of the outer abdominal wall.[6] Based on their findings, the following section outlines the course of the plexus nerves within these anatomical zones, identifies locations at which nerve injuries typically occurred, and suggests how to avoid these injuries in clinical practice.

14.2 L1/L2

14.2.1 Subcostal Nerve

The subcostal nerve emerges from the T12 nerve root and runs along the inferior border of the 12th rib before it pierces through the outer abdominal muscles. At L1/L2, it is only encountered within the outer abdominal muscles (zone III) and the subcutaneous tissue (zone IV). This nerve was injured in zone III and zone IV.[6]

Surgical Considerations

Careful blunt dissection through the subcutaneous and muscle tissues, without excessive monopolar coagulation, could avoid such injuries. The fasciae of the abdominal muscles should be opened bluntly in the direction of their muscle fibers.

14.2.2 Ilioinguinal and Iliohypogastric Nerves

Emerging from the T12/L1 nerve root, the iliohypogastric and ilioinguinal nerves run posterior to or within the psoas major

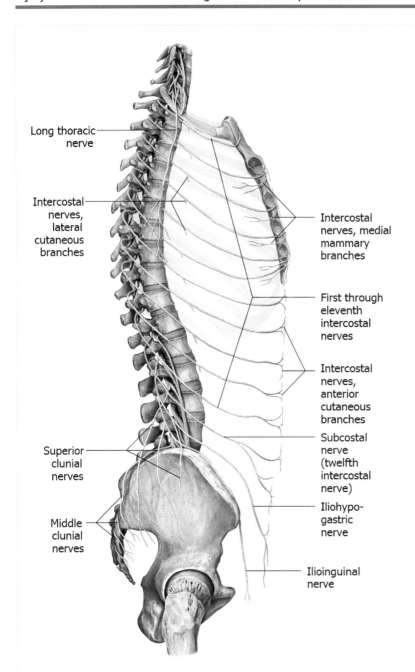

Long thoracic nerve

Intercostal nerves, lateral cutaneous branches

Superior clunial nerves

Middle clunial nerves

Intercostal nerves, medial mammary branches

First through eleventh intercostal nerves

Intercostal nerves, anterior cutaneous branches

Subcostal nerve (twelfth intercostal nerve)

Iliohypo-gastric nerve

Ilioinguinal nerve

Fig. 14.1 Schematic drawing of the right-sided segmental nerves and their course from a lateral position. The subcostal, iliohypogastric, and ilioinguinal nerves are seen in their superficial course around the anterolateral abdominal wall. (Reproduced with permission from Schuenke M, Schulte E, Schumacher U, Ross LM, Zeberg H, Atlas of Anatomy. New York, NY: Thieme Medical Publishers; 2015. Illustration by Karl Wesker)

muscle (zone I). Leaving the psoas major, both nerves continue their oblique descent on the anterior surface of the quadratus lumborum, along the posterior abdominal wall (zone II). As it reaches the outer abdominal muscles (zone III), small branches pierce the surrounding abdominal muscles until they reach the subcutaneous tissue (zone IV). At L1/L2 level, these nerves can potentially be injured in all anatomical zones.[6]

Surgical Consideration

Careful blunt dissection should be performed as described for the subcostal nerve. The retroperitoneal space is typically not dissected under direct visualization, making both nerves difficult to encounter. However, injuries at this anatomical zone

were typically found on the anterior surface of the quadratus lumborum muscle, which builds the lateral wall of the retroperitoneal space.[6] The muscle can be located by finger palpation prior to tube insertion—this could help preclude retractor placement in tight spaces.

Surgeons tend to choose a more posterior docking point or over-retract at L1/L2 as it is considered a "safe level," since there are no lower extremity motor fibers in this area and is, therefore, usually "silent" on electromyogram (EMG) monitoring. This practice should be avoided as both L1 and L2 nerve roots carry motor fibers for the outer abdominal muscles,[10] and denervation with potential anterolateral abdominal wall hernia[11] can result from injuries to these nerves. The authors therefore recommend "safe zone" retractor placement as

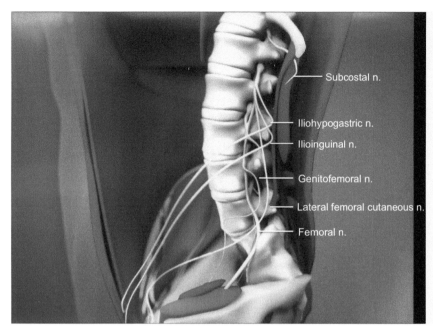

Fig. 14.2 Schematic drawing of the left-sided lumbar plexus from a lateral perspective.

Subcostal n.

Iliohypogastric n.

Ilioinguinal n.

Genitofemoral n.

Lateral femoral cutaneous n.

Femoral n.

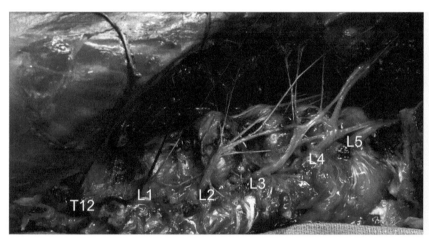

Fig. 14.3 Right-sided, lateral approach to the lumbar spine. The psoas major has been retracted anteriorly to illustrate the many branches of the lumbar plexus. Labeled are the ventral rami of T12–L5. Note how the branches of the lumbar plexus are draped over the lateral vertebral bodies of the lumbar spine.

T12   L1   L2   L3   L4   L5

described by Uribe et al[4]: limited retraction and avoidance of quadratus lumborum muscle compression while the retractor is being placed and dilated.[6]

14.2.3 Genitofemoral Nerve

The genitofemoral nerve originates from the L1 and L2 nerve roots; traveling obliquely in a cephalocaudal direction, it pierces through the psoas major muscle from posterior to anterior before continuing its descent on the anterior surface of the muscle. From previous cadaveric studies, it is generally accepted that the nerve typically pierces the psoas major muscle at the level between L3 and L4[4,8,9]; however, Grunert et al found anatomical variations where the nerve pierces the muscle more superiorly at L1/L2, and injuries were found to occur at this site.[6]

Surgical Consideration

With conventional transtubular techniques, the surface of the psoas major muscle is usually not visible. Tender and Serban and

Acosta et al described a "shallow docking" technique that allows the nerve to be visualized by docking on the surface of the muscle prior to dilating it. The genitofemoral nerve can then be placed out of the visual field behind the retractor blades.[12,13]

14.3 L2/L3

14.3.1 Lateral Femoral Cutaneous Nerve

The lateral femoral cutaneous nerve originates from the L2/L3 nerve roots. It runs caudally within the psoas muscle, emerging laterally from the muscle around L4 to enter the retroperitoneum and continue its oblique descent toward the anterior superior iliac spine, lying anterior to the surface of the iliacus muscle.[9] Corresponding to its anatomical course, injury to the nerve at this level occurred within the psoas major muscle.[6]

Surgical Consideration

When conventional transtubular techniques are used, not all intramuscular nerves are visible during retractor placement.

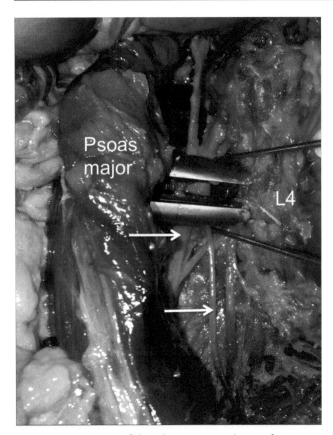

Fig. 14.4 Anterior view of the right retroperitoneal space after a transpsoas, lateral approach to the L4 vertebra. The psoas major has been retracted laterally to illustrate the docking location placed under fluoroscopy. The juxtaposition of the lumbar plexus is obvious and seen posterior to the instrument. The femoral (*upper arrow*) and obturator (*lower arrow*) nerves are seen extending from L2–L4.

Grunert et al recommend limiting cauterization and avoiding extensive muscle resection over the intervertebral disc.

14.3.2 L2 Nerve Root

After exiting the neural foramen and before entering the psoas major muscle, all lumbar nerve roots run within the retroperitoneal space. This space is typically more posterior than the disc space, so the nerve is less likely to be encountered in that anatomical zone. Injury to this nerve was observed within the psoas muscle, shortly before the nerve root split into plexus nerves.[6]

Surgical Consideration

As with L1/L2, the L2/L3 level is considered relatively safe and is silent on EMG monitoring. However, for the same reasons described for the L1/L2 level, safe zone docking and limited retraction (especially posteriorly) are also suggested.

The obturator nerve originates from the L2–L4 ventral rami and is located in the posterior aspect of the intervertebral disc.[4] There were no injuries observed to this nerve.[6]

14.4 L3/L4

14.4.1 Lateral Femoral Cutaneous Nerve

In contrast to the intramuscular injury (zone I) at L2/L3, the injury at L3/L4 was observed in the retroperitoneal space (zone II), on the anterior surface of the psoas major muscle.[6] This confirms the anatomical course described by Dakwar et al.[9]

Surgical Consideration

The aforementioned technique of "shallow docking" could also be applied for the lateral femoral cutaneous nerve.

14.4.2 Femoral Nerve

The femoral nerve is formed from the L2–L4 spinal nerves. At L3/L4, it runs in the posterior aspect of the intervertebral disc/vertebral bodies and tends to migrate anteriorly at L4/L5, close to the midline of the intervertebral disc.[14] From L3 to L5, the nerve can only be encountered within the psoas major muscle, where its injuries were also found.[6]

Surgical Consideration

Despite "safe zone" retractor placement, femoral nerve injuries still occurred. This could be explained either by anatomical variations of the nerve running more anterior, close to midline at that level, or by extensive posterior retraction. Grunert et al recommend, in addition to intraoperative monitoring, careful inspection of the visual field after retractor placement on top of the disc space.[6] Interestingly, despite the obturator nerve's proximity to the femoral nerve at this level, no injuries to this nerve were found.[6] This could be because it lies medial to the femoral nerve.[4]

14.5 L4/L5

No nerve injuries were found at this level; however, as stated in Grunert et al's study, this result could be due to the study's sample size.

14.5.1 Cutaneous Nerve Injuries

Clinical outcome studies have demonstrated that sensory nerve deficits or alterations are common status post lateral approaches.[2,10] However, it has been difficult to assess which sensory nerves are affected since many sensory fields, specific to the iliohypogastric, ilioinguinal, genitofemoral, and subcostal nerves, overlap and are therefore difficult to distinguish clinically.[10] In light of this limitation, Ahmadian et al summarized the sensory fields of these nerves into sensory cutaneous zones in the upper ventral and lateral thigh.[10] Grunert et al suggest that, at least in a cadaver spine model, all the aforementioned nerves are prone to injury during these procedures, with most injuries occurring at the level of L1/L2.[6]

14.5.2 Monitoring

Intraoperative EMG-based neuromonitoring allows for geographic "mapping" of the lumbar plexus, which improves the safety of lateral approaches.[15,16] Current monitoring techniques use insulated tubes with an isolated stimulation source at the tip.[15] This allows for focused stimulation within the psoas major muscle. Given the course of the obturator and femoral nerves and the largest portion of the nerve roots, these monitoring techniques can detect those nerves intraoperatively. The disadvantage of focused stimulation is that motor fibers lateral to the psoas muscle (zones II–IV) are not detected. Although not routinely monitored, motor fibers of the ilioinguinal and iliohypogastric nerves could only be stimulated within their relatively short course in the psoas muscle at the L1/L2 level, and not in their retroperitoneal course, where injuries were observed.

14.5.3 Type and Mechanism of Nerve Injuries

The incidence of sensory or motor deficits after lateral fusion procedures is reported in the literature as between 6 and 33.6%.[2] Despite extensive studies, the types and mechanisms of nerve injury occurring after lateral approaches remain unknown. Most types of injury proposed in the literature are injuries without structural changes to the nerve, such as nerve compression, traction, transient irritation,[2] or ischemic injuries.[10] These types of injury can be classified as Sunderland I: impaired nerve conduction without detectable histological change.[17,18] However, studies have suggested that structural nerve injuries can occur. In Grunert et al's study, both partial and complete transections were observed.[6] Partial transections can be rated as Sunderland grades IV–V; complete transections are all rated as Sunderland V.[17,18] The Sunderland grade positively correlates with the time of nerve function recovery. Over 90% of neurological deficits after lateral fusion resolve.[2,3,19] However, the time required for significant improvement ranges from 6 weeks to 24 months.[2,3] Given the differing lengths of recovery time exhibited, it is plausible that various Sunderland grades can result from these approaches. Permanent deficits are likely to be related to complete or partial transection injuries, as they seldom recover without surgical repair.[17] In this regard, surgical repair of long-term motor deficits after lateral approaches could be suggested.

Intraoperative crush injuries typically result from acute traumatic compression by a blunt object (such as retractor blades or cages) causing partial or complete nerve transections.[17] This description of injuries matches those observed by Grunert et al.[6] Additionally, Banagan et al described laceration from Kirschner wire placement as a mechanism of injury.[7] In their cadaver study, Kirschner wires were placed in the disc space without the protection of dilator tubes. Given that standards of practice differ within each institute, these factors should be kept in mind when evaluating potential mechanisms of injury. Lastly, some of the weakness the psoas major after lateral lumbar approaches might be attributed to direct injury to the muscle from retraction versus nerve injury.

14.6 Conclusion

Lumbar plexus nerve injuries can occur throughout the mediolateral approach to the lumbar spine. Nerve injuries lateral to the psoas major muscle were observed predominantly at L1/L2 and L2/L3. Structural nerve injuries (Sunderland IV–V) can also occur from lateral approaches. These can be classified as intraoperative crush injuries from blunt objects. Awareness of mediolateral anatomical zones and the topographic anatomy of the lumbar plexus nerves within these zones can help reduce the risk of injuries in patients undergoing lateral approaches to the lumbar spine.

References

[1] Arnold PM, Anderson KK, McGuire RA, Jr. The lateral transpsoas approach to the lumbar and thoracic spine: A review. Surg Neurol Int. 2012; 3 Suppl 3: S198–S215

[2] Pumberger M, Hughes AP, Huang RR, Sama AA, Cammisa FP, Girardi FP. Neurologic deficit following lateral lumbar interbody fusion. Eur Spine J. 2012; 21 (6):1192–1199

[3] Rodgers WB, Gerber EJ, Patterson J. Intraoperative and early postoperative complications in extreme lateral interbody fusion: an analysis of 600 cases. Spine. 2011; 36(1):26–32

[4] Uribe JS, Arredondo N, Dakwar E, Vale FL. Defining the safe working zones using the minimally invasive lateral retroperitoneal transpsoas approach: an anatomical study. J Neurosurg Spine. 2010; 13(2):260–266

[5] Benglis DM, Vanni S, Levi AD. An anatomical study of the lumbosacral plexus as related to the minimally invasive transpsoas approach to the lumbar spine. J Neurosurg Spine. 2009; 10(2):139–144

[6] Grunert P, Drazin D, Iwanaga J, et al. Injury to the lumbar plexus and its branches following lateral fusion procedures: a cadaver study. World Neurosurg. 2017; 105:519–525

[7] Banagan K, Gelb D, Poelstra K, Ludwig S. Anatomic mapping of lumbar nerve roots during a direct lateral transpsoas approach to the spine: a cadaveric study. Spine. 2011; 36(11):E687–E691

[8] Moro T, Kikuchi S, Konno S, Yaginuma H. An anatomic study of the lumbar plexus with respect to retroperitoneal endoscopic surgery. Spine. 2003; 28 (5):423–428, discussion 427–428

[9] Dakwar E, Vale FL, Uribe JS. Trajectory of the main sensory and motor branches of the lumbar plexus outside the psoas muscle related to the lateral retroperitoneal transpsoas approach. J Neurosurg Spine. 2011; 14(2):290–295

[10] Ahmadian A, Deukmedjian AR, Abel N, Dakwar E, Uribe JS. Analysis of lumbar plexopathies and nerve injury after lateral retroperitoneal transpsoas approach: diagnostic standardization. J Neurosurg Spine. 2013; 18(3):289–297

[11] Cahill KS, Martinez JL, Wang MY, Vanni S, Levi AD. Motor nerve injuries following the minimally invasive lateral transpsoas approach. J Neurosurg Spine. 2012; 17(3):227–231

[12] Acosta FL, Jr, Drazin D, Liu JC. Supra-psoas shallow docking in lateral interbody fusion. Neurosurgery. 2013; 73(1) Suppl Operative:ons48–ons51, discussion ons52

[13] Tender GC, Serban D. Genitofemoral nerve protection during the lateral retroperitoneal transpsoas approach. Neurosurgery. 2013; 73(2) Suppl Operative:ons192–ons196, discussion ons196–ons197

[14] Davis TT, Bae HW, Mok JM, Rasouli A, Delamarter RB. Lumbar plexus anatomy within the psoas muscle: implications for the transpsoas lateral approach to the L4-L5 disc. J Bone Joint Surg Am. 2011; 93(16):1482–1487

[15] Uribe JS, Vale FL, Dakwar E. Electromyographic monitoring and its anatomical implications in minimally invasive spine surgery. Spine. 2010; 35(26) Suppl: S368–S374

[16] Ozgur BM, Aryan HE, Pimenta L, Taylor WR. Extreme Lateral Interbody Fusion (XLIF): a novel surgical technique for anterior lumbar interbody fusion. Spine J. 2006; 6(4):435–443

[17] Sunderland S. The anatomy and physiology of nerve injury. Muscle Nerve. 1990; 13(9):771–784

[18] Menorca RM, Fussell TS, Elfar JC. Nerve physiology: mechanisms of injury and recovery. Hand Clin. 2013; 29(3):317–330

[19] Lykissas MG, Aichmair A, Hughes AP, et al. Nerve injury after lateral lumbar interbody fusion: a review of 919 treated levels with identification of risk factors. Spine J. 2014; 14(5):749–758

15 Lumbar Plexus Anatomy with Application to Lateral Approaches to the Lumbar Spine

Chidinma Nwaogbe, R. Shane Tubbs

Abstract

Injuries to the lumbar plexus during lateral approaches to the spine are not uncommon and may result in permanent deficits. This chapter reviews the lateral approach and the anatomy of the lumbar plexus in relation to surgery of the transpsoas approach to the lumbar spine.

Keywords: anatomy, spine, vertebral column, lumbar, complications, nerve injury

15.1 Introduction

The minimally invasive lateral retroperitoneal transpsoas approach for fusion of the lumbar spine has become a popular surgical technique. However, potential complications include injury to the bowel, vasculature, and, most commonly, the lumbar plexus.[1,2,3,4] The incidence of motor deficits following lateral transpsoas spine surgery has been reported to range between 0.7 and 33.6%, while sensory deficits following such approaches can be as high as 75%.[1]

The lumbar plexus is a network of nerve fibers located on the posterior abdominal wall, much of it lying within the substance of the psoas major muscle. The plexus is formed by the ventral rami of the first through the fourth lumbar spinal nerves. It also receives minor contributions from the 12th thoracic spinal nerve (i.e., the subcostal nerve). It produces branches that innervate structures of the lower abdomen, genitalia, and parts of the lower limb. A brief review of the salient anatomy of each branch of the lumbar plexus follows.

15.2 Anatomy

The subcostal nerve is the ventral ramus of the 12th thoracic spinal nerve. Laterally, it pierces the transversus abdominis and travels between it and the internal oblique muscle. It terminates above the terminal midline fibers of the iliohypogastric nerve and sends a lateral cutaneous branch over the iliac crest. The iliohypogastric nerve usually originates from the ventral ramus of the L1 spinal nerve. It emerges from the upper lateral border of the psoas major and crosses obliquely in front of the quadratus lumborum. It is distributed to the posterolateral gluteal skin. The anterior cutaneous branch runs between the internal oblique and transversus abdominis and innervates both muscles. It passes through the internal oblique muscle approximately 3 cm above the superficial inguinal ring and is then distributed to the suprapubic skin. The ilioinguinal nerve arises from the first lumbar ventral ramus. It emerges from the lateral border of the psoas major, along with or just inferior to the iliohypogastric nerve, passes obliquely across the quadratus lumborum and the upper part of the iliacus, and enters the transversus abdominis near the anterior end of the iliac crest. It pierces and innervates the internal oblique muscle inferior to the iliohypogastric before traversing the inguinal canal to innervate the skin of the anterior scrotum or labia majora. The lateral femoral cutaneous nerve usually arises from the posterior divisions of L2 and L3. It emerges from the lateral border of the psoas major and crosses the iliacus obliquely toward the anterior superior iliac spine (ASIS) to supply the skin of the lateral thigh. The genitofemoral nerve is formed within the substance of the psoas major, originating from the L1 and L2 ventral rami. The genital branch crosses the lower part of the external iliac artery, entering the inguinal canal through its deep ring. It supplies the cremaster and the skin of the scrotum in males. In females, it accompanies the round ligament and ends in the skin of the mons pubis and labium majus. The femoral branch provides sensory innervation to the medial upper thigh and the skin over the femoral vessels. The femoral nerve is a motor and sensory nerve derived from the posterior divisions of the ventral rami of the L2–L4 spinal nerves. Distally, in the pelvis, it is located lateral to the psoas major muscle, in the cleavage between this muscle and the iliacus. It travels deep to the inguinal ligament and lies lateral to the femoral artery. It innervates the quadriceps femoris, pectineus, sartorius, and the skin over the anterior thigh and medial leg down to the medial foot. The obturator nerve arises from the anterior divisions of the second to fourth lumbar ventral rami. It descends through the psoas major and emerges from its medial border at the pelvic brim running down between this muscle and the lumbar vertebral column to exit via the obturator foramen into the thigh.

15.2.1 Anatomical Landmarks

Anatomical landmarks are very useful surgically and can be critical for success with minimally invasive procedures.[5,6,7,8,9] Interestingly, there are few reports in the medical literature describing surgical landmarks with which to identify the branches of the lumbar plexus on the posterior abdominal wall. In an earlier cadaveric study and in regard to open retroperitoneal procedures, we[7] measured the distances between the branches of the lumbar plexus and various regional bone landmarks. The mean distances from the midline to the subcostal, iliohypogastric, ilioinguinal, lateral femoral cutaneous, genitofemoral, and femoral nerves as they emerged through or lateral to the psoas major muscle were 5.5, 6.0, 6.5, 6.0, 4.5, and 4.5 cm, respectively. The obturator nerve had a mean distance of 3.0 cm lateral to the midline and the lateral femoral cutaneous had a mean distance of 1.5 cm inferomedial to the ASIS. Although these landmarks can assist the surgeon during larger, more invasive openings, they have less application to minimally invasive procedures, especially those that approach the lumbar spine via a lateral trajectory. Moreover, this earlier study measured distances to the main trunk of the nerves and did not take the entire intra-abdominal courses of the nerve branches into account.

15.2.2 Nerves at Risk

In an magnetic resonance imaging (MRI) study, Kepler et al[10] found that the percentages of patients with neurovascular structures that were at risk during lateral transpsoas interbody fusion procedures differed between left and right sides and level. They found that for left sides the percentages were 2.3% at L1–L2, 7.0% at L2–L3, 4.7% at L3–L4, and 20.9% at L4–L5. For right sides, the percentages were 7.0% at L1–L2, 7.0% at L2–L3, 9.3% at L3–L4, and 44.2% at L4–L5.

Regev et al[11] found that the L4–L5 level was at greatest risk for injury. Lu et al,[12] using a virtual human dataset, concluded that the anterior two-thirds of the psoas major can be exposed without harming the lumbar plexus. However, some branches (e.g., the genitofemoral nerve) usually traverse the psoas major muscle, so these landmarks would not be useful for all branches of the plexus. For endoscopic approaches to the lumbar spine and in regard to minimizing injury to the lumbar plexus, Moro et al[6] found a relative safety zone from L2–L3 and above. In another cadaveric study, Benglis et al[5] found that the lumbosacral plexus moves from a posterior to an anterior location descending from the L1 to L5 intervertebral disc spaces.

Rodgers et al[13] performed a prospective analysis of 600 patients treated with a lateral approach for fusion of degenerative spinal conditions. The overall incidence of perioperative complications was 6.2%, with four patients (0.7%) found to have transient postoperative neurological deficits. Even when electromyogram (EMG) is used during lateral approaches to the lumbar spine, false-positive or false-negative responses can occur.[1] Therefore, fluoroscopic identification of bony landmarks to localize the branches of the lumbar plexus, as identified in this study, could be useful for the surgeon who operates on the lumbar spine, especially from a lateral approach.

Injury to the subcostal and iliohypogastric nerves can result in abdominal wall paresis and sensory deficit over the iliac crest and above the pubic bone. Injury to the ilioinguinal nerve can result in absent cremaster reflex or pain in the anterior scrotum or labia majora. Injury to the genitofemoral nerve can result in absent cremaster reflex and sensory loss over the femoral triangle and inferior pole of the scrotum. In our earlier study,[7] at a vertical line through the midpoint between the ASIS and the midline, the subcostal, iliohypogastric, and ilioinguinal nerves were superior to the supracristal plane at mean distances of 8, 4, and 5 cm, respectively.

Injury to the lateral femoral cutaneous nerve results in sensory loss over the lateral thigh. Injury to the femoral can result in loss of knee extension and some hip flexion (iliacus, pectineus, and sartorius) and sensory deficits over the anterior thigh and medial leg and foot. Injury to the obturator nerve results in weakness or loss of adduction of the thigh. Weakness in external rotation of the thigh accompanies a slight loss of hip flexion. Pain and numbness of the medial thigh result from injuries to the obturator nerve. From an earlier study,[7] but with less application from a lateral approach, inferior to the supracristal plane and in a vertical line through a midpoint between the anterior inferior iliac spine and the midline, the lateral femoral and femoral nerves were found to have mean distances of 5 and 5.5 cm, respectively.

References

[1] Ahmadian A, Deukmedjian AR, Abel N, Dakwar E, Uribe JS. Analysis of lumbar plexopathies and nerve injury after lateral retroperitoneal transpsoas approach: diagnostic standardization. J Neurosurg Spine. 2013; 18(3):289–297

[2] Ahmadian A, Abel N, Uribe JS. Functional recovery of severe obturator and femoral nerve injuries after lateral retroperitoneal transpsoas surgery. J Neurosurg Spine. 2013; 18(4):409–414

[3] Beveridge TS, Power A, Johnson M, Power NE, Allman BL. The lumbar arteries and veins: quantification of variable anatomical positioning with application to retroperitoneal surgery. Clin Anat. 2015; 28(5):649–660

[4] Prats-Galino A, Reina MA, Mavar Haramija M, Puigdellivol-Sánchez A, Juanes Méndez JA, De Andrés JA. 3D interactive model of lumbar spinal structures of anesthetic interest. Clin Anat. 2015; 28(2):205–212

[5] Benglis DM, Vanni S, Levi AD. An anatomical study of the lumbosacral plexus as related to the minimally invasive transpsoas approach to the lumbar spine. J Neurosurg Spine. 2009; 10(2):139–144

[6] Moro T, Kikuchi S, Konno S, Yaginuma H. An anatomic study of the lumbar plexus with respect to retroperitoneal endoscopic surgery. Spine. 2003; 28 (5):423–428, discussion 427–428

[7] Tubbs RS, Salter EG, Wellons JC, III, Blount JP, Oakes WJ. Anatomical landmarks for the lumbar plexus on the posterior abdominal wall. J Neurosurg Spine. 2005; 2(3):335–338

[8] Van Schoor AN, Bosman MC, Bosenberg AT. Descriptive study of the differences in the level of the conus medullaris in four different age groups. Clin Anat. 2015; 28(5):638–644

[9] van Schoor A, Bosman MC, Bosenberg AT. The value of Tuffier's line for neonatal neuraxial procedures. Clin Anat. 2014; 27(3):370–375

[10] Kepler CK, Bogner EA, Herzog RJ, Huang RC. Anatomy of the psoas muscle and lumbar plexus with respect to the surgical approach for lateral transpsoas interbody fusion. Eur Spine J. 2011; 20(4):550–556

[11] Regev GJ, Chen L, Dhawan M, Lee YP, Garfin SR, Kim CW. Morphometric analysis of the ventral nerve roots and retroperitoneal vessels with respect to the minimally invasive lateral approach in normal and deformed spines. Spine. 2009; 34(12):1330–1335

[12] Lu S, Chang S, Zhang YZ, Ding ZH, Xu XM, Xu YQ. Clinical anatomy and 3D virtual reconstruction of the lumbar plexus with respect to lumbar surgery. BMC Musculoskelet Disord. 2011; 12:76

[13] Rodgers WB, Gerber EJ, Patterson J. Intraoperative and early postoperative complications in extreme lateral interbody fusion: an analysis of 600 cases. Spine. 2011; 36(1):26–32

16 The Subcostal Nerve during Lateral Approaches to the Lumbar Spine

Garrett Ng, R. Shane Tubbs

Abstract

Lateral approaches to the spine have recently gained popularity. However, details of the innervation pattern of the abdominal oblique muscles with the initial dissection for this procedure have not been well studied. Knowledge of the specific innervation and nerve dominance pattern for the lateral approach to the spine might help decrease postoperative complications such as sensory deficits or abdominal wall hernias. The subcostal nerve is the dominant nerve in regard to both size and innervation of the oblique muscles in the lateral position approach.

Keywords: lateral approach, anatomy, innervation, complications, surgery, spine

16.1 Introduction

There has been a recent increase in minimally invasive spine surgery. One approach utilized is the lateral transpsoas approach, first described by Ozgur et al in 2006.[1] Intraoperative monitoring is used in accessing the space between the 12th rib and iliac crest. Lumbar lateral interbody fusion procedures have gained popularity due to several advantages: low blood loss, preservation of the posterior musculature and ligamentous chain, the ability to perform an extensive discectomy, and placement of a large intervertebral graft across the apophyseal ring leading to indirect decompression.[2] As the use of lateral transpsoas approaches continues to increase, it is important for surgeons to remain aware of procedural complications such as postoperative nerve palsies.[3]

The corridor used to gain access to the retroperitoneal space during the lateral transpsoas approach lies between the 12th rib and the iliac crest, which is primarily supplied by the 11th intercostal and subcostal nerves with lesser contributions from the 10th intercostal nerve and L1.[4] Minimal access lateral spine exposure involves dissection through the abdominal musculature in addition to possible resection of the rib. However, details of the innervation pattern of the abdominal oblique muscles with the initial dissection for this procedure have not been well studied, particularly in relation to lateral abdominal hernia. Most literature on iatrogenic abdominal wall hernias resulting from lateral approaches has been derived from renal and thoracic approaches.[5,6,7] Such deformities significantly affect quality of life, especially in patients younger than 60 years, and may be a result for up to 50% of patients who undergo a flank incision.[6]

In an earlier anatomical study of the subcostal nerve in relation to the lateral approach, we found that it was the predominant nerve in regard to abdominal oblique muscle innervation (▶ Fig. 16.1).[8] Regarding size, the subcostal nerve was the largest (average diameter 6 mm) nerve in this region and had a wider field of distribution with more branches (average eight) compared to the L1 (average four) and 11th intercostal nerves

(average two). L2 only contributed small branches to the lateral abdominal wall musculature on two sides. The average diameter of the L1 and L2 nerves was 4.2 (range, 3–4.8 mm) and 3.8 mm (range, 2.8–4.4 mm), respectively. The proximal 6 to 10 cm of each of these nerves had few, if any, branches. Additionally, the subcostal nerve was often found (75%) up to 5 cm inferior to the 12th rib in its initial course. The area of least concentration (i.e., "safe" zone) was located in the direct lateral position at an approximate midpoint between the lower edge of the 12th rib and the superior-most aspect of the iliac crest. At the direct lateral approach region, the subcostal nerve and its branches comprised, on average, approximately two-thirds of the superior nerves located between the iliac crest and 12th rib. Additionally, a previously undescribed branch of the subcostal nerve was found to travel posterior to the quadratus lumborum and anastamose with the remaining normally placed subcostal nerve at or near the direct lateral position on 15% (two right sides and one left side) of studied sides. Laterally, extensive neural interconnections were found between the subcostal, intercostal, and L1 nerve fibers.

The intercostal nerves are composed of four branches: muscular, collateral, lateral cutaneous, and anterior cutaneous. The collateral branch arises at the angle of the ribs and supplies the intercostal muscles and parietal pleura as it courses closely with the subcostal vessels.[9] The subcostal nerve, which was found in our study to be the dominant nerve in the incision for a lateral transpsoas approach, travels with the subcostal vein and the subcostal artery in the inferior aspect of the 12th rib. While the subcostal vein and artery travel superiorly to the nerve in the grove of the 12th rib, the nerve is often exposed along its inferior margin. Knowledge of this anatomical pattern

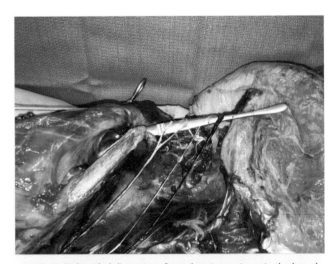

Fig. 16.1 Right-sided dissection of a cadaveric specimen in the lateral decubitus position between the right rib and iliac crest noting the nerves of this region. The subcostal (yellow), iliohypogastric (white), and ilioinguinal (black) nerves are seen.

can help prevent aggressive dissection inferior to the rib, with subsequent damage, during surgical approaches. The subcostal nerve then courses posterior to the lateral arcuate ligament and kidney and anterior to the quadratus lumborum. In 15% of cadaver sides, however, the following unusual, previously unde-scribed anatomical nerve pattern was observed: a large branch of the subcostal nerve travels posterior to the quadratus lumbo-rum muscle, and then joins the main part of the subcostal nerve more laterally. The subcostal nerve continues between the transversus abdominis and the internal oblique muscles and assists in innervating the lateral abdominal wall muscles.[10] The subcostal nerve assists with respiration by innervating the rectus abdominus, the transversus abdominis, and the inferior portion of the external oblique.[10,11,12]

Naturally, one might be inclined to assume that because the subcostal nerve gives muscular branches to the muscles of the anterior wall, damage to the subcostal nerve might also reduce the function of these muscles. However, Standring[10] stated that the anterolateral wall of the abdomen is innervated by several branches of segmented spinal nerves. Therefore, damage to one spinal nerve is very unlikely to produce any notable loss in muscle tone. Effective reduction in anterolateral wall muscle function would require damage to multiple spinal nerves or their branches. The lateral cutaneous branch innervates the skin of the anterolateral abdomen at its respective thoracic level. The subcostal nerve travels over the anterior superior iliac spine and pierces the rectus sheath, giving branches to the skin over the anterior region inferior to the umbilicus.[9,10] A few fibers from the subcostal nerve may travel inferior to the greater trochanter of the femur. It also has smaller contribu-tions to the parietal peritoneum and diaphragm.[10] The iliohypo-gastric nerve often receives a branch from the subcostal nerve.

Intercostal neuralgia, pain over the corresponding derma-tome, may be caused by tumor, nerve entrapment, thoracot-omy, or herpes zoster virus.[8,13] In a study of 68 patients who experienced postoperative abdominal pain and upper thigh numbness ipsilateral to the site of percutaneous nephrolithot-omy, it was found that the most commonly affected area was innervated by the subcostal nerve.[14] A neuroma of the 12th nerve may occur after a nephrectomy.[15] Rib fracture leading to pseudohernia as a result of subcostal nerve damage has been reported.[16] A postoperative abdominal wall flank bulge may occur with damage to the subcostal nerve or with extensive damage to the abdominal musculature.[11]

In order to access the retroperitoneal space, three muscle layers must be traversed—the external oblique, internal oblique, and transversus abdominis. They support the abdominal viscera and provide core strength.[17] Each of these muscular layers is sup-plied by the primary rami of the lower six intercostal nerves (T7–T12) and L1. The lower intercostal nerves divide and give off an anterior branch that supplies the skin and the external obli-que, and a posterior branch that supplies the internal oblique and the transversus abdominis muscles. The main trunk of the intercostal nerve runs between the internal oblique and the transversus abdominis. The intercostal nerves are classically described as lying along the subcostal groove.[18,19] Few reports have found them running through a midintercostal trajectory.[5,20] One study found them running caudal in the intercostal space.[21] The transversalis fascia is encountered deep to the transversus muscle and is thinner over the lateral abdominal wall closest to

the peritoneum and becomes more pronounced in thickness as it travels and attaches in the transverse process.[17] A study on the development of postoperative abdominal bulges after abdominal aortic aneurysm repair through a retroperitoneal approach found an incidence of 11%. The incidence increased to 19.4% if the incision extended into the 11th intercostal space.[5]

Use of specially made dilator systems allows access to the lumbar spine using a relatively narrow corridor through the lat-eral abdominal wall. More available data regarding hernias come from other lateral approaches, such as nephrectomy, where it has been reported to occur in 3% of cases after a classical flank inci-sion and in 3.6% after a mini-flank incision, although up to 50% of patients may develop flank bulging after a flank incision.[6] Dener-vation of the abdominal wall musculature as a result may lead to subsequent sagging of the abdomen.[22] In the urology literature, patients who undergo laparoscopic partial nephrectomy have been found to have smaller flank muscle volume changes and a flank bulge incidence of 12%, compared to 57% in patients who undergo an open procedure.[23] The incidence of flank bulges may be higher than reported due to poor postoperative examination, the development of a hernia months after surgery (possibly after the postsurgical follow-up period), and the patient's body habitus, which may impair visibility of small abdominal flank bulges.

16.2 Surgical Technique

Typically, the subcostal nerve is encountered during approaches to the thoracolumbar junction. For example, an L2 corpectomy may require resection of the T12 rib. An incision is made at the curvature of the rib, and the subcutaneous tissue is bluntly dis-sected without the use of electrocautery. The latissimus dorsi, serratus anterior, and intercostal muscles are dissected to expose the rib. We recommend dissection with the use of a moist sponge, as described by Brown and Petrou.[24] The sponge is used to protect the rib as the inferior neurovascular bundle is separated. It avoids the use of sharper instruments and decreases the risk of a pleurotomy in addition to intercostal nerve injury. We have slightly modified this technique by applying thrombin foam to the sponge while the dissection is being performed. This has decreased our use of the bipolar, and places the subcostal nerve at a lower risk from thermal injury. The internal and external abdominal oblique muscles are sepa-rated to expose the transversus abdominis and underlying transversalis fascia. After it is divided, the retroperitoneal space is accessed; this is easily recognized by the yellow glistening retroperitoneal fat. For minimally invasive procedures, a dilator is inserted. The dilator needs to be opened gently, until the minimal required window for visibility is achieved. Since more superficial nerves may not be visualized, overexpansion of the retractor may lead to a crush injury or ischemia of the nerve. Shorter retraction times should theoretically lead to a decrease in nerve manipulation and subsequent injury.

16.3 Lateral Lumbar Spine Approach Complications

There have been a few reports of incisional hernia following the lateral spine approach.[3,17,25] More commonly reported consequen-ces and complications of the lateral lumbar approach include weakness, thigh numbness, and dysesthesias, which occur in approximately 30% of patients.[26] A study has estimated that thigh sensory symptoms may occur in up to 60% of patients.[27]

In a retrospective study of 201 lumbar levels that had undergone the lateral lumbar approach procedure, there were two femoral nerve injuries at the L4–L5 level, representing a 4.8% incidence of injury of the femoral nerve at the L4–L5 disc space.[3] All femoral nerve injuries occurred at the L4–L5 level. Five patients (4.2%) in their series had a postoperative abdominal flank bulge.[3] Among patients with abdominal flank bulges, two underwent a single level lateral lumbar approach, two underwent a two-level lateral lumbar approach, and one underwent a three-level lateral lumbar approach. The levels experiencing abdominal flank bulges ranged from L1–L2 to L3–L4, with no abdominal bulges seen with approaches to L4–L5. It is easy to assume that interventions at the thoracolumbar and upper lumbar levels will be more likely to cause damage to the subcostal nerve due to its proximity. However, a cadaveric study showed that the lateral cutaneous branch of the subcostal nerve may be encountered as close as 6 cm from the anterior superior iliac spine.[28]

Fahim et al[12] suggested that sources of injury to the subcostal nerve distal to the rib that can lead to the development of a hernia include heat-induced injury as a result of electrocautery use, direct sharp transection, or through nerve entrapment as the abdominal wall is closed.[3] Additional sources of injury may include tension of the subcostal nerve due to overdistraction of the dilator and prolonged traction.

In our dissections, we found that the lateral wall abdominal musculature is largely innervated by the subcostal nerve with only a minor contribution from T11.[8] Based on our anatomical study, high-risk areas for subcostal nerve injuries include resection of the 12th rib, L1–L2, and thoracolumbar corpectomies necessitating a longer incision, larger fascial openings, and prolonged retraction times. When a partial resection of the 12th rib is necessary for exposure to the retroperitoneal space, we elect not to resuture the 12th rib in order to avoid movement of the fractured segment, which could strangulate the subcostal nerve.

16.4 Conclusion

Knowledge of the specific innervation and nerve dominance pattern for the lateral approach to the spine may help decrease postoperative complications such as sensory deficits or abdominal wall hernias. The subcostal nerve is the dominant nerve regarding both size and innervation of the oblique muscles in the lateral position approach.

References

[1] Ozgur BM, Aryan HE, Pimenta L, Taylor WR. Extreme Lateral Interbody Fusion (XLIF): a novel surgical technique for anterior lumbar interbody fusion. Spine J. 2006; 6(4):435–443

[2] Dakwar E, Cardona RF, Smith DA, Uribe JS. Early outcomes and safety of the minimally invasive, lateral retroperitoneal transpsoas approach for adult degenerative scoliosis. Neurosurg Focus. 2010; 28(3):E8

[3] Cahill KS, Martinez JL, Wang MY, Vanni S, Levi AD. Motor nerve injuries following the minimally invasive lateral transpsoas approach. J Neurosurg Spine. 2012; 17(3):227–231

[4] van der Graaf T, Verhagen PCMS, Kerver ALA, Kleinrensink GJ. Surgical anatomy of the 10th and 11th intercostal, and subcostal nerves: prevention of damage during lumbotomy. J Urol. 2011; 186(2):579–583

[5] Gardner GP, Josephs LG, Rosca M, Rich J, Woodson J, Menzoian JO. The retroperitoneal incision. An evaluation of postoperative flank 'bulge'. Arch Surg. 1994; 129(7):753–756

[6] Chatterjee S, Nam R, Fleshner N, Klotz L. Permanent flank bulge is a consequence of flank incision for radical nephrectomy in one half of patients. Urol Oncol. 2004; 22(1):36–39

[7] Timmermans L, Klitsie PJ, Maat AP, de Goede B, Kleinrensink GJ, Lange JF. Abdominal wall bulging after thoracic surgery, an underdiagnosed wound complication. Hernia. 2013; 17(1):89–94

[8] Alonso F., Graham R., Rustagi T., Drazin D., Loukas M., Oskouian R.J., Chapman J.R., Tubbs R.S.. The subcostal nerve during lateral approaches to the lumbar spine: an anatomical study with relevance for injury avoidance and postoperative complications such as abdominal wall hernia. World Neurosurg. 2017; 104:669–673

[9] Moore KL, Dalley AF, Agur AMR. Nerves of the thoracic wall. In: Clinically Oriented Anatomy. 6th ed. Philadelphia, PA: Wolters Kluwer Health/Lippincott Williams & Wilkins; 2010

[10] Standring S. Abdomen and pelvis. In: Gray's Anatomy: The Anatomical Basis of Clinical Practice. 41st ed. New York, NY: Elsevier Health Sciences; 2015

[11] Tubbs RS, Rizk E, Shoja MM, Loukas M, Barbaro N, Spinner RJ. Surgical exposure/anatomy of the lateral lumbar spine and plexus. In: Nerves and Nerve Injuries, Vol. 2: Pain, Treatment, Injury, Disease, and Future Directions. 1st ed. New York, NY: Elsevier; 2015

[12] Fahim DK, Kim SD, Cho D, Lee S, Kim DH. Avoiding abdominal flank bulge after anterolateral approaches to the thoracolumbar spine: cadaveric study and electrophysiological investigation. J Neurosurg Spine. 2011; 15(5):532–540

[13] Chiu HY, Lin SJ. A painful bulge in the left flank. JAMA. 2013; 310(6):639–640

[14] Nasseh H, Pourreza F, Saberi A, Kazemnejad E, Kalantari BB, Falahatkar S. Focal neuropathies following percutaneous nephrolithotomy (PCNL)–preliminary study. Ger Med Sci. 2013; 11(11):Doc07

[15] Williams EH, Williams CG, Rosson GD, Heitmiller RF, Dellon AL. Neurectomy for treatment of intercostal neuralgia. Ann Thorac Surg. 2008; 85(5):1766–1770

[16] Butensky AM, Gruss LP, Gleit ZL. Flank pseudohernia following posterior rib fracture: a case report. J Med Case Reports. 2016; 10(1):273

[17] Galan TV, Mohan V, Klineberg EO, Gupta MC, Roberto RF, Ellwitz JP. Case report: incisional hernia as a complication of extreme lateral interbody fusion. Spine J. 2012; 12(4):e1–e6

[18] Davies F, Gladstone RJ, Stibbe EP. The anatomy of the intercostal nerves. J Anat. 1932; 66(Pt 3):323–333

[19] Aubert J, Koumare K, Dufrenot A. Anatomical study of the twelfth intercostal nerve and oblique lumbotomies [author's transl; in French]. J Urol (Paris). 1981; 87(5):283–289

[20] Hardy PA. Anatomical variation in the position of the proximal intercostal nerve. Br J Anaesth. 1988; 61(3):338–339

[21] Court C, Vialle R, Lepeintre JF, Tadié M. The thoracoabdominal intercostal nerves: an anatomical study for their use in neurotization. Surg Radiol Anat. 2005; 27(1):8–14

[22] Loos MJ, Scheltinga MR, Mulders LG, Roumen RM. The Pfannenstiel incision as a source of chronic pain. Obstet Gynecol. 2008; 111(4):839–846

[23] Crouzet S, Chopra S, Tsai S, et al. Flank muscle volume changes after open and laparoscopic partial nephrectomy. J Endourol. 2014; 28(10):1202–1207

[24] Brown JA, Petrou SP. Use of a surgical sponge facilitates rib resection in flank incisions. Urology. 1997; 49(6):946–947

[25] Plata-Bello J, Roldan H, Brage L, Rahy A, Garcia-Marin V. Delayed abdominal pseudohernia in young patient after lateral lumbar interbody fusion procedure: case report. World Neurosurg. 2016; 91:671.e13–671.e16

[26] Wang MY, Mummaneni PV. Minimally invasive surgery for thoracolumbar spinal deformity: initial clinical experience with clinical and radiographic outcomes. Neurosurg Focus. 2010; 28(3):E9

[27] Cummock MD, Vanni S, Levi AD, Yu Y, Wang MY. An analysis of postoperative thigh symptoms after minimally invasive transpsoas lumbar interbody fusion. J Neurosurg Spine. 2011; 15(1):11–18

[28] Chou D, Storm PB, Campbell JN. Vulnerability of the subcostal nerve to injury during bone graft harvesting from the iliac crest. J Neurosurg Spine. 2004; 1(1):87–89

17 Surgical Techniques for Approaching the Lumbosacral Plexus

Amgad Hanna, Vikas Parmar, Susan I. Toth

Abstract

Pathologies can present in and around the lumbosacral plexus in various ways. A needle biopsy may be prudent in situations of large neoplasms. Also, benign asymptomatic tumors could be followed with serial imaging. However, if pathology, symptoms, or growth on imaging predicts surgical resection, there are several approaches that can be used to provide a surgical corridor. The posterior[1] approach, traditionally an approach used for lateral disc herniation, can also be used for proximal plexus pathologies. The lateral transpsoas approach is also used for proximal lumbosacral plexus pathology but is chosen over the Wiltse approach when the pathology is more lateral and caudal and less posterior. The anterior muscle-splitting retroperitoneal approach gains the surgeon access to the proximal lateral femoral cutaneous, ilioinguinal, genitofemoral, and femoral nerves. Finally, the presacral (pelvic) approach is used for complex pathology that extends often into the retroperitoneal (presacral) and sacral space. As our surgical finesse with handling pathologies of the lumbosacral plexus continue to grow, laparoscopic techniques will certainly play a crucial role in this evolution.

Keywords: lumbosacral plexus, posterior Wiltse approach, lateral transpsoas approach, anterior muscle-splitting approach, presacral approach, laparoscopic approach to lumbosacral plexus

17.1 Introduction

Owing to the large craniocaudal extent of the lumbosacral plexus, pathologies can occupy different anatomical spaces in the abdomen and/or pelvis. Different approaches can be used to access those lesions depending on which anatomical compartment they mostly occupy. This offers a wide variety of options for surgeons. The choice should be based mainly on which approach will provide best access to deal with the lesion. It should also consider the surgeon's comfort level with different approaches. Most of these procedures usually require the help of an access surgeon.

17.2 Posterior (Wiltse) Approach

The posterior[1] surgery (► Fig. 17.1) is a paraspinal approach that was originally described as an alternative conduit to the lumbar spine. It went between the lateral board of the erector spinae muscles and the quadratus lumborum muscle and was first described in 1959 by Watkins.[2] However, in 1973, Wiltse modified it via a muscle-splitting sacrospinalis technique. The approach has largely been used for far lateral disc herniations, instrumented lumbar fusion, or foraminal decompression. Here, it is described in regard to pathologies of the lumbosacral plexus.

17.2.1 Indications

The Wiltse approach allows the proximal aspect of the lumbosacral plexus (i.e., the spinal nerves) to be visualized. Thus, the indications are for proximal pathologies. This often primarily involves tumors, but can also include traumatic avulsions.

17.2.2 Case Example:

A 33-year-old woman had a 2-month history of left anterior thigh pain in an L2 and L3 distribution. Her pain was shooting and shocklike, but did not reach her knee. These episodes of pain occurred 20 to 30 times a day. Motor examination revealed left iliopsoas with a Medical Research Council (MRC) grade 4 and left quadriceps 4, otherwise 5 throughout. Sensation was intact to light touch. Deep tendon reflexes were symmetric at 2 + for the ankle jerk and 3 + for the knee jerk. Magnetic resonance imaging (MRI) of the lumbar spine as shown in ► Fig. 17.2 revealed a left L2–L3 nerve sheath tumor extending from the L2 foramen. The mass was enhanced with contrast. The patient was scheduled for surgery via a left posterior paramedian approach for resection of what appeared to be a nerve sheath tumor. Another small intradural tumor was considered asymptomatic and was left for surveillance.

17.2.3 Surgical Technique

General anesthesia was induced with the airway secured via an endotracheal tube. The left lower extremities were monitored by electromyography (EMG). The patient's head was placed in pins and she was positioned prone on a Jackson table. The level was localized using a spinal needle and lateral fluoroscopy. The

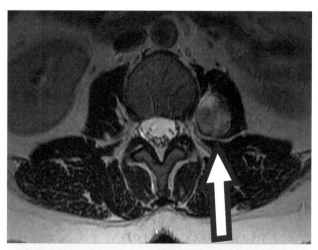

Fig. 17.1 Axial T2-weighted MRI showing a mass within the left psoas muscle. The mass can easily be approached via a left paraspinal[1] approach (*arrow*).

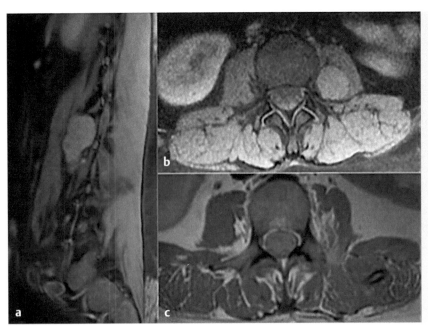

Fig. 17.2 (a, b) Sagittal and axial T2-weighted MRI demonstrating a left nerve sheath tumor extending from the L2–L3 foramen. **(c)** Axial and sagittal T2-weighted MRI shows complete surgical resection.

incision was marked to the left of midline overlying the area of the transverse processes of L2 and L3. The back was prepped and draped in the usual sterile fashion.

An incision was made and dissection proceeded with monopolar electrocautery down to the level of the dorsal lumbar fascia. The fascia was divided sharply with a 15 blade through both layers, and then the cut was completed with scissors. Serial dilators were then used to dissect through the paraspinal muscles and an expandable tubular retractor was used to dock on the left L2–L3 facet. Fluoroscopy was used to confirm positioning of the tube, and then it was secured to the operating table. Alternatively, other deep self-retaining retractors can be used.

The transverse processes of L2 and L3 were exposed using monopolar electrocautery and the intertransverse membrane was opened. Soft-tissue dissection revealed the tumor. Stimulation was used to test for functional nerve fascicles. Only fascicles entering and exiting the tumor were sacrificed and the tumor was dissected free from the remaining nerves. Kerrison punches were used to take portions of the L2 left transverse processes to facilitate exposure of the tumor and nerve root.

Once the tumor was adequately circumferentially dissected, it was removed and sent to pathology for a permanent specimen. The surgical field was copiously irrigated with antibiotic saline and meticulous hemostasis was obtained. The layers of the lumbodorsal fascia were then closed together and the skin and subcutaneous tissues were closed in multiple layers with interrupted sutures.

Postoperative MRI demonstrated complete surgical resection as demonstrated in ▶ Fig. 17.2. Clinically, the patient no longer had any shooting pain in her left thigh. She did complain of burning pain in the left anterior thigh, as well as allodynia that responded to medication. Motor examination was more stable after than before surgery. She had new diminished light touch sensation over the left anterior thigh in an L2 distribution.

17.3 Transpsoas Approach

Lateral approaches through the psoas muscle have primarily been used for both open and minimally invasive spine surgery. The same approach can be used for lumbosacral plexus pathologies. The technique is a lateral retroperitoneal exposure of the psoas muscle and within it the lumbosacral plexus, as shown in ▶ Fig. 17.3.

17.3.1 Indications

Traditionally, the lateral transpsoas approach has been used for various spinal disorders such as disc degeneration, deformity, lateral disc herniation, and interbody fusion surgery. In terms of use for lumbosacral plexus pathology, it should be chosen for proximal lesions near the psoas muscle. In contrast to the posterior Wiltse approach, the lateral approach is chosen for pathology that is less posterior and has a notably lateral/caudal extension.

17.3.2 Case Example

A 49-year-old man presented to the Neurosurgery Clinic following the discovery of a left-sided mass associated with his lumbosacral plexus, as demonstrated in ▶ Fig. 17.4. At the time, he was asymptomatic. Additional imaging revealed a mass in the left internal auditory canal suggesting a schwannoma. On general examination, he had multiple subcutaneous masses but full strength throughout and sensation was grossly intact. On the basis of all these findings, it was believed that he had neurofibromatosis type 2. Surgery was recommended for resection of the left lumbosacral mass owing to its large size.

17.3.3 Surgical Technique

The patient was placed under general endotracheal anesthesia supine on the operating room table. A bump was placed under the patient's left buttock and back. This could also be done in a full lateral position. Needles were placed for EMG monitoring during surgery.

Although a direct lateral approach could have been performed, the access surgeon here opted for an oblique approach.

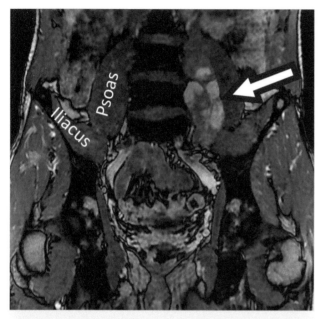

Fig. 17.3 Coronal T1-weighted MRI with contrast reveals a multifocal nerve sheath tumor of the left lumbosacral plexus. This was best approached via a left retroperitoneal transpsoas approach (*arrow*). This case would not be well served by a posterior approach since the tumor extends caudally in front of the sacroiliac joint.

An oblique incision approximately 10 cm long was made over the left part of the lower abdomen. Scarpa's fascia was opened. The anterior rectus sheath was divided. The rectus muscle was mobilized medially. The abdominal wall was divided into layers and the retroperitoneum entered. Retroperitoneal contents were retracted medially including the left colon, left kidney, left ureter, left iliac artery, and left iliac vein. Care was taken to identify all these structures and avoid injuring them. At this point, retractors were placed using the wishbone-type table-affixed general surgery retractor. It was then easy to identify the spine and the tumor within the psoas muscle. This was first identified by palpation through the psoas muscle, and then once the muscle fibers had been split, the tumor was easily visualized. We then started to dissect it.

Initially, we focused on the most rostral and medial of the five masses. We dissected around the tumor, stimulating intermittently with the nerve stimulator. The capsule surrounding the tumor was opened, and then we dissected circumferentially. The most rostral aspect of the tumor was removed piecemeal. We then proceeded from rostral to caudal, resecting each tumor in the same fashion, dissecting around them, stimulating intermittently any time we had to cut. After we had dissected around all the masses and resected them, we palpated throughout the psoas muscle. No other masses could be palpated.

The psoas muscle did not need reapproximation. The abdominal contents were returned to their anatomical locations. The abdominal wall was closed in layers with 0 PDS suture (Polydioxanone, Ethicon, Johnson & Johnson) and 3–0 Vicryl (Ethicon, Johnson & Johnson) for the subcutaneous Scarpa's fascia and 4–0 PDS for the skin. Steri-Strips (3M) were applied. A routine postoperative abdominal X-ray was obtained and ruled out any retained instruments.

Postoperatively, the patient's strength in the left iliopsoas was 4/5 but improved over time to 5/5. He also developed decreased light touch sensation over the left L4 distribution. Pathology revealed schwannomas.

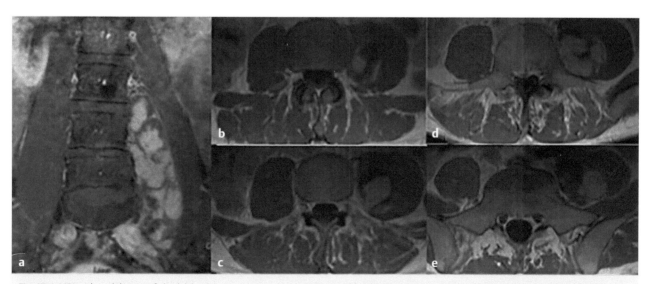

Fig. 17.4 MRI with gadolinium of the **(a)** lumbar spine coronal and various axial levels: **(b)** L3, **(c)** L4, **(d)** L5, **(e)** S1. These demonstrate what are probably multiple left paraspinal masses coalescing into one large mass with involvement of the left L3–L4, L4–L5, and L5–S1 nerve roots into the neural foramina without intradural extension.

17.4 Anterior Muscle-Splitting Approach

17.4.1 Introduction

The anterior approach began with approaches to the lumbar spine by Müller in 1906, while anterior lumbar interbody fusion was introduced during the 1930s.[3,4] These were first described as anterior transperitoneal approaches. These anterior approaches had soon evolved to be retroperitoneal, very much like the lateral approach. The difference between these two approaches is the trajectory as depicted in ▶ Fig. 17.5. With the anterior approach, the ventral aspect of the spine and lumbosacral plexus can be identified. This approach has been adopted for surgical treatment for patients with meralgia paresthetica who have failed lateral femoral cutaneous nerve decompression. Alberti et al[5] depict a suprainguinal, anterior, retroperitoneal approach for these pathologies.

17.4.2 Indications

The indications for an anterior approach have traditionally been related to spinal disorders. However, in relation to the lumbosacral plexus, this approach can be used to expose the lateral femoral cutaneous, ilioinguinal, genitofemoral, and proximal femoral nerves. It is therefore typically used to visualize the proximal aspect of the terminal branches and divisions of the lumbosacral plexus anterior or lateral to the psoas muscle.

17.4.3 Case Example

A 40-year-old woman with left-sided meralgia paresthetica had undergone decompression approximately 3 months earlier, which gave her about 70% pain relief for approximately 1.5 months. Unfortunately, the left-sided pain recurred in the same distribution as before. The patient then opted for surgical transection of the left lateral femoral cutaneous nerve.

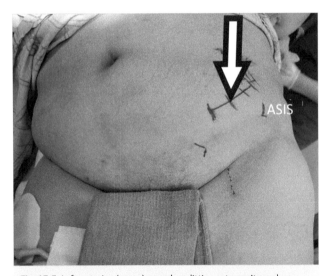

Fig. 17.5 Left anterior (*arrow*) muscle-splitting retroperitoneal approach to the lateral femoral cutaneous nerve. ASIS, anterior superior iliac spine.

17.4.4 Surgical Technique

The patient was intubated with general anesthesia and placed in the supine position with a bump under the left hip. The left lower abdomen and upper thigh was prepped and draped in the usual sterile fashion. With the help of an access surgeon, we first identified the landmark of the anterior superior iliac spine (ASIS) and the pubic symphysis, marking out the approximate location of the inguinal ligament. An incision approximately 3 to 4 cm long was made just superior to the inguinal ligament. The dissection continued down to the level of the Scarpa's fascia where the fascia was sharply dissected. The external oblique fascia was identified and entered sharply, and then opened in the line of its fibers. The internal oblique was then bluntly separated with Army-Navy retractors and the transversalis was opened sharply. The retroperitoneum was entered. The peritoneum and the intraperitoneal structures were swept medially until we encountered the iliacus and psoas muscles. The left ureter was identified and retracted out of the field along with the peritoneal structures. The left iliac artery was identified. Along the length of its exposure, it was soft and there were no calcifications. We placed the remainder of the retractors for viewing the retroperitoneal space within which we were working.

The femoral nerve (the largest nerve) was located between the psoas and iliacus muscles. Just lateral to it was the lateral femoral cutaneous nerve, and then the ilioinguinal nerve. Medial to the femoral nerve and anterior to the psoas muscle was the genitofemoral nerve. The femoral nerve was confirmed with the nerve stimulator. Then we proceeded to transect the segment of the left lateral femoral cutaneous nerve. The proximal end of the nerve was electrocauterized using a bipolar to minimize risk for development of neuromas.

The wound was then irrigated with bacitracin solution. Our retractors were removed one at a time, confirming no evidence of bleeding in the retroperitoneal space. There was a strong palpable pulse in the left iliac artery. The peritoneal structures were allowed to fall back into place. The fascial layers were then closed in two layers with running 0 PDS suture (Ethicon, Johnson & Johnson). Scarpa's fascia was closed with a running 2–0 Vicryl (Ethicon, Johnson & Johnson). Deep dermal interrupted 3–0 Vicryl (Ethicon, Johnson & Johnson) sutures were placed. The skin was then closed with a running 4–0 Monocryl (Ethicon, Johnson & Johnson). Steri-Strips and sterile dressings were applied.

The patient was extubated without complications. Postoperatively, the patient had loss of sensation in the distribution of the left lateral femoral cutaneous nerve as expected and reported no further pain.

17.5 Presacral (Pelvic) Approach

17.5.1 Introduction

The approach for discussion of lumbosacral plexus surgeries is related to the sacral component of the plexus, for example, in cases of sacral and presacral tumors. The area of the presacral space can be accessed by a retroperitoneal approach; before proceeding, it is essential to understand the anatomy of this region. The anterior boundary is marked by the mesorectum, while the posterior border is limited by the anterior aspect of

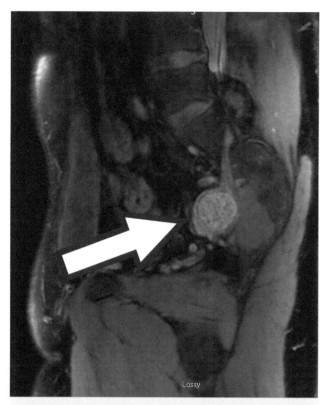

Fig. 17.6 Sagittal, proton-density, fat-suppressed MRI revealing a left S1 tumor extending into the pelvis. This tumor is best approached by an anterior suprapubic approach (*arrow*). The incision can be vertical midline or horizontal (Pfannenstiel).

the sacrum. Inferiorly, the space extends to the rectosacral fascia and superiorly the peritoneum. It is important to note that the lateral extent of the presacral space encompasses the common, internal and external iliac vessels, ureters, and sacral nerve roots. The median sacral artery can also be a primary feeder to pathologies in this area.

17.5.2 Indications

The indication for using this approach is for lesions found primarily in the presacral space, as marked out on a sagittal MRI in ► Fig. 17.6. However, chordomas, chondrosarcomas, giant cell tumors, plasmacytomas, lymphomas, and aneurysmal bone cysts have also been reported in this location.[6,7] In particular, schwannomas of the sacral roots have only been reported a handful of times in the literature. Klimo et al[8] classified these tumors on the basis of primary location.[8] They defined class I as tumors primarily confined to the sacrum, class II as tumors that delve anterior and posterior of the sacral walls, and class III as tumors mainly in the presacral or retroperitoneal space.

17.5.3 Case Example

A 35-year-old man presented with pelvic pain, increased urinary frequency, and intermittent constipation. MRI (► Fig. 17.7) revealed left pelvic mass, thought to be associated with the S1 nerve.

17.5.4 Surgical Technique

The patient was placed supine with the arms abducted at 90 degrees, under general anesthesia. The skin was prepped and draped in a sterile fashion. The EMG needles had been placed in the lower extremities, and a midline incision was made from the pubis to below the umbilicus. Alternatively, a horizontal Pfannenstiel incision could have been used. The midline fascia was divided, the abdomen was entered, and a Bookwalter retractor was placed. The sigmoid colon was retracted medially and was released from its peritoneal attachments such that the sigmoid could be retracted in a right lateral and cephalad fashion, completely exposing the pelvic mass. The dissection was continued around the tumor capsule, lateralizing the left common iliac artery and vein, the internal iliac artery and vein, and the ureter, all of which were identified and retracted laterally and protected.

Once the mass was exposed, the capsule was divided sharply. The EMG was monitored throughout this period and we had no definitive EMG activity. Once the capsule was opened, it was dissected circumferentially around the large mass. The mass was adherent to the capsule but it was possible to dissect it in a reasonably clean plane with some persistence and blunt dissection. We found that the mass most likely extended from the S2 foramen. There was significant venous bleeding toward the foramen that was easily tamponaded. Gross total resection was achieved.

A piece of Surgicel (Ethicon, Johnson & Johnson) was placed down in the resection bed. We put the sigmoid back into its natural anatomical position, closed the midline fascia with looped #1 PDS (Ethicon, Johnson & Johnson), and closed the skin with interrupted dermal Vicryl (Ethicon, Johnson & Johnson) sutures, followed by Dermabond (Ethicon, Johnson & Johnson).

Alternatively, a retroperitoneal approach could have achieved the same exposure. An incision is made paramedian along the left side from the umbilicus to the pubic symphysis. The anterior rectus sheath is cut vertically through. The peritoneum is dissected free from the abdominal wall. The iliac vessels and ureter are visualized and retracted medially. The tumor appears just slightly deeper in the surgical field. Often, the superior gluteal vessels are splayed around the lesion and should be checked on preoperative imaging. Once the tumor is removed, the anterior rectus sheath followed by the deep dermal layer and skin are then closed after hemostasis and copious irrigation. Pathology revealed schwannoma.

17.6 Laparoscopic Approach to the Lumbosacral Plexus

17.6.1 Introduction

Classically, entrapment of the lateral femoral cutaneous nerve, a spectrum of meralgia paresthetica, is a potential complication of laparoscopic inguinal hernia repair. The typical cause is neural entrapment due to staples or mesh fibrosis. However, the rate of meralgia paresthetica has decreased since surgical techniques were improved by laparoscopic approaches. There are a few recent case reports of primary treatment of meralgia paresthetica via a laparoscopic approach.[9,10] Chopra et al described

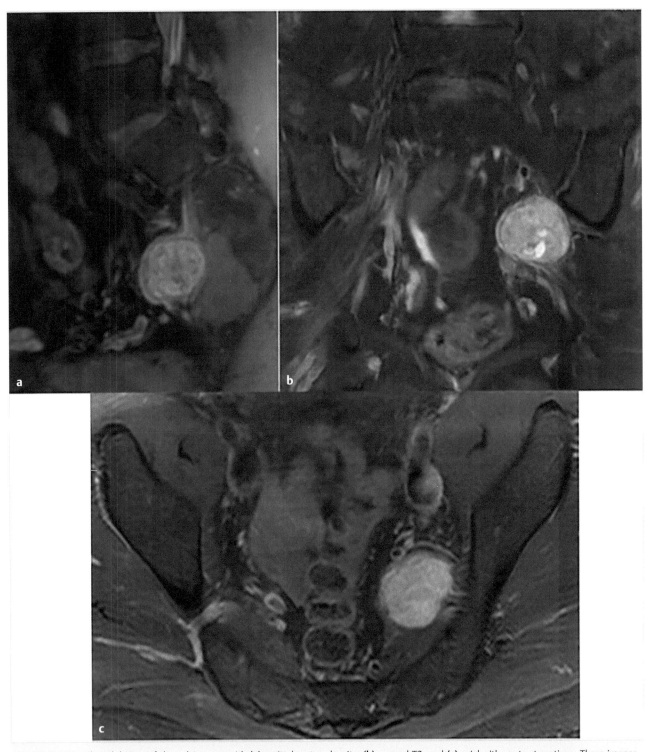

Fig. 17.7 MRI with gadolinium of the pelvic space with **(a)** sagittal proton density, **(b)** coronal T2, and **(c)** axial with contrast sections. These images demonstrate a left T2 hyperintense and enhancing mass with small areas of cystic degeneration projecting medially from the left sciatic nerve in the left hemipelvis adjacent to the piriformis muscle, measuring approximately 3.3 × 3.4 × 3.3 cm.

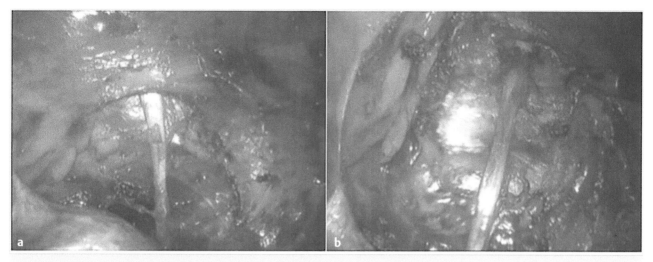

Fig. 17.8 Intraoperative laparoscopic pictures of lateral femoral cutaneous nerve prior to **(a)** decompression and with inguinal ligament entrapment, and **(b)** after release of the nerve from below via a hook diathermy. (Reprinted with permission from Bhardwaj and Lloyd.[10])

its use for a patient who had both symptomatic cholelithiasis and meralgia paresthetica.[9]

17.6.2 Details of Procedure

After successful intubation, the patient is positioned supine and three ports are made, a 10 mm infraumbilical and two 5 mm ports, as if performing an initial hernia repair. The nerve is often visible through the translucent parietal peritoneum. The peritoneum is opened with a small incision 2 cm below and medial to the ASIS. The nerve is released by dividing the posterior leaflet of the inguinal ligament and any fibrous attachments to the nerve using a hook diathermy as seen in ▶ Fig. 17.8. The nerve could also be transected in the event of recurrence after decompression.

17.6.3 Complications

Complications entailed in the anterior surgical approach to the lumbosacral plexus can be minimized by adhering to the principles of safe surgical technique. Complications will nevertheless occur, even in the most skilled and experienced hands. Pelvic surgery is associated with a distinct set of complications, in addition to those common to any abdominal surgery requiring general anesthesia. The rates of these complications can be minimized by following national guidelines for prevention and treatment.

There are two approaches for anterior surgical exposure of the lumbosacral region: *extraperitoneal* and *transabdominal*. Depending on the location of neurosurgical intervention, the extraperitoneal approach is most preferred if the tissue planes have not previously been exposed/injured, e.g., with preperitoneal hernia mesh placement, colorectal surgery, or radiation therapy.

Intraoperative complications during an *extraperitoneal* approach include bleeding from the epigastric vessels while exposing the preperitoneal space; injury to the genitofemoral nerve on the psoas muscle; injury to the ureter; bleeding from

the iliac vessels (usually from the internal iliac vein and its branches); bleeding from the presacral arteries/veins; injury to the sacral sympathetic trunks and pelvic splanchnic nerves, which include sympathetic and parasympathetic innervation to the bladder, anal and urinary sphincters, rectum, and genital organs such as the prostate, seminal vesicles, penis, uterus/cervix, and ovaries; and injury to the rectum.

Intraoperative complications during a *transabdominal* approach include injury to the small bowel or colon/rectum, injury to the ureter, bleeding from the iliac vessels, bleeding from the presacral vessels, and injury to the sacral sympathetic trunks and pelvic splanchnic nerves.

Postoperative complications include limb ischemia from arterial thromboembolism, wound infection, ileus (which would be expected with a transabdominal approach), small bowel obstructions from pelvic adhesions, which mostly occur after a transabdominal approach, fistula formation from the small bowel or rectum resulting from inadvertent bowel injury, ureteral obstruction/stricture from traction or crush injury, pelvic abscess, peripheral neuropathy, retrograde ejaculation, and impotence. Incisional hernia can occur especially with the muscle-cutting techniques.

Common complications after any major abdominal procedure include deep venous thrombosis/pulmonary embolism, myocardial infarction, cerebrovascular accident, and pneumonia.

17.7 Conclusion

Several approaches can be used to access the lumbosacral plexus. The choice depends on the location of the epicenter of the pathology, the surgeon's comfort level, and the availability of an access surgeon. In cases of large neoplasms, it could be prudent to order a computed tomography (CT)-guided needle biopsy to obtain a histological diagnosis prior to definitive surgery. Keep in mind that some benign asymptomatic tumors could be followed with serial imaging. The complication rate is lower with retroperitoneal approaches than the more traditional intraperitoneal ones.

References

[1] Wiltse LL. The paraspinal sacrospinalis-splitting approach to the lumbar spine. Clin Orthop Relat Res. 1973(91):48–57

[2] Watkins MB. Posterolateral bonegrafting for fusion of the lumbar and lumbosacral spine. J Bone Joint Surg Am. 1959; 41-A(3):388–396

[3] Ito H, Tsuchiya J, Asami G.. A new radical operation for Pottw disease report of ten cases. J Bone Joint Surg. 1934; 16:499–515

[4] Müller W. Transperitoneale Freilegung der Wirbelsäule bei tuberkulöser Spondylitis. Langenbecks Arch Surg. 1906; 85:128–135

[5] Alberti O, Wickboldt J, Becker R. Suprainguinal retroperitoneal approach for the successful surgical treatment of meralgia paresthetica. J Neurosurg. 2009; 110(4):768–774

[6] Domínguez J, Lobato RD, Ramos A, Rivas JJ, Gómez PA, Castro S. Giant intrasacral schwannomas: report of six cases. Acta Neurochir (Wien). 1997; 139 (10):954–959, discussion 959–960

[7] Ozdemir N, Bezircioğlu H, Akar O. Giant erosive spinal schwannomas: surgical management. Br J Neurosurg. 2010; 24(5):526–531

[8] Klimo P, Jr, Rao G, Schmidt RH, Schmidt MH. Nerve sheath tumors involving the sacrum. Case report and classification scheme. Neurosurg Focus. 2003; 15 (2):E12

[9] Chopra PJ, Shankaran RK, Murugeshan DC. Meralgia paraesthetica: Laparoscopic surgery as a cause then and a cure now. J Minim Access Surg. 2014; 10 (3):159–160

[10] Bhardwaj N, Lloyd DM. Laparoscopic relief of meralgia paraesthetica. Ann R Coll Surg Engl. 2011; 93(6):491

18 Nerve Root Anomalies with Application to the Lumbar Plexus

Cameron Schmidt, Chidinma Nwaogbe, R. Shane Tubbs

Abstract

Nerve root anomalies are a set of well-described congenital irregularities for which several classification systems have been devised over the years. This comprehensive review examines the anatomy and characteristics of these anatomical variants and relates them to the lumbar plexus.

Keywords: spine, spinal nerve, variations, anatomy, imaging, duplicated, nerve roots

18.1 Introduction

18.1.1 Anatomy

Spinal nerves originate in the spinal column as a set of ventral and dorsal rootlets. Emerging from the spinal cord, these rootlets converge to form the ventral and dorsal roots, respectively. Unlike cervical and thoracic regions, lumbosacral nerve roots must descend distal to the conus medullaris within the dural sac to reach their appropriate root sleeves. At their respective pedicle, nerve roots diverge inferolaterally, traversing the inferior surface of the corresponding pedicle before exiting through the intervertebral foramen. As nerve roots diverge, they remained bound by a meningeal sheath.[1] Continuing laterally, the subarachnoid extension is terminated near or on the dorsal root ganglion (DRG). Distally, the dorsal and ventral roots join to become the very short spinal nerve, before diverging again into dorsal and ventral rami.

18.2 Congenital Nerve Root Anomalies

18.2.1 Conjoined Nerve Roots

Conjoined nerve roots (CNRs) are defined as two adjacent nerve roots that, at some point during their course from the thecal sac, share a common dural sheath (▶ Fig. 18.1, ▶ Fig. 18.2, ▶ Fig. 18.3, ▶ Fig. 18.4, ▶ Fig. 18.5). Remaining

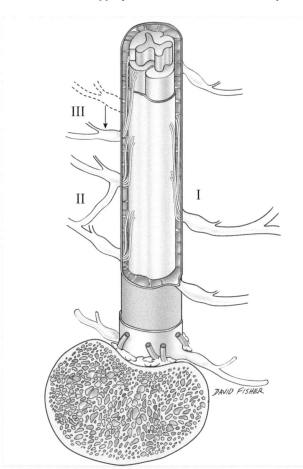

Fig. 18.1 Cannon et al classification: (I) conjoined nerve root, (II) extradural anastomosis, (III) caudal origin (transverse root)

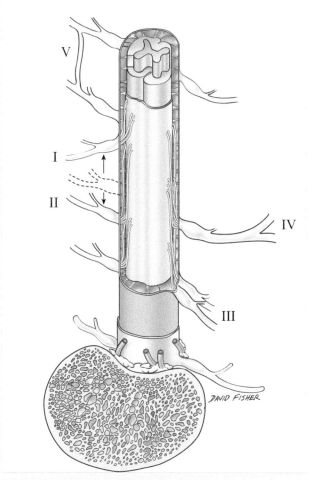

Fig. 18.2 Postacchini et al classification: (I) cranial origin, (II) caudal origin (transverse root), (III) closely adjacent nerve roots, (IV) conjoined nerve root, (V) extradural anastomosis

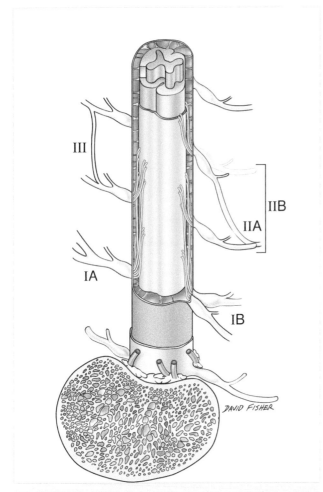

Fig. 18.3 Neidre and MacNab classification: (IA) conjoined nerve root, (IB) closely adjacent nerve roots, (IIA) two nerve roots exit through common foramen leaving one foramen unoccupied, (IIB) nerve roots in all foramina, but one foramen contains two separate roots, (III) extradural anastomosis.

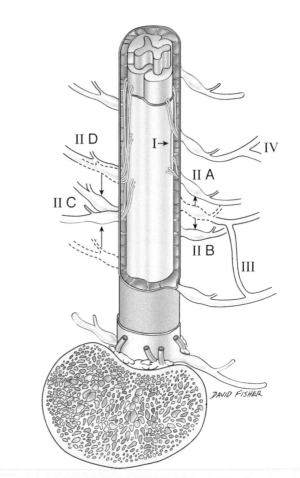

Fig. 18.4 Kadish and Simmons classification: (I) intradural anastomosis, (IIA) cranial origin, (IIB) caudal origin, (IIC) closely adjacent nerve roots, (IID) conjoined nerve roots, (III) extradural anastomosis, (IV) extradural division of nerve root.

conjoined for a variable course, the two roots separate, following independent courses either through the same or separate foramina. This anomaly tends to display no disturbance of any adjacent segments. CNRs are the most commonly reported anomaly in the literature, generally involving the L5 and S1 nerve roots.[2,3,4,5,6,7,8] These anomalies tend to appear unilaterally, although there are reports of bilateral CNRs.[9]

The L5–S1 level has unique characteristics, interesting considering its role as the locale of so many CNRs. The L5 nerve root has the greatest amount of space in the spinal canal and the narrowest lateral recess and intervertebral foramen, and S1 and L5 dorsal roots have the largest overall diameters.[2] Taken together, along with knowledge of the root sleeves attachments to surrounding structures within the lateral recess and neural foramen, L5 spinal nerves have a significantly susceptibility to entrapment and compression.[2,10,11]

18.2.2 Closely Adjacent Nerve Roots

A similar variant of the CNR anomaly occurs when two nerve roots arise through closely adjacent openings in the dural sac.

In many cases, these closely adjacent nerves are tightly adherent to one another, each contained within an individual dural sheath requiring careful dissection to separate.

18.2.3 Caudal/Cranial Nerve Root Origin

Nerve roots are sometimes found arising from the dura in an abnormally cranial or caudal location, resulting in an exceedingly oblique or transverse course from the dural sac, respectively. In these cases, there is no abnormality associated with the nerve or its dural sheath. It is simply the root's abnormal origin of emergence from the dural sac which gives rise to its atypical course.

18.2.4 Anastomosed Nerve Roots

Nerve interconnections (anastomoses) have been found to occur both intradurally and extradurally. The anomaly consists of a nerve fiber connection between two adjacent nerve roots. Cadaveric studies have revealed a greater number of anastomoses between sacral roots.[12]

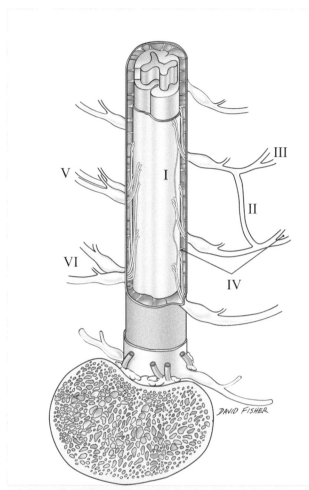

Fig. 18.5 Chotigavanich and Sawangnatra classification: (I) intradural anastomosis, (II) extradural anastomosis, (III) extradural division of nerve root, (IV) intradural anastomosis and extradural division of nerve root, (V) intradural and extradural division of nerve root, (VI) closely adjacent nerve roots

18.3 Embryology

Knowledge of the embryologic fault underlying these anomalies is imprecise. It has been suggested that the emergence of nerve roots from an abnormally caudal location, as well as the presence of conjoined and/or closely adjacent nerve roots, likely results from defective migration of nerve roots during embryonic development[13,14] Emergence of nerve roots from an abnormally cranial location, as well as bilateral anomalies, has been suggested to result from defective emergence of affected roots from the spinal cord.[14] Finally, abnormal connections between two roots have been suggested to result from the abnormal exit of a root from the dural pouch during fetal development.[15,16]

18.4 Prevalence

Nerve root anomalies (NRAs) have been detected in patients between the ages of roughly 15 and 73.[5,10,17,18] The mean patient age is approximately 38 years.[5,18] NRAs most frequently involve the L5 and S1 nerve roots, routinely accounting for 50 to 70% of reported NRAs.[3,4,6,7,8,14,19,20,21,22] Various case series have reported either L4 or S2 to be the next most commonly involved nerve root, present in approximately one-third of cases.[3,7,23,24] NRAs are apparently equally common on left and right sides.[3,4,7,10,13,14,24]

Despite broad reporting in the literature, these anomalies remain underdiagnosed, best appreciated by the significant differences in reported prevalence rates.

18.4.1 Surgical Prevalence

Prevalence rates of intraoperatively discovered CNR anomalies range from 0.32 to 5.8%,[6,23] averaging around 2.38% (► Table 18.1). Most cases of intraoperative discovery involve patients undergoing surgery for diagnosed intervertebral disc herniations.[18,23,25,26] These cases demonstrate the ease with which anomalies are overlooked in preoperative imaging. Concern has been raised over increasingly minimal invasive surgical techniques diminishing a surgeon's likelihood of intraoperative identification of anomalous roots, thus increasing prevalence of surgical failure.[16,27] However, among patients undergoing microendoscopic discectomy, Morishita et al reported an intraoperative discovery rate for CNR anomalies of 3.6%, a relatively large figure among the surgical literature.[28]

A surgical case series by Pamir et al, detailing intraoperatively discovered anomalies among patients undergoing lumbar disc herniation surgery, reported a prevalence rate of 3%.[5] Of interest, over the 3-year period of this study 2.5% of all patients required reexploration. Among this group, secondary exploration revealed anomalies in 20% of cases.[5] One-third of Cannon et al's patients underwent secondary surgery before their anomalies were discovered and half of Neidre and MacNab's patients only had their anomalies discovered at repeat exploration for failed disc surgery.[4,13]

18.4.2 Radiologic Prevalence

Reported prevalence rates of NRAs from radiologic studies also display significant variability. Importantly, these prevalence rates must be teased apart for appropriate comparison (► Table 18.2). For instance, magnetic resonance imaging (MRI) studies have reported prevalence rates ranging from 0.25 to 6.7%.[15,29] The 0.25% prevalence rate reported by Artico et al specifically described the prevalence of CNR anomalies.[15] In contrast, the 6.67% prevalence rate reported by Aota et al included four types of extradural anomalies.[29] Of the 300 patients examined, 7 patients had CNR anomalies (2.33% prevalence), 7 patients had closely adjacent nerve roots (2.33% prevalence), 5 patients had two separate nerve roots in a single foramen (1.67% prevalence), and 1 patient had anastomosed nerve roots (0.33% prevalence). These distinctions are frequently unnoted in the literature, leading to improper prevalence comparisons. One such example is a cited 17.3% prevalence of anomalous nerve roots, originally reported by Haijiao et al.[27] Teased apart, there is merely a 0.53% prevalence of CNR anomalies, a 1.6% prevalence of nerve roots of abnormally cranial or caudal origin, and a 15.1% prevalence of furcal nerve roots.

Using metrizamide myelography, Peyster et al reported CNR anomalies in 2% of 8,000 lumbar computed tomography (CT)

Table 18.1 Surgical prevalence of nerve root anomalies, sorted by author and anomaly type

		Ethelberg and Riishede (1952)	Epstein et al (1981)	Pamir et al (1992)	Prestar (1996)	Scuderi et al (2004)	Kang et al (2008)	Song et al (2008)	Lotan et al (2010)	Morishita et al (2012)	Kessely et al (2016)	Mean
Postdural sac	Anastomosis between roots			0.25	0.08							0.17
	Closely adjacent nerve roots			0.25		1.25					0.16	0.55
	Root exit from dural sac at abnormally cranial level				0.02							0.02
	Root exit from dural sac at abnormally caudal level; transverse root											
	Conjoined nerve roots - arise from dural sac in common trunk (intra/extraforaminal division)	0.34	1.13	1	0.22	2.50	1.80	2.19	5.80		0.16	1.68
	Extradural division of nerve root											
	Two nerve roots exit one foramen (a) leaving one foramen unoccupied			0.5		1.25				3.70		1.82
	Two nerve roots exit one foramen (b) nerve roots in all foramina, but one foramen contains two separate roots			0.5							0.16	0.33
Intradural	Anastomosis between rootlets at different levels											
	Anastomosis between rootlets at different levels, external division of nerve root											
	Intradural and extradural division of nerve root											
Total		0.34	1.13	3	0.32	5.00	1.80	2.19	5.80	3.70	0.49	2.38

Note: All values are expressed as percentages.

Table 18.2 Radiographic prevalence of nerve root anomalies, sorted by author and anomaly type

		Myelography				CT		CT/MRI	MRI				Mean
		McCormick (1982)	Postacchini et al (1982)	Coughlin and Miller (1983)	Kadish and Simmons (1984)	Peyster et al (1985)	Torricelli et al (1987)	Artico et al (2006)	Aota et al (1997)	Haijiao et al (2001)	Song et al (2008)	Can et al (2017)	
Postdural sac	Anastomosis between roots		0.05						0.33				0.19
	Closely adjacent nerve roots		0.71		2.00				2.33				1.68
	Root exit from dural sac at abnormally cranial level		0.38							0.27			0.32
	Root exit from dural sac at abnormally caudal level; transverse root		0.24							1.33			0.78
	Conjoined nerve roots—arise from dural sac in common trunk (intra/extraforaminal division)	3.50	0.80	1.77	2.00	2.00	1.93	0.25	2.33	0.53	0.81	2.12	1.64
	Extradural division of nerve root												
	Two nerve roots exit one foramen (a) leaving one foramen unoccupied											1.14	1.14
	Two nerve roots exit one foramen (b) nerve roots in all foramina, but one foramen contains two separate roots								1.67			0.16	0.92
Intradural	Anastomosis between rootlets at different levels												
	Anastomosis between rootlets at different levels, external division of nerve root												
	Intradural and extradural division of nerve root												
Total		3.50	2.17	1.77	4.00	2.00	1.93	0.25	6.67	2.13	0.81	3.43	2.60

Note: All values are expressed as percentages.

scans.[21] Postacchini et al report an overall prevalence of 2.17% for NRAs.[14] In that study, the prevalence of CNR anomalies was 0.8%, while roots of abnormally cranial or caudal origin had a prevalence of 0.62%, closely adjacent nerve roots were at 0.71%, and anastomosed nerve roots had a prevalence of 0.05%.

Of interest, in a parallel metrizamide myelography and cadaveric investigation, Kadish and Simmons reported preva-

lence rates of 14 and 4%, respectively, clearly demonstrating the limitations of imaging techniques in identifying these anomalies (▶ Table 18.2 and ▶ Table 18.4).[3]

Further, it is interesting to note, considering many assertions regarding the improved diagnostic value of MRI over CT and myelography, that MRI studies do not boast prevalence rates significantly higher than those of myelography studies (▶ Table 18.3).

Table 18.3 Radiographic prevalence of nerve root anomalies, sorted by imaging modality and nerve type. All values expressed as percentages

		Myelography	CT	CT/MRI	MRI
Postdural sac	Anastomosis between roots	0.05			0.33
	Closely adjacent nerve roots	1.35			2.33
	Root exit from dural sac at abnormally cranial level	0.38			0.27
	Root exit from dural sac at abnormally caudal level; transverse root	0.24			1.33
	Conjoined nerve roots—arise from dural sac in common trunk (intra/extraforaminal division)	2.02	1.97	0.25	1.45
	Extradural division of nerve root				
	Two nerve roots exit one foramen (a) leaving one foramen unoccupied				1.14
	Two nerve roots exit one foramen (b) nerve roots in all foramina, but one foramen contains two separate roots				0.92
Intradural	Anastomosis between rootlets at different levels				
	Anastomosis between rootlets at different levels, external division of nerve root				
	Intradural and extradural division of nerve root				
Mean total		2.86	1.97	0.25	3.26

Note: All values are expressed as percentages.

Table 18.4 Cadaveric prevalence of nerve root anomalies, sorted by author and anomaly type

		d'Avella and Mingrino (1979)	Kadish and Simmons (1984)	Kikuchi (1984)	Chotigavanich and Sawangnatra (1992)	Mean
Postdural sac	Anastomosis between roots		5.00	1.69	5.00	3.90
	Closely adjacent nerve roots				1.67	1.67
	Root exit from dural sac at abnormally cranial level		2.00			2.00
	Root exit from dural sac at abnormally caudal level; transverse root					
	Conjoined nerve roots - arise from dural sac in common trunk (intra/extraforaminal division)		8.00	6.78	11.67	8.82
	Extradural division of nerve root				5.00	
	Two nerve roots exit one foramen (a) leaving one foramen unoccupied					
	Two nerve roots exit one foramen (b) nerve roots in all foramina, but one foramen contains two separate roots					
Intradural	Anastomosis between rootlets at different levels	20.46	8.00		6.67	11.71
	Anastomosis between rootlets at different levels, external division of nerve root					
	Intradural and extradural division of nerve root					
Total		20.46	23.00	8.47	30.00	20.48

Note: All values expressed as percentages.

Table 18.5 Summary of mean reported nerve root anomaly prevalence, sorted by setting of discovery and anomaly type. All values expressed as mean percentages

		Surgical	Radiographic	Cadaveric
Postdural sac	Anastomosis between roots	0.17	0.19	3.90
	Closely adjacent nerve roots	0.55	1.68	1.67
	Root exit from dural sac at abnormally cranial level	0.02	0.32	2.00
	Root exit from dural sac at abnormally caudal level; transverse root		0.78	
	Conjoined nerve roots - arise from dural sac in common trunk (intra/extraforaminal division)	1.68	1.64	8.82
	Extradural division of nerve root			5.00
	Two nerve roots exit one foramen (a) leaving one foramen unoccupied	1.82		
	Two nerve roots exit one foramen (b) nerve roots in all foramina, but one foramen contains two separate roots	0.33	1.14	
Intradural	Anastomosis between rootlets at different levels		0.92	11.71
	Anastomosis between rootlets at different levels, external division of nerve root			
	Intradural and extradural division of nerve root			
Mean total		2.38	2.60	20.48

Note: All values expressed as percentages.

18.4.3 Cadaveric Prevalence

Cadaveric studies have reported NRA rates of 8.47 to 30%,[2,9] averaging at a rate of approximately 20.48% (▶ Table 18.4). For CNR anomalies, Kadish and Simmons reported an 8% prevalence,[3] Chotigavanich and Sawangnatra an 11.67% prevalence,[9] and Hasue et al a 6.78% prevalence.[2]

Intrathecal anastomotic connections were found to have a 20.46% prevalence, with 221 out of 1,080 possible anastomoses found across all bodies.[12] The study reported a greater prevalence of a connection in sacral roots with 65% of these found within 1 to 2 cm of the spinal cord, 34% found within the cauda equina, and 11% found peripherally or close to the DRG. These anastomoses were described as appearing in parallel pairs or intersecting in an X pattern. Finally, it was found that a connection occurred between posterior roots at a significantly higher rate, almost three times more often, than between anterior roots.[12,30] Such anastomoses may translate into misleading clinical findings, due to a loss of dermatomal organization.

▶ Table 18.5 provides an overview of the surgical, radiographic, and cadaveric prevalence rates reported in the literature. Note the greater prevalence rates reported in during cadaveric studies compared to the similar radiographic and surgically reported rates. These differences suggest a large proportion of NRAs remain either asymptomatic or undiscovered during radiographic and/or surgical exploration.

18.5 Clinical Presentation

The diagnosis of NRAs remains challenging given its atypical clinical profile. Resultantly, many cases are intraoperatively diagnosed or otherwise overlooked. Generally, anomalies remain asymptotic until affected by an associated pathology which results in roots compression, entrapment, or tension.[14] It is noted that roots of an abnormally caudal origin are rarely symptomatic, tending to be incidental findings.[27] Instead, it is CNRs, with their size and intractability, which hold the greatest susceptibility to trauma.

In the presence of space-occupying comorbidities such as lateral recess stenosis or disc herniations, the effects on a CNR or two nerve roots passing through a single foramen are amplified as the little remaining reserve space is lost. Other associated findings include neural arch defects, spondylolysis or spondylolisthesis, spina bifida occulta, and other bony abnormalities. For example, the pedicle of a vertebra might be a factor in the pathogenesis of neuropathy in a CNR.[13] Tethered to a common origin, increased irritation and tension may result as roots branch around this feature, producing significant neuropathy.

Importantly, due to the space-occupying nature of CNRs, an associated pathology need not progress far before manifesting symptoms. As such, any symptomology greater in intensity than what would be expected from the associated pathology should heighten a clinician's suspicion of a CNR. However, radicular symptoms in the presence of NRAs without an associated pathology have been reported.[3,9,13,19,21,22,31] Excessive nerve root traction resulting in a strain effect, manifested through normal movement of the spine, may be at fault in these cases.

The pathology of NRAs often mimics, and frequently occurs with, herniated intervertebral discs.[17,19] However, surgical exploration in patients with a diagnosis of disc herniation has revealed no or minimal abnormal disc pathology, or disc protrusion at another level.[21,22,32] Such cases are frequently associated with NRAs consisting of two closely adjacent nerve roots exiting through a single foramen.[14,22,33]

Most commonly, patients present with a long history of either consistent or intermittent pain, originating in the lower back and radiating to the hips, buttocks, and legs.[19,34,35] In roughly half of cases, an aggravating event, such as heavy lifting or strain, is associated with either the increase or radiation of low back pain.[13,35] Typically, younger patients present with lower back pain and radiculopathy, while older patients demonstrate a progressive sciatica.[36]

In differentiating an NRA from a disc herniation, it has been observed that claudicant pains, concurrent with or preceding radiculopathy, should heighten a physician's suspicion of an NRA.[23,26] Lotan et al found statistically significant differences in symptomology between patients with a CNR and those with herniated discs.[23] CNR patients demonstrate significantly higher rates of claudicant and radicular symptoms, while presenting with fewer neurological deficits such as motor weakness or hypoesthesia.

The straight leg raise (SLR) test is commonly utilized as a diagnostic indicator. The lack of a positive SLR test has been hailed as the most prominent distinguishing feature between NRAs and disc herniations.[13,19] However, elsewhere this claim has been strongly refuted, with some NRA case series of predominantly presenting with positive SLR tests[10] or presenting with positive rates identical to those of a matched cohort of disc herniation patients.[23] Additional studies have revealed inconsistent patterns of presentation.[5,7,8,16,18,28] As such, the SLR test appears an unreliable clinical indicator.

In over 50% of cases, symptomatic NRAs are in fact associated with disc herniations. These patients tend to present with more marked neurological deficits than typical disc herniation patients.[7,8,15] A comorbidity with a herniated disc may cause additional discrepancies, including symptomatic indications at an incorrect level or side. Comorbidities include stenosis of the lumbar canal, narrowing of the lateral recess and/or intervertebral foramen, spondylolisthesis and spondylolysis, and spina bifida.

18.6 Imaging

On myelography, CNR anomalies are characterized by asymmetry of the roots as they exit the thecal sac on myelography. A broader dural sheath will be present at the site of the anomaly, exiting midway between the upper and lower nerve root sheaths of the contralateral side. This finding will be associated with a widening of the axillary pouch, and is best observed on the straight anteroposterior view.[16,20,37] A "gun barrel" appearance has also been observed in the presence of a CNR.[35] Anastomotic connections can almost never be appreciated via myelography.[29]

CT imaging was the next standard of imaging nerve roots. CT affords slightly enhanced definition of individual roots, compared to MRI.[38] Greater detection of root sleeve filling and bony alterations of the spinal canal are also provided by CT myelography, compared to metrizamide myelography.[39] It has been suggested that CT imaging has up to an 83% rate of CNR diagnosis.[5] However, considering discrepancies in reported prevalence rates, this claim is difficult to substantiate.

Bony changes of the spinal canal may also serve some diagnostic value. Asymmetry of the lateral recess has been noted in cases of CNR, with widening of the lateral recess ipsilateral to the CNR.[40] This asymmetry is postulated to result from either slow erosion by cerebrospinal fluid pulsations or from an accommodating developmental response to the abnormal mass. It is noted that NRAs are on occasion associated with complex bony anomalies such as dysplastic laminae, transverse processes, and facets.

Additional or conjoined roots will present as increased soft-tissues masses, decreasing epidural fat in the ipsilateral lateral recess, or neuroforamen.[41] CNRs can mimic an extruded disc fragment given the resulting asymmetry of epidural space. Estimation of the material's attenuation value, a measure of density, has been demonstrated to aid in the differentiation of NRAs from disc herniations. Helms et al proposed the use of the "identify" or "blink" mode to identify subtle differences in material's densities.[41] The density of a CNR is similar or slightly greater than that of the adjacent thecal sac, "blinking" around 10 to 20 HU, whereas an extruded disc fragment would present with a significantly higher attenuation coefficient, around 40 to 50 HU.[21,40,41] As such, if isodense or mildly hyperdense tissues are identified in the anterolateral area of epidural space, a CNR should be suspected.[36,42]

An additional difference exists in the location of these densities. Whereas extruded disc fragments generally migrate away from the disc space, CNR anomalies are usually found at the pedicle level, in the anterolateral aspect of the spinal canal, adjacent and contiguous with the thecal sac.[21]

NRAs sit 90 degrees to sagittal or transaxial images, resulting in a high potential for misdiagnosis, specifically misinterpretation of NRAs for disc herniations. As such, correlation between myelographic and CT-myelography findings remains essential. It has been suggested the myelography is superior for the diagnosis of CNRs, which can be misidentified as disc herniations on CT.[43] There are some limitations to this imaging technique, primarily revolving around false-positives for disc protrusion, neural foraminal extrusion, or dumbbell tumors. When associated with large posterolateral disc herniations and/or stenosis of the lateral recess, NRAs may remain concealed.

MRI is currently held as the "gold standard" in imaging for the diagnosis of NRAs. T1-weighted images (T1WI) are preferred due to the greater contrast between the dural sac and intervening epidural fat, aiding in the identification of certain secondary signs, while imaging on the coronal plane permits tracking of anomalies, both allowing for a more definitive diagnosis.[24] Several secondary signs have proved useful in the diagnosis of NRAs. Song et al in a retrospective review of intraoperatively discovered CNRs found three reliable signs, best seen on axial T1WI: (1) the "corner sign" is described as an asymmetric morphology of the anterolateral corner of the dural sac and was noted in all cases. Song et al noted that (1) while this "sign" was highly selective, it was nonspecific and can be seen in other conditions such as spinal stenosis and epidural lipomatosis; as such, this sign requires corroboration with additional features; (2) the "fat crescent sign" is characterized by intervening extradural fat tissue between the asymmetric dural sac and the CNR; this sign was present in two-thirds of reviewed case; (3) finally, the "parallel sign" described the parallel course of the entire nerve root at the disc level and was present in half of all reviewed cases.[24] It is in the identification of these signs that the elevated contrast between the dural sac and the intervening epidural fat afforded by T1WI is most useful.

Kang et al identified two additional signs to aid in the diagnosis of CNRs. The "sagittal shoulder sign" is described as a vertical structure connecting two consecutive nerve roots and the overlying disc on the sagittal MR images. A retrospective analysis of 10 cases of CNR anomalies found the presence of the sign in 90.9% of cases.[25] The "axial common passage" sign is noted by the presence of the common passage of two consecutive nerve roots through the neural foramen on axial MR images. The sign requires the presence of a broader dural sheath at the point of convergence of the roots or the presence of confluent roots taking off a level halfway between contralateral roots. Kang et al's retrospective analysis found this sign to be present in over 50% of cases. Recently, MR neurography has been used to demonstrate CNRs.[44] However, resolution limitations remain the most significant impediment to this imaging technique's diagnostic value.

18.7 Surgery

Preoperative identification of NRAs is vital to avoid negative surgical outcomes. A lack of preoperative diagnosis and failure to intraoperatively identify an NRA dramatically increases the chance of damage to neural elements. Without knowledge of existing anomalies, excessive retraction may result in dural tears, accidental incision, damage to the nerve rootlets, or a nerve root avulsion, leading to postoperative neurological deficits and neuropathic pain.

White et al described several clues for intraoperative diagnosis.[8] When difficulty is encountered during attempts to mobilize a nerve root medially, an NRA should be expected and further lateral exposure must be obtained. Undiagnosed NRAs should be suspected in all cases of failed disc surgery and are not infrequently found in secondary operations.[4,5,13]

The principal goals of surgery in the setting of an NRA include visualization, mobilization, and decompression of the involved roots to avoid persistent compression and traction. The common dural sleeve of CNRs is often located above a ruptured disc and attempts to extract the disc frequently result in excessive surgical trauma. Additionally, migration of disc material into the secondary axilla may increase the technical difficulty of disc extraction.

To this end, it was initially suggested that wide exposure via a hemilaminectomy is ideal, minimizing the risk of excess traction or lacerations.[10,13,14,15,45] Cannon et al further recommended laterally positioning patients during the procedure to allow for larger exposure of the nerve root, disc, and foramen.[13] Other authors suggested the use of a laminectomy and foraminotomy before removing the disc.[46] However, White et al reported only 30% of patients treated via hemilaminectomy and discectomy achieved successful reductions in pain.[8,10,13] In a postoperative analysis, Stambough et al found that the more extensive the foraminotomy and total decompression, via removal of the medial portion of the superior facet and as much removal of the pedicle as necessary to free the anomalous nerve root, the greater the chance symptom relief.[47] This finding, that the extent of decompression is correlated with patient's pain reduction, supports the notion of NRA symptomology arising in part due to decreased mobility.

White et al noted that the close approximation of the bifurcating CNR to the pedicle was a significant challenge in root mobilization. Seven out of eight patients who underwent the hemilaminectomy combined with a pediculectomy prior to discectomy had reductions in pain and returned to work.[8] The authors posited that the pathogenesis of neuropathy is dependent on the topographical relationship between the secondary axilla and intervening pedicle. As such, discretionary removal of the pedicle prevents excessive surgical trauma incurred by attempts to extract a ruptured disc from beneath a fixed CNR.

Given the goals of maximizing nerve root mobilization and decompression, it is now commonly suggested to perform a hemilaminectomy with the potential extension to a facetectomy and partial pediculectomy to prevent over-retraction.[5,7] A foraminotomy and/or pediculectomy have also been stated as necessary during initial discectomy when two nerve roots occupy a single foramen or in the case of anastomoses between roots to obtain appropriate decompression.[4] Pediculectomy can cause spinal instability, back pain, and may warrant fusion. Alternatively, it has been suggested that successful decompression can be achieved via a laminectomy which maintains stability and appropriate mobility of the spinal canal.[48] Otherwise, the removal of a herniated disc through a contralateral laminectomy may be advised when an abnormal nerve configuration/fixation prevents adequate exposure.[15]

Spinal stenosis is often associated with a herniated disc. In these settings, unroofing of the lateral recess, foraminotomy, and medial facetectomy are usually required to attain adequate decompression and mobilization.[10,15] Authors have commented that in these cases hemilaminectomy and discectomy procedures do not provide sufficient decompression, instead recommending a laminectomy and facetectomy with excision of the pedicle and all compressive tissue.[5,49,50] Ultimately, the choice of procedure is determined by the requirements associated with achieving maximum nerve root mobilization and decompression.

18.7.1 Review of Classification Systems

There exist several overlapping classification systems for NRAs (▶ Table 18.6).

Cannon et al originally classified NRAs into three general morphologically determined categories.[13]

- Type I (conjoined roots): Two adjacent root sleeves show a common origin when exiting the dural sac. They may either exit through the same or independent foramina.
- Type II (extradural anastomoses): A nerve which branches shortly after emitting from the dural sac, joining the root immediately below.
- Type III (caudal origin): a root which originates from the dural sac at a more caudal level than average, forming an approximately right angle with the dural sac.

From their case series, Postacchini et al divided NRAs into five major types[14]:

- Type I: One or more nerve roots emerge from the dural sac at an abnormally cranial level.
- Type II: One nerve root emerges from the dural sac at an abnormally caudal level.
- Type III: Two or more nerve root emerge through closely adjacent openings in the dural sac.
- Type IV: Two nerve roots emerge from the dural sac in a common nerve trunk. The CNRs either remain joined, leaving through a single foramen, or separated before exiting through their appropriate foramen.
- Type V: An interconnection between two nerve roots distal to the dural sac.

Table 18.6 Summary of nerve root anomaly classification systems

		Cannon et al (1962)	Postacchini et al (1982)	Neidre and MacNab (1983)	Kadish and Simmons (1984)	Chotigavanichand Sawangnatra (1992)
Postdural sac	Anastomosis between roots	Type II	Type V	Type III	Type III	Type II
	Closely adjacent nerve roots		Type III	Type I (B)	Type II (C)	Type VI
	Root exit from dural sac at abnormally cranial level		Type I		Type II (A)	
	Root exit from dural sac at abnormally caudal level; transverse root	Type III	Type II		Type II (B)	
	Conjoined nerve roots - arise from dural sac in common trunk (Intra/extraforaminal division)	Type I	Type IV	Type I (A)	Type II (D)	
	Extradural division of nerve root				Type IV	Type III
	Two nerve roots exit though one foramen (a) leaving one foramen unoccupied or (b) nerve roots in all foramina, but one foramen contains two separate roots			Type II (A)/(B)		
Intradural	Anastomosis between rootlets at different levels				Type I	Type I
	Anastomosis between rootlets at different levels, external division of nerve root					Type IV
	Intradural and extradural division of nerve root					Type V

Elaborating on the three-category classification system of Cannon et al, Neidre and MacNab added subtypes for types I and II[4]:

- Type I (A): Two nerve roots arise from the dural sac in a common dural sheath.
- Type I (B): Two nerve roots are almost conjoined, resulting in a nerve exiting the dural sac at a right angle, similarly to cervical nerve roots.
- Type II (A): Two nerve roots exiting through one foramen, leaving one root canal unoccupied.
- Type II (B): There are nerve roots in all foramina, but one foramen has two individual roots.
- Type III: Adjacent nerve roots interconnected.

Kadish and Simmons classified NRAs in four general types, containing several subtypes[3]:

- Type I: Intradural connection between rootlets at different levels.
- Type II: Anomalous origin of nerve roots: (a) cranial origin; (b) caudal origin; (c) combination of (a) and (b) affecting more than one nerve root (closely adjacent roots); and (d) CNRs.
- Type III: Extradural connection between nerve roots.
- Type IV: Extradural division of the nerve root.

Chotigavanich and Sawangnatra classified NRAs into six fundamental groups, based on findings from their 60-cadaver study[9]:

- Type I: Intradural connection between rootlets at different levels.
- Type II: Extradural connection between nerve roots.
- Type III: Extradural division of the nerve root.
- Type IV: Intradural connection between rootlets and extradural division of nerve root.

- Type V: Intradural and extradural division of nerve root.
- Type VI: Closely adjacent nerve roots.

18.8 Conclusion

We have herein discussed the major NRAs, their anatomy, prevalence rates, clinical and radiographic presentations, surgical management, and various classification systems. Surgical and radiographic investigations boast low prevalence rates, yet cadaveric investigations reveal meaningfully higher rates highlighting the percentage of NRAs which remain unappreciated. Given its atypical clinical profile and unreliable radiographic detection, NRAs are largely diagnosed intraoperatively. While all NRAs may produce symptomology, the susceptibility of CNRs to trauma increases the likelihood of related symptomology. While clinical findings are variable, NRAs tend to mimic and are often misdiagnosed as herniated intervertebral discs. There exist several radiographic signs to suggest the presence of an NRA, but resolution remains the most significant limitation.

Surgical aims involve achieving maximum decompression and mobilization, which correlate with greater reductions in patient pain. Unappreciated NRAs represent a major potential for neurologic injury if they undergo excessive traction during attempts at routine mobilization. Given the frequency with which NRAs are not observed preoperatively, surgeons should maintain a high intraoperative index of suspicion for these features.

There is significant overlap between the five reviewed classifications. This is not ideal and a consolidation into a standardized system would be of benefit for clinical reporting and analysis.

References

[1] Hogan Q, Toth J. Anatomy of soft tissues of the spinal canal. Reg Anesth Pain Med. 1999; 24(4):303–310

[2] Hasue M, Kikuchi S, Sakuyama Y, Ito T. Anatomic study of the interrelation between lumbosacral nerve roots and their surrounding tissues. Spine. 1983; 8(1):50–58

[3] Kadish LJ, Simmons EH. Anomalies of the lumbosacral nerve roots. An anatomical investigation and myelographic study. J Bone Joint Surg Br. 1984; 66 (3):411–416

[4] Neidre A, MacNab I. Anomalies of the lumbosacral nerve roots. Review of 16 cases and classification. Spine. 1983; 8(3):294–299

[5] Pamir MN, Ozek MM, Ozer AF, Keleş GE, Erzen C. Surgical considerations in patients with lumbar spinal root anomalies. Paraplegia. 1992; 30(5):370–375

[6] Prestar FJ. Anomalies and malformations of lumbar spinal nerve roots. Minim Invasive Neurosurg. 1996; 39(4):133–137

[7] Taghipour M, Razmkon A, Hosseini K. Conjoined lumbosacral nerve roots: analysis of cases diagnosed intraoperatively. J Spinal Disord Tech. 2009; 22 (6):413–416

[8] White JG, III, Strait TA, Binkley JR, Hunter SE. Surgical treatment of 63 cases of conjoined nerve roots. J Neurosurg. 1982; 56(1):114–117

[9] Chotigavanich C, Sawangnatra S. Anomalies of the lumbosacral nerve roots. An anatomic investigation. Clin Orthop Relat Res. 1992(278):46–50

[10] Epstein JA, Carras R, Ferrar J, Hyman RA, Khan A. Conjoined lumbosacral nerve roots. Management of herniated discs and lateral recess stenosis in patients with this anomaly. J Neurosurg. 1981; 55(4):585–589

[11] Hogan Q. Size of human lower thoracic and lumbosacral nerve roots. Anesthesiology. 1996; 85(1):37–42

[12] d'Avella D, Mingrino S. Microsurgical anatomy of lumbosacral spinal roots. J Neurosurg. 1979; 51(6):819–823

[13] Cannon BW, Hunter SE, Picaza JA. Nerve-rootanomalies in lumbar-disc surgery. J Neurosurg. 1962; 19(3):208–214

[14] Postacchini F, Urso S, Ferro L. Lumbosacral nerve-root anomalies. J Bone Joint Surg Am. 1982; 64(5):721–729

[15] Artico M, Carloia S, Piacentini M, et al. Conjoined lumbosacral nerve roots: observations on three cases and review of the literature. Neurocirugia (Astur). 2006; 17(1):54–59

[16] Bouchard JM, Copty M, Langelier R. Preoperative diagnosis of conjoined roots anomaly with herniated lumbar disks. Surg Neurol. 1978; 10(4):229–231

[17] Davidson D, Rowan R, Reilly C. Lumbosacral nerve root anomaly associated with spondylolisthesis in an adolescent: a case report and review of the literature. Spine. 2006; 31(19):E718–E721

[18] Can H, Kircelli A, Kavadar G, et al. Lumbosacral conjoined root anomaly: anatomical considerations of exiting angles and root thickness. Turk Neurosurg. 2017; 27(4):617–622

[19] Ethelberg S, Riishede J. Malformation of lumbar spinal roots and sheaths in the causation of low backache and sciatica. J Bone Joint Surg Br. 1952; 34-B (3):442–446

[20] McCormick CC. Developmental asymmetry of roots of the cauda equina at metrizamide myelography: report of seven cases with a review of the literature. Clin Radiol. 1982; 33(4):427–434

[21] Peyster RG, Teplick JG, Haskin ME. Computed tomography of lumbosacral conjoined nerve root anomalies. Potential cause of false-positive reading for herniated nucleus pulposus. Spine. 1985; 10(4):331–337

[22] Scuderi GJ, Vaccaro AR, Brusovanik GV, Kwon BK, Berta SC. Conjoined lumbar nerve roots: a frequently underappreciated congenital abnormality. J Spinal Disord Tech. 2004; 17(2):86–93

[23] Lotan R, Al-Rashdi A, Yee A, Finkelstein J. Clinical features of conjoined lumbosacral nerve roots versus lumbar intervertebral disc herniations. Eur Spine J. 2010; 19(7):1094–1098

[24] Song SJ, Lee JW, Choi JY, et al. Imaging features suggestive of a conjoined nerve root on routine axial MRI. Skeletal Radiol. 2008; 37(2):133–138

[25] Kang CH, Shin MJ, Kim SM, et al. Conjoined lumbosacral nerve roots compromised by disk herniation: sagittal shoulder sign for the preoperative diagnosis. Skeletal Radiol. 2008; 37(3):225–231

[26] Kessely YC, Ibrahima T, Sakho MG, Mbaye M, Meidal MA, Traore Y, Diop AA, Sakho Y. Diagnostic and therapeutic implications of conjoined nerve root anomalies: a senegalese study of three cases. Iranian Journal of Neurosurgery. 2016; 1(3):21–25

[27] Haijiao W, Koti M, Smith FW, Wardlaw D. Diagnosis of lumbosacral nerve root anomalies by magnetic resonance imaging. J Spinal Disord. 2001; 14(2): 143–149

[28] Morishita Y, Ohta H, Matsumoto Y, Shiba K, Naito M. Intra-operative identification of conjoined lumbosacral nerve roots: a report of three cases. J Orthop Surg (Hong Kong). 2012; 20(1):90–93

[29] Aota Y, Saito Y, Yoshikawa K, Asada T, Kondo S, Watanabe K. Presurgical identification of extradural nerve root anomalies by coronal fat-suppressed magnetic resonance imaging: a report of six cases and a review of the literature. J Spinal Disord. 1997; 10(2):167–175

[30] Hauck EF, Wittkowski W, Bothe HW. Intradural microanatomy of the nerve roots S1-S5 at their origin from the conus medullaris. J Neurosurg Spine. 2008; 9(2):207–212

[31] Kitab SA, Miele VJ, Lavelle WF, Benzel EC. Pathoanatomic basis for stretch-induced lumbar nerve root injury with a review of the literature. Neurosurgery. 2009; 65(1):161–167, discussion 167–168

[32] Keon-Cohen B. Abnormal arrangement of the lower lumbar and first sacral nerves within the spinal canal. J Bone Joint Surg Br. 1968; 50(2):261–265

[33] Goldstein B. Anatomic issues related to cervical and lumbosacral radiculopathy. Phys Med Rehabil Clin N Am. 2002; 13(3):423–437

[34] Akbasak A, Biliciler B, Vatansever M, Baysal T, Toksoz M.. Conjoined lumbosacral nerve roots: report of two cases. Turk Neurosurg. 1995; 5(3–4):57–61

[35] Gomez JG, Dickey JW, Bachow TB. Conjoined lumbosacral nerve roots. Acta Neurochir (Wien). 1993; 120(3–4):155–158

[36] Böttcher J, Petrovitch A, Sörös P, Malich A, Hussein S, Kaiser WA. Conjoined lumbosacral nerve roots: current aspects of diagnosis. Eur Spine J. 2004; 13 (2):147–151

[37] Coughlin JR, Miller JD. Metrizamide myelography in conjoined lumbosacral nerve roots. J Can Assoc Radiol. 1983; 34(1):23–25

[38] Cohen MS, Wall EJ, Kerber CW, Abitbol J-J, Garfin SR. The anatomy of the cauda equina on CT scans and MRI. J Bone Joint Surg Br. 1991; 73(3):381–384

[39] Meyer JD, Latchaw RE. Conjoined lumbosacral nerve roots-metrizamide myelography and CT findings. J Comput Assist Tomogr. 1983; 7(1):202

[40] Hoddick WK, Helms CA. Bony spinal canal changes that differentiate conjoined nerve roots from herniated nucleus pulposus. Radiology. 1985; 154 (1):119–120

[41] Helms CA, Dorwart RH, Gray M. The CT appearance of conjoined nerve roots and differentiation from a herniated nucleus pulposus. Radiology. 1982; 144 (4):803–807

[42] Torricelli P, Spina V, Martinelli C. CT diagnosis of lumbosacral conjoined nerve roots. Findings in 19 cases. Neuroradiology. 1987; 29(4):374–379

[43] Cail WS, Butler AB. Conjoined lumbosacral nerve roots. Diagnosis with metrizamide myelography. Surg Neurol. 1983; 20(2):113–119

[44] Engar C, Wadhwa V, Weinberg B, Chhabra A. Conjoined lumbosacral nerve roots: direct demonstration on MR neurography. Clin Imaging. 2014; 38(6): 892–894

[45] Aziz A, Kazmi A, Khan S, Shoaib S. Conjoined lumbosacral nerve roots: a case report and review of literature. Pak J Surg. 2012; 28(2):160–162

[46] Rask MR. Anomalous lumbosacral nerve roots associated with spondylolisthesis. Surg Neurol. 1977; 8(2):139–140

[47] Stambough JL, Balderston RA, Booth RE, Rothman RH. Surgical management of sciatica involving anomalous lumbar nerve roots. J Spinal Disord. 1988; 1 (2):111–114, discussion 114–115

[48] Houra K, Beroš V, Kovač D, Sajko T, Gnjidić Z, Rotim K. Accidental finding of an anomalous spinal nerve root during lumbar-disc surgery: a case report and a review of literature. Coll Antropol. 2010; 34(3):1105–1108

[49] Goffin J, Plets C. Association of conjoined and anastomosed nerve roots in the lumbar region. A case report. Clin Neurol Neurosurg. 1987; 89(2):117–120

[50] Jokhi VH, Ponde SV, Sonawane C, Bansal SS, Chavhan A. Conjoint lumbosacral nerve root-a case report. J Orthop Case Rep. 2015; 5(4):14–16

[51] Kikuchi S, Hasue M, Nishiyama K, Ito T. Anatomic and clinical studies of radicular symptoms. Spine. 1984; 9(1):23–30

19 Lumbar Dorsal Root Ganglia

Mohammad W. Kassem, R. Shane Tubbs

Abstract

The dorsal root ganglia (or spinal ganglia) are described as nodulelike structures found on the posterior root of each spinal nerve, which contains the soma (or cell bodies) of the afferent sensory nerves carrying signals back to the central nervous system. There is a dorsal root ganglion associated with each spinal nerve, and their ability to execute their function of receiving afferent nerve signals can be impeded by numerous pathologies. Here, we discuss the ganglionopathies caused by inflammatory, congenital, and traumatic conditions.

Keywords: dorsal root ganglion, herpes simplex, tangier disease, radiculopathy, cholesterol esters, Sjogren's

19.1 Introduction

The dorsal root ganglia (or spinal ganglia) (▶ Fig. 19.1) are described as nodulelike structures found on the posterior root of each spinal nerve, which contains the soma (or cell bodies) of the afferent sensory nerves carrying signals back to the central nervous system.[1] These structures develop from neural crest cells migrating into the rostral mesoderm, and each is described as oval and reddish in nature with size depending on its root for the corresponding level.[2] Histologically, the ganglia are described as containing the cell bodies of the pseudounipolar sensory neurons, which are spherical and lack dendrites. Since the cell bodies have no dendrites and are not directly involved in conducting sensory signals, the ganglion also has glial cells (satellite cells) within it to insulate the cell bodies electrically. Nerve fibers and connective tissue are also noted on histology, but the predominant image is the circular cell bodies of the sensory nerves with the glial cells interspersed between them.[3]

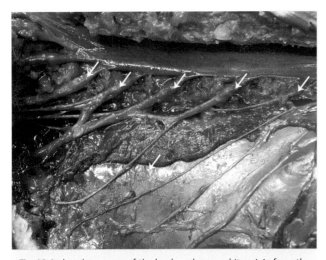

Fig. 19.1 dorsal exposure of the lumbar plexus and its origin from the thecal sac. Note the dorsal root ganglia (*arrows*) within their meningeal sheaths just lateral to the dura mater of the thecal sac.

There is a dorsal root ganglion (DRG) associated with each spinal nerve, the only possible exception being the C1 spinal nerve, which is primarily a motor neuron. The DRG of the C1 spinal nerve may be rudimentary or absent.[4] The pseudounipolar nature of the sensory nerves in the peripheral nervous system means that the cell body is located between the two branches, which act as axons. These branches can be labeled the distal and proximal processes. Signals in these nerves begin in the distal process via communication between sensory cells, travel proximally, can bypass the soma, and continue into the spinal cord via the posterior root into the posterior (or dorsal) horn to synapse in one of the sensory pathway tracts.[2]

19.2 Location

The locations of DRG depend on the level at which the corresponding nerve is found. From the cervical down to the lumbar spine, the DRG for these nerves are generally located in or marginally outside the midpoints of the intervertebral foramina, immediately lateral to the perforation of the dura mater by the dorsal root. However, in the lower lumbar, sacral, and coccygeal regions they can be intraspinal or within the dura mater itself.[5] One consequence of the positioning of these ganglia is clinical manifestations with compression. Proximally located DRG is more likely to be associated with radicular syndromes.[6] This is especially true in L4 and L5 radiculopathy as DRG become more proximal the further caudal they are. These ganglia are vulnerable to compression owing to the narrow epiradicular space, larger size, and risk of compression from spinal disc herniation. They can also have indentations.[6] Kikuchi et al noted variations in the appearance of these indentations, which were more common in older patients and patients with radiculopathy and were absent in the S1 nerve roots.[7] These findings suggest that the main causes of ganglionic indentation are compression by the superior facets at the intervertebral foramina and bulging discs causing compression. The highest incidence for indentation was in the intraspinal DRG; more distal DRG had a lower incidence.[8]

19.3 Blood Supply

The DRG receive their blood supply from nutrient arteries that branch directly from the dorsal division of each spinal segmental artery.[9] Compression of the spinal nerve distal to a DRG decreased blood flow by up to 45%, while compression proximal to it caused only a 10 to 15% decrease.[10] The ganglion has more abundant intrinsic vessels than the nerve root, consisting of continuous and fenestrated capillaries. The association of such capillaries with the DRG suggests the blood–nerve barrier around the ganglion is not as impervious as originally thought, similar to peripheral nerves, so the DRG could be subject to more hemodynamic stress and/or injury. This is especially true for patients with diabetes mellitus, who in postmortem studies had statistically significantly thicker DRG perineural capillary basement membranes than nondiabetics.[11] This finding is not surprising in view of findings with diabetic peripheral neuropathy, but could implicate DRG pathology in neuropathic manifestations of dysesthesia and anesthesia in diabetics.

19.4 Lumbar Dorsal Root Ganglion

The lumbar DRG are clinically important owing to their proximal position in the foraminal spaces from which the nerves exit. This set of ganglia has been proved to be important in lower back pain and sciatica because of their susceptibility to mechanical irritation from injury.[12]

Studies to visualize the lumbar DRG have elucidated their role in pain when they are subject to compression through lumbar disc herniation.[7] In one study, the location of the DRG from the L1–L3 nerves were found to be extraforaminal or foraminal, while the L4 DRG were in the foraminal region, and the L5 DRG were predominantly in the foraminal region with the possibility of being intraspinal.[13] Only at the L5 level were intraspinal ganglia noted, more in females than males, though there was no statistically significant difference.[14] The same studies showed the more caudally located ganglia to be wider and longer. The architecture of the lumbar DRG proved unique. The L5 and L2 DRG have a trigangliar architecture, which is considered an anatomical variant as they are predominantly singular at those levels. The L3 and L4 DRG tend to show a near 1:1 ratio of singular and bigangliar architecture, and the L1 DRG is almost always single.[7]

19.5 Pathologies of the Dorsal Root Ganglia

19.5.1 Sensory Ganglionopathies

Sensory ganglionopathies (or sensory neuronopathies) are a distinct group of peripheral neuropathies that affect the cell bodies of sensory neurons. They can occur in a DRG or in the trigeminal ganglia and lead to the degeneration and destruction of both their central and peripheral sensory projections. This pathological process causes degeneration of both short and long axons. The clinical presentation of a sensory ganglionopathy entails severe sensory loss in the effect region of the ganglion. An assortment of disease conditions can cause ganglionopathies especially since, as discussed earlier, the blood–nerve barrier around the DRG is permeable, rendering the ganglion vulnerable to infection, tumor metastasis, autoimmune disorders, and toxins. Hereditary disorders such as Tay–Sachs can also be implicated in sensory ganglionopathies. Ganglionectomy of the DRG can be used to diagnose the condition causing the sensory ganglionopathy.[15,16]

A sensory ganglionopathy can begin with patchy, asymmetrical sensory loss involving proximal regions. As it progresses, it can involve more distal regions and become more symmetrical. This is different from peripheral neuropathy, where distal sensory loss precedes proximal sensory loss.[17] Necrosis of the sensory cell bodies within the ganglia results in the degeneration of the axons, which is important as the patients show clinical symptoms of gait ataxia (due to denervation of the muscle spindles), loss of vibratory sense, loss of tendon reflexes, and dysesthesias. Ganglionopathies have been dubbed "ataxic neuropathies" in view of the gait ataxia, but this title is misleading as ataxic

neuropathies also include other conditions such as demyelinating neuropathies, where ataxia is the main symptom.

Various conditions can cause sensory ganglionopathies. Paraneoplastic syndromes, especially with small cell lung cancer, can be causes. Patients present with a rapidly progressive and painful neuropathy resulting in loss of all sensory modalities when neoplastic syndromes are causal. On histology, the DRG can show marked inflammation, loss of ganglion cell bodies, and gliosis. Symptoms usually present in the upper limbs first. Over time, the sensory loss can extend to all limbs, face, neck, chest, and abdomen. Tendon reflexes are reduced or absent, and patients become bedridden owing to severe ataxia and unsteady gait. Two antibodies have been associated with paraneoplastic sensory ganglionopathies: antineuronal nuclear autoantibodies type 1 (ANNA-1), and collapsin response mediator protein-5 (CRMP-5).[18]

Chronic inflammatory conditions such as Sjogren's can also cause sensory ganglionopathy. In Sjogren's-related ganglionopathy, sensory disturbances are unilateral and asymmetric and predominantly involve the upper limbs. Symptoms include sensory loss and inability to use the limb, but with normal strength retained by the muscle, and eventually progress to symmetrical sensory loss along with the other clinical manifestations characteristic of Sjogren's.

Familial and inherited diseases such as Tangier's disease (familial analphalipoproteinemia) can also cause sensory ganglionopathy. Tangier's disease is an inborn error of metabolism due to a mutation in the adenosine triphosphate (ATP)–binding cassette transporter 1, which is involved in the passage of cholesterol from within the cells to outside the cells (efflux). Tangier's disease is categorized by the absence of or extremely low number of high density lipoproteins (HDLs) in the plasma and with elevated levels of cholesterol esters in most of the tissues throughout the body including tonsils, liver, spleen, lymph node, thymus, intestinal mucosa, peripheral nerves, and cornea.[19] In Tangier's-related ganglionopathy, there is predominantly axonal sensorimotor polyneuropathy with signs of chronic and active denervation and mild to moderate demyelination. Some patients are described as having a syrinx-like distribution of the neuropathies that is proximal to distal with peripheral neuropathy. As the cholesterol esters accumulate in the tissues, including the DRG, more symptoms begin to arise, such as radiculopathies and disruptions to the reticuloendothelial system.

Medications such as chemotherapeutic agents and pyridoxine have been implicated in causing sensory ganglionopathies. Pyridoxine intoxication is said to be a reversible cause, and there can be partial recovery when chemotherapeutic agents are discontinued.[17]

Chemotherapeutic agents that are platinum based, such as cisplatin, are known to cause apoptosis of the DRG neurons in vitro and in vivo. Cisplatin binds to neuronal DNA preferentially by an unknown mechanism; however, it is thought that DRG DNA has less shielding by binding proteins and histones. Roughly 20% of patients treated with platinum-based chemotherapeutic agents are unable to finish the regimen due to the severe neuropathic side effects.[20]

Other underlying conditions that can result in sensory ganglionopathies include herpes zoster infection (to be discussed separately), rabies, and human immunodeficiency virus (HIV).

HIV infection has been noted for causing ganglionopathies. Postmortem examination of the DRG revealed a considerable increase in nodules of Nageotte, causing sensory neuropathy in the patients.[21] The ganglia were also infiltrated with lymphocytes, which could also have injured the cell bodies of the sensory neurons.

One condition that can lead to ganglionopathy, specifically in the lumbar DRG, is via the effects of a subarachnoid hemorrhage (SAH) causing vasospasm of the artery of Adamkiewicz (AKA), the main artery that supplies blood to the lower portion of the spinal cord. SAH can occur for a number of reasons, with the leading causes being trauma and spontaneity. Arterial vasospasm typically occurs in more than 33% of patients following a SAH. The vasospasm of AKA that occurs after an SAH event will cause ischemic changes and lead to neurodegeneration of the lumbar 4 DRG (L4DRG).[22]

19.5.2 Herpes Zoster and Changes in the Dorsal Root Ganglion

Herpes zoster is a viral infection that usually begins with chickenpox, the clinical manifestation of the primary varicella zoster virus infection. During the course of chickenpox, the virus spreads through sensory nerves from the skin and travels along the sensory pathway to infect the cell bodies in either the DRG or the cranial sensory ganglia. The sensory nerve cell bodies become a latent store of infection as the genomic DNA of the virus survives in the nuclei, potentially reoccurring at any time. When reactivation occurs, usually in immunocompromised or elderly (immunosenescent) patients, the virus multiplies and infects the other cell bodies within the ganglion.[23] The reinfection process causes an inflammatory reaction resulting in pain in the dermatome.[24] The ganglia in which infection recurs have also been known to suffer necrotic changes, appearing pale and fibrinoid on postmortem examination.[25] The viral spread down the sensory neurons back to the dermatome results in the characteristic clinical rash manifestation, affecting only a single dermatome rather than the diffuse spread in the initial zoster infection (chickenpox).

Even after the clinical manifestation is resolved, postherpetic neuralgia has been reported in patients lasting for months to years after the herpetic rash has healed. The cause of the neuralgia is injury to the primary afferent nociceptors in the cutaneous tissue, or to the DRG if it has suffered necrosis and fibrosis. As a result, patients can suffer from persistent burning pain and allodynia, which interferes with sleep and decreases the quality of life. Treatment can include tricyclic antidepressants, topical analgesics, and topical capsaicin.[24]

19.5.3 Sensory Ganglioneuromas

Ganglioneuromas are rare benign tumors that arise from neural crest cell-derived ganglionic progenitor cells and can contain a combination of small round cells and large cells with eccentric nuclei.[26] Most ganglioneuromas grow in the autonomic nervous system, usually the sympathetic ganglia, but very rarely, tumors have been seen to grow from sensory ganglia. They grow in children and young adults and can be associated with hereditary conditions such as neurofibromatosis type 1 (von Recklinghausen disease), though it is very rare. They can grow in a dumbbell shape into the cervical spinal canal extradurally. Cervical ganglioneuromas are unilateral and single. They cause sensory deprivation and can lead to progressive limb ataxia and/or gait disturbance depending on location and size. However, there have been cases where they present multiply and bilaterally with symmetry. In a case reported in Japan, a 35-year year-old male with von Recklinghausen disease had bilateral cervical ganglioneuromas at the C2–C3 root levels, which caused gait disturbance and clumsiness in both hands along with a history of numbness.[27] In another case, a female patient with von Recklinghausen presented with bilateral and symmetrical ganglioneuromas of the entire spine.[28] Other peculiar locations for ganglioneuromas have included the filum terminale-cauda equina region and brachial plexus.

Ganglioneuroblastomas involving the DRG are even rarer than sensory ganglioneuromas. These malignant tumors are usually associated with autonomic ganglia and can be located in the mediastinum and retroperitoneal tissues of pediatric patients. They consist of neuroblastic cells at various stages of maturation into ganglionic cells. Involvement of the spinal cord is exceptionally rare. However, a case of a ganglioneuroblastoma with sensory involvement located intradurally in the cauda equina region has been reported.[29] Treatment for ganglioneuromas and ganglioneuroblastoma is surgical excision with regimental chemotherapy and/or radiotherapy as needed.

Phantom limb pain (PLP) is another area of interest when ganglionopathies are mentioned. Nearly all amputees still have a feeling of their limbs that are amputated, and experience chronic pain, known as PLP. There are multiple theories as to the origin of the source of pain, with the majority of the field believing that it comes from top down, meaning that the loss of sensory and feedback inputs from the limb's afferents, causes maladaptive cortical plasticity. However, more recently studies suggest that there is mounting evidence for a bottom-up theory of signal generation. This is thought to be generated in the DRG causing an excess of input by the axotomized afferent neurons that previously belonged to the amputated limb. It was noted that when 2% lidocaine (~100 mM) is applied to the dorsal root axons, nerve directly, or the DRG, there is a total cessation of spike propagation, leading to pain relief. In the DRG, significantly lower concentrations, ~10 µM, are sufficient to reach the same result, blocking all pain. Therapeutic considerations for this model are important since we are able to use low concentrations of lidocaine via a small diameter to rid patients of their PLP. In addition, it may be possible to research and target other neuropathies where the DRG is centrally involved in ectopic signal production.[30]

References

[1] Standring S. Gray's Anatomy- The Anatomical Basis of Clinical Practice. 40th ed. Edinburgh: Churchill Livingstone; 2008:41–65, 225–236

[2] Tubbs RS, Loukas M, Slappey JB, Shoja MM, Oakes WJ, Salter EG. Clinical anatomy of the C1 dorsal root, ganglion, and ramus: a review and anatomical study. Clin Anat. 2007; 20(6):624–627

[3] Robinson N. Histochemistry of human cervical posterior root ganglion cells and a comparison with anterior horn cells. J Anat. 1969; 104(Pt 1):55–64

[4] Yabuki S, Kikuchi S. Positions of dorsal root ganglia in the cervical spine. An anatomic and clinical study. Spine. 1996; 21(13):1513–1517

[5] Bergman RA, Thompson SA, Afifi AK. Compendium of Human Anatomic Variation: Text, Atlas, and World Literature. Baltimore: Urban & Schwarzenberg; 1988

[6] Kikuchi S, Sato K, Konno S, Hasue M. Anatomic and radiographic study of dorsal root ganglia. Spine. 1994; 19(1):6–11

[7] Hasegawa T, Mikawa Y, Watanabe R, An HS. Morphometric analysis of the lumbosacral nerve roots and dorsal root ganglia by magnetic resonance imaging. Spine. 1996; 21(9):1005–1009

[8] Miller AN, Routt ML, Jr. Variations in sacral morphology and implications for iliosacral screw fixation. J Am Acad Orthop Surg. 2012; 20(1):8–16

[9] Bergman L, Alexander L. Vascular supply of the spinal cord. Arch Neurol Psychiat. 1941; 46:761–782

[10] Yoshizawa H, Kobayashi S, Hachiya Y. Blood supply of nerve roots and dorsal root ganglia. Orthop Clin North Am. 1991; 22(2):195–211

[11] Johnson PC. Thickening of the human dorsal root ganglion perineurial cell basement membrane in diabetes mellitus. Muscle Nerve. 1983; 6(8):561–565

[12] Baron R. Post-herpetic neuralgia case study: optimizing pain control. Eur J Neurol. 2004; 11 Suppl 1:3–11

[13] Ebraheim NA, Lu J. Morphometric evaluation of the sacral dorsal root ganglia. A cadaveric study. Surg Radiol Anat. 1998; 20(2):105–108

[14] Shen J, Wang HY, Chen JY, Liang BL. Morphologic analysis of normal human lumbar dorsal root ganglion by 3D MR imaging. AJNR Am J Neuroradiol. 2006; 27(10):2098–2103

[15] Colli BO, Carlotti CG, Jr, Assirati JA, Jr, et al. Dorsal root ganglionectomy for the diagnosis of sensory neuropathies. Surgical technique and results. Surg Neurol. 2008; 69(3):266–273, 273

[16] Weigel R, Capelle HH, Schmelz M, Krauss JK. Selective thoracic ganglionectomy for the treatment of segmental neuropathic pain. Eur J Pain. 2012; 16 (10):1398–1402

[17] Sheikh SI, Amato AA. The dorsal root ganglion under attack: the acquired sensory ganglionopathies. Pract Neurol. 2010; 10(6):326–334

[18] Kuntzer T, Antoine JC, Steck AJ. Clinical features and pathophysiological basis of sensory neuronopathies (ganglionopathies). Muscle Nerve. 2004; 30(3): 255–268

[19] Sinha S, Mahadevan A, Lokesh L, et al. Tangier disease–a diagnostic challenge in countries endemic for leprosy. J Neurol Neurosurg Psychiatry. 2004; 75(2): 301–304

[20] McDonald ES, Randon KR, Knight A, Windebank AJ. Cisplatin preferentially binds to DNA in dorsal root ganglion neurons in vitro and in vivo: a potential mechanism for neurotoxicity. Neurobiol Dis. 2005; 18(2):305–313

[21] Scaravilli F, Sinclair E, Arango JC, Manji H, Lucas S, Harrison MJ. The pathology of the posterior root ganglia in AIDS and its relationship to the pallor of the gracile tract. Acta Neuropathol. 1992; 84(2):163–170

[22] Turkmenoglu ON, Kanat A, Yolas C, Aydin MD, Ezirmik N, Gundogdu C. First report of important causal relationship between the Adamkiewicz artery vasospasm and dorsal root ganglion cell degeneration in spinal subarachnoid hemorrhage: An experimental study using a rabbit model. Asian J Neurosurg. 2017; 12(1):22–27

[23] Oxman MN. Herpes zoster pathogenesis and cell-mediated immunity and immunosenescence. J Am Osteopath Assoc. 2009; 109(6) Suppl 2:S13–S17

[24] Johnson RW, Wasner G, Saddier P, Baron R. Herpes zoster and postherpetic neuralgia: optimizing management in the elderly patient. Drugs Aging. 2008; 25(12):991–1006

[25] Dayan AD, Ogul E, Graveson GS. Polyneuritis and herpes zoster. J Neurol Neurosurg Psychiatry. 1972; 35(2):170–175

[26] Shankar GM, Chen L, Kim AH, Ross GL, Folkerth RD, Friedlander RM. Composite ganglioneuroma-paraganglioma of the filum terminale. J Neurosurg Spine. 2010; 12(6):709–713

[27] Kyoshima K, Sakai K, Kanaji M, et al. Symmetric dumbbell ganglioneuromas of bilateral C2 and C3 roots with intradural extension associated with von Recklinghausen's disease: case report. Surg Neurol. 2004; 61(5):468–473, discussion 473

[28] Bacci C, Sestini R, Ammannati F, et al. Multiple spinal ganglioneuromas in a patient harboring a pathogenic NF1 mutation. Clin Genet. 2010; 77(3):293–297

[29] Tripathy LN, Forster DM, Timperley WR. Ganglioneuroblastoma of the cauda equina. Br J Neurosurg. 2000; 14(3):264–266

[30] Vaso A, Adahan H-M, Gjika A, et al. Peripheral nervous system origin of phantom limb pain. Pain. 2014; 155(7):1384–1391

20 History of the Dermatomes with Focus on the Contributions from the Lumbar Plexus

Lexian McBain, R. Shane Tubbs

Abstract

Our current knowledge of the human dermatome map has a long history based on clinical observations and scientific experimentation. This chapter reviews the history of these areas of skin supplied by segmental nerves and focuses on the areas that the lumbar plexus serves. A good working knowledge of the human dermatome system is essential for clinical practice.

Keywords: skin, sensation, sensory, anatomy, historical

20.1 Introduction

A dermatome is defined as an area of skin innervated by a single dorsal nerve root.[1] Knowledge of dermatomes is derived from the work of Sir Henry Head, Otfrid Foester,[2] Jay Keegan, Frederic Garrett, and others.[3] Many different methods were used by these authors and have contributed to the variable findings and representations of what is understood as "the precise boundaries" of dermatomes. The differences could have also arise because several of these methods were based on physiology rather than anatomy.[6] The ability of the central nervous system to suppress, facilitate, and reorganize the activities of primary sensory neurons may also account for differences in mapping.[4] Additionally, sensory neurons with a ganglion cell at one level through intersegmental anastomoses among posterior spinal rootlets are allowed to enter the spinal cord at another level,[4,5,6,7,8] resulting in differences in skin supply by the dorsal roots, dorsal root ganglia, and spinal nerves.[4] In this chapter, the history of the discovery of dermatomes is explored.

In 1893, William Thorburn, a surgical registrar in the Manchester Royal Infirmary, after observing patients with spinal cord lesions published detailed maps of the lumbar and sacral dermatomes (▶ Fig. 20.1).[4,9,10,11,12] Thorburn speculated that the dermatomes existed because of contributions from "certain serial sections of the nervous system." He went on to state that "it remains to be proved that these 'sections' are spinal segments, nerve roots, or other serial arrangements."[4,12]

In 1892, maps of the dermatomes was also constructed by Professor M. Allen Starr of the College of Physicians and Surgeons in New York after examining patients with cauda equina syndrome (▶ Fig. 20.2).[4,13]

From identifying the locations of afflicted skin in herpes zoster patients and from monitoring patients with visceral nonneurological disorders and spinal cord injuries, Sir Henry Head also constructed dermatomal maps (▶ Fig. 20.3).[4] His initial work on the association between cutaneous tenderness and visceral disease began in 1893, and he created charts outlining what others refer to as "Head's zones," which show the distribution of cutaneous tenderness in many diseases.[14] Through examining cases of herpes zoster, Head observed that the areas of herpetic eruptions matched the "area of tenderness" he had described.[4,14] Consequently, he made the deduction that the "areas of tenderness" corresponded to spinal cord segments.[4]

By observing a case of sensory loss due to a "fracture of the 1st and 2nd lumbar vertebrae" L1 was determined.[14] Head found that the upper border of L1 matched the upper border of the sensory loss and that this area coincided with the upper border of the "gluteocrural area," one of his proposed "areas of tenderness." He inferred that these areas were the same and that the lower border of L1 must be the lower border of the "gluteocrural area." After deriving such conclusions at L1 and later S1 to S5, Head noticed that the lateral area of the leg had no designated dermatome. He deduced that this area must be L5 because it was located next to the sacral skin segments. Using a case of presumed spinal cord injury, L4 was determined and a case of herpes zoster rash determined L3. The three dermatomes L3–L5 were proposed by Head to be involved after observing the pattern of the rash. As a result, L3 was assigned to the area outside the already determined areas, L4 and L5. Later, he speculated that L2 must be between L1 and L3. In 1900, Head and Campbell studied 500 cases of shingles and sketched a map showing the distribution of cutaneous lesions.[15] They also found that there were overlaps between adjacent nerve territories and considered that body shape influences differences in the shape of the affected skin.[16] The roots involved in most cases of herpes zoster could not be identified; however, they were able to identify them in 16 autopsy cases. Eight segments in those 16 cases (between T1 and L1) were represented. Head had no confirmation for C5 to C8 or areas below L1, and therefore there were uncertainties when it came to mapping the arm and leg.[4,15]

Using the "method of remaining sensibility," Sir Charles Scott Sherrington studied the dermatomes in monkeys and produced dermatomal maps in 1893 and 1898.[4] Sherrington found that after many roots above and below a given nerve root had been sectioned the remaining areas of sensation in the skin indicated input from the unsectioned root.[4,17,18] Sherrington also found evidence to support Herringham's ventral axial line.[19] He found gaps where contiguous dermatomes were missing in the proximal portions of the dorsal and ventral parts of both the upper and the lower limbs. According to Sherrington, "the gap" formed an axial line that coursed downwards from the midline at the level of the sternal angle to the forearm.[16,17]

Otfrid Foester, a German neurologist and neurosurgeon, adopted Sherrington's approach but applied it to humans. He severed multiple nerve roots and electrically stimulated the distal end of the divided root that resulted in vasodilatation in the dermatomal area.[1] One of the shortcomings of Foester was his lack of awareness that removing a nerve most likely resulted in pain due to input to the central nervous system, probably resulting in death in his patients.[1] In the words of Dr. Robert Wartenburg, "he helped his patients, but they had to pay the price by being subjected to physiological experimentation."[20] Foester found from his research that removing a single root did not result in loss of sensibility, so he made the deduction that dermatomes in humans overlap. He also observed that only one rootlet from the entire posterior root was needed for sensibility

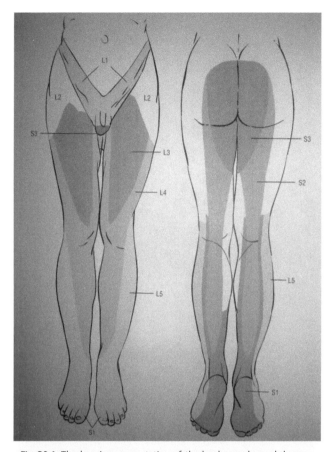

Fig. 20.1 Thorburn's representation of the lumbar and sacral dermatomes. L4 is extended proximally and S1 is assigned to the medial foot. (Reproduced with permission from Thorburn.[12])

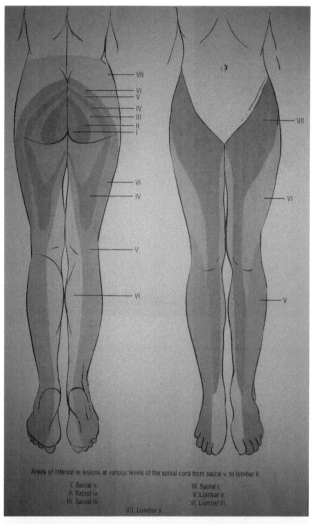

Areas of interest in lesions at various levels of the spinal cord from sacral v. to lumbar ii.

I. Sacral v.	IV. Sacral i.
II. Sacral iv.	V. Lumbar v.
III. Sacral iii.	VI. Lumbar iii.
	VII. Lumbar ii.

Fig. 20.2 M. Allen Starr's representation of the lumbar and sacral dermatomes. L2 (labeled VII) extends distally and S1 does not extend below the knee. (Reproduced with permission from Starr.[13])

within a dermatome and identified different dermatomes for different sensory modalities.[4] He found that the areas of vasodilatation matched the dermatomes determined by anesthesia. This finding presented similarities in distribution to the map drawn by Head from his studies of shingles.[16]

Following the association made between disc herniation and back and leg pain in 1934,[21] Keegan and Garrett contradicted Sherrington and Foester's hypothesis about nerve roots and cutaneous sensibility. They proposed that decreased sensibility of the skin resulted from disc compression of a single nerve root.[22,23,24,25,26,27] They observed patients with different herniations of the cervical and lumbar areas and made maps reflecting the areas of decreased sensibility on the limbs. From the upper limbs studied in 165 cases, 47 cases showed that a single root was affected. Note that 707 cases showed that a single nerve root was affected out of 1,264 cases of the lower limb studied. They also used Novacain injection to test a single lower cervical nerve root in 10 medical students volunteers.[16] The maps constructed by Keegan and Garrett, like Head's maps, showed no overlap of dermatomes (▸ Fig. 20.4).[4] Keegan and Garrett dismissed Foester's claim that removing a single nerve root caused no sensory loss.[16,22] They also disagreed with Sherrington and concluded that "dermatomic loops" and "dorsal axial lines do not exist."[22] Last[28] analyzed Keegan and Garrett's publications and found the following limitations in their findings:

"(1) The subjective method of mapping a dermatome by hypoalgesia must be open to wide error. (2) The lack of overlap of adjacent dermatomes is difficult to accept in face of the almost unanimous opinions of countless observers. (3) No mention is made of variability yet prefixation and post fixation of the plexuses are known to be common. (4) Their claim that an isolated nerve root is affected in their case of disc protrusions or injected medical students is not convincing; there may well have been some involvement of adjacent nerve roots."[28]

Several textbooks continue to use Keegan and Garrett's sketch of the dermatome map despite the lack of significant supporting evidence. Faleiros et al used nerve conduction studies, electromyography (EMG) data, neurosurgical findings, and computed tomography (CT), and magnetic resonance imaging (MRI) images to investigate the dermatomes. Their findings support Head and Foester's view about L4 but oppose Keegan and Garrett's view. They found that L4 is most likely to be found in the medial part of the leg distal to the knee.[16,29] Davis et al also obtained findings that opposed Keegan and Garrett.

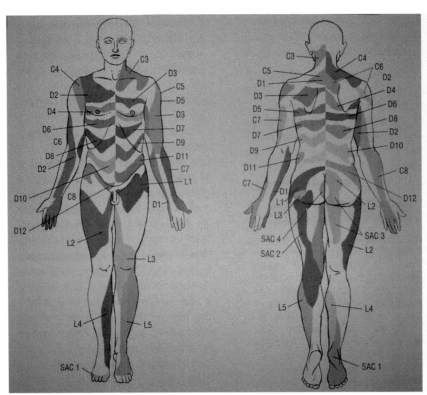

Fig. 20.3 Sir Henry Head's dermatomal maps. (Reproduced with permission from Head.[14])

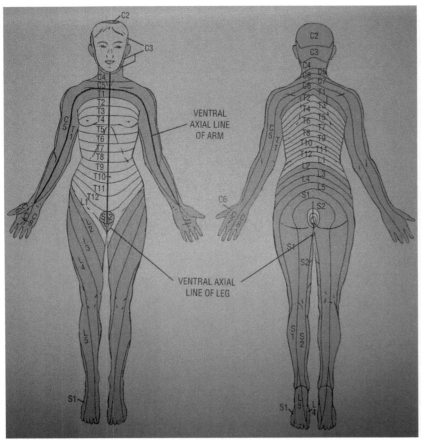

Fig. 20.4 Keegan and Garrett's dermatome maps. (Reproduced with permission from Keegan and Garrett.[22])

Investigating 500 cases of herniated nucleus pulposus, they found changes in sensation in 327 with different sensory patterns. They concluded that the lack of consistency in the sensory pattern made the method used by Keegan and Garrett to create dermatome maps inadequate.[16,30]

The "method of remaining sensibility" was used by another group of researchers, Denny-Brown, Kirk, and Yanagisawa, who studied monkeys and assigned dermatomes to "areas of sensibility" that remained after three roots above and below the root of interest had been dissected.[31] The roots proximal and distal to the ganglia were sectioned in other experiments. They found that dermatomes corresponding to dorsal roots differed from those corresponding to dorsal root ganglia. They also found that one ganglion was responsible for sensory function of an area of the skin corresponding to seven roots, and that the dermatomes in the proximal section were larger than those in the distal section. Consequently, they deduced that adjacent ganglia with an intact spinal cord allowed sensation to be transmitted to a given ganglion, and thus increased the dermatome size. From these studies, Denny-Brown, Kirk, and Yanagisawa concluded that hyposensitivity of the dermatomes depended on the presence of multiple adjacent ganglia, the anatomical and physiological features of large areas of nervous tissue, and the neighboring spinal cord.[4]

Maigne et al demonstrated that the lateral buttock/iliac crest is innervated by the dorsal rami of T12 and L1 and sometimes by L3 opposed to L5 and S1 dermatomes proposed by Keegan.

Nitta et al examined 71 patients undergoing lumbar spinal anesthetic block who had lumbar sacral radicular symptoms. They mapped areas of hyposensitivity after recognition of the nerve root using radiculography, also under fluoroscopy. They found significant overlap between adjacent dermatomes and differences in sensory impairment among patients. Findings consistent with Keegan and Garrett were obtained in under 50% of cases by Nitta et al[32] whereby there was hyposensitivity across the buttock and posterior thigh from blocking L4 and L5 .

In 2008, Lee et al[33] researched the sources of variation in anatomy books and found that some books used Keegan and Garrett's models of dermatome maps while others used Foester's model. Evidence-based study of the methods used in dermatome mapping conducted by Lee et al found that the nerve isolation method used by Foester; the method of recording action potentials in mixed spinal nerves by Inouye and Buchthal[34]; the studies of herpes zoster by Head and Campbell; and the studies of nerve blocking Poletti et al,[35] Nitta et al,[32] and Wolf et al[36] were all clinically relevant and yielded "good" quality evidence. Observations of disc compression by Keegan[26] and Keegan and Garret[22]; methods of removing nerve roots by Sherrington and Kirk and Denny-Brown; and human dissections by Maigne et al[37] were "intermediate" quality evidence. Observations of sensory loss after spinal cord injuries by Thorburn[9,10,11,12] were "poor" quality evidence. Lee et al compiled information and sketched a modern map of dermatomes.

References

[1] Butler DS, Matheson J. Manual Assessment of Nerve Conduction. The Sensitive Nervous System. Adelaide: Noigroup Publications; 2000:219–220

[2] Foester O. The dermatomes in man. Brain. 1933; 56(part 1):1–39

[3] Williams RP, Sugars W. Lumbar foot innervation of the medial foot and ankle region. Aust N Z J Surg. 1998; 68(8):565–567

[4] Greenberg SA. The history of dermatome mapping. Arch Neurol. 2003; 60(1):126–131

[5] Moriishi J, Otani K, Tanaka K, Inoue S. The intersegmental anastomoses between spinal nerve roots. Anat Rec. 1989; 224(1):110–116

[6] Pallie W. The intersegmental anastomoses of posterior spinal rootlets and their significance. J Neurosurg. 1959; 16(2):188–196

[7] Pallie W, Manuel JK. Intersegmental anastomoses between dorsal spinal rootlets in some vertebrates. Acta Anat (Basel). 1968; 70(3):341–351

[8] Schwartz HG. Anastomoses between cervical nerve roots. J Neurosurg. 1956; 13(2):190–194

[9] Thorburn W. Cases of injury to the cervical region of the spinal cord. Brain. 1886; 9:510–543

[10] Thorburn W. On injuries of the cauda equina. Brain. 1887–1888; 10:381–407

[11] Thorburn W. Spinal localization as indicated by spinal injuries. Brain. 1888–1889; 11:289–324

[12] Thorburn W. The sensory distribution of the spinal nerves. Brain. 1893; 16(3):355–374

[13] Starr MA. Local anesthesia as a guide in the diagnosis of the lower spinal cord. Am J Med Sci. 1892; 104:14–35

[14] Head H. On disturbances of sensation with especial reference to the pain of visceral disease 1. Brain. 1893; 16(1–2):1–133

[15] Head H, Campbell AW. The pathology of herpes zoster and its bearing on sensory localisation. Brain. 1900; 23(3):353–362

[16] Downs MB, Laporte C. Conflicting dermatome maps: educational and clinical implications. J Orthop Sports Phys Ther. 2011; 41(6):427–434

[17] Sherrington CS. Experiments in examination of the peripheral distribution of the fiber of the posterior roots of some spinal nerves. Philos Trans R Soc Lond B Biol Sci. 1893; 184:641–763

[18] Sherrington CS. Experiments in examination of the peripheral distribution of the fibers of the posterior roots of some spinal nerves. Philos Trans R Soc Lond B Biol Sci. 1898; 190B:45–187

[19] Herringham W. The minute anatomy of the brachial plexus. Proc R Acad 1886;41:423–441

[20] Haymaker W, Schiller F. The Founders of Neurology. 2nd ed. Springfield, IL: Charles C Thomas; 1970:555

[21] Mixter WJ, Barr JS. Rupture of the intervertebral disc with involvement of the spinal canal. N Engl J Med. 1934; 211:210–215

[22] Keegan JJ, Garrett FD. The segmental distribution of the cutaneous nerves in the limbs of man. Anat Rec. 1948; 102(4):409–437

[23] Keegan JJ. Dermatome hypalgesia associated with herniation of intervertebral disk. Arch Neur Psych. 1943; 50:67–83

[24] Keegan JJ. Diagnosis of herniation of the lumbar intervertebral disks by neurological signs. JAMA. 1944; 126:868–873

[25] Keegan JJ. Neurological interpretation of dermatome hypalgesia with herniation of the lumbar intervetebral disc. J Bone Joint Surg. 1944; 26:238–248

[26] Keegan JK. Dermatome hypalgesia with posterolateral herniation of lower cervical intervertebral disc. J Neurosurg. 1947; 4(2):115–139

[27] Keegan JJ. Relations of nerve roots to abnormalities of lumbar and cervical portions of the spine. Arch Surg. 1947; 55(3):246–270

[28] Last RJ. Innervation of the limbs. J Bone Joint Surg Br. 1949; 31B(3):452–464

[29] Faleiros AT, Resende LA, Zanini MA, Castro HA, Gabarra RC. L4-L5-S1 human dermatomes: a clinical, electromyographical, imaging and surgical findings. Arq Neuropsiquiatr. 2009; 67 2A:265–267

[30] Davis L, Martin J, Goldstein SL. Sensory changes with herniated nucleus pulposus. AMA Arch Neurol Psychiatry. 1952; 67(3):408–411

[31] Liguori R, Krarup C, Trojaborg W. Determination of the segmental sensory and motor innervations of the lumbosacral spinal nerves. Brain. 1992; 115:915–934

[32] Nitta H, Tajima T, Sugiyama H, Moriyama A. Study on dermatomes by means of selective lumbar spinal nerve block. Spine. 1993; 18(13):1782–1786

[33] Lee MW, McPhee RW, Stringer MD. An evidence-based approach to human dermatomes. Clin Anat. 2008; 21(5):363–373

[34] Inouye Y, Buchthal F. Segmental sensory innervation determined by potentials recorded from cervical spinal nerves. Brain. 1977; 100(4):731–748

[35] Poletti CE. C2 and C3 pain dermatomes in man. Cephalalgia. 1991; 11(3):155–159

[36] Wolff AP, Groen GJ, Crul BJ. Diagnostic lumbosacral segmental nerve blocks with local anesthetics: a prospective double-blind study on the variability and interpretation of segmental effects. Reg Anesth Pain Med. 2001; 26(2):147–155

[37] Maigne JY, Lazareth JP, Guerin SH, Maigne R. The lateral cutaneous branches of the dorsal rami of the thoracolumbar junction. Surg Radiol Anat. 1989; 11:289–293

21 Dermatomes and the Lumbar Plexus

Chidinma Nwaogbe

Abstract

The skin can be divided into regions innervated by the segmental nerves of the body called dermatomes. This chapter briefly discusses the general map of each dermatome and their clinical significance. This chapter will also describe three dermatome maps that have been regarded as the primary sources for the various dermatome maps, as well as a recently proposed evidence-based dermatome map.

Keywords: skin, sensation, physical examination, anatomy, disease

21.1 Introduction

The skin can be divided into several areas that are served by the segmental nerves of the body called dermatomes. During embryogenesis of the vertebrate, somites give rise to the sclerotome, myotome, and the dermatome. The sclerotome gives rise to the vertebrae, the myotome forms the skeletal muscle, and the dermatomes result in patches of skin innervated segmentally.

There are various proposed models that mark the distributions for these dermatomes. As such, significant variations exist in the literature. In this chapter, we will briefly describe the general map of each dermatome and their clinical significance. We will discuss further three dermatome maps that have been regarded as the primary sources for the various dermatome maps in circulation today: Foerster's, Head and Campbell's, and Keegan and Garrett's maps. Dermatome maps in general are inconsistent. The segmental pattern typically presented leads to areas of overlap between consecutive spinal nerves. More recently, Lee et al conducted a literature review comparing various dermatome maps and proposed an evidence-based dermatome map that is discussed below.[1]

21.2 Lower Extremity and Genitalia

The skin distribution over the lower extremity and the genitalia are covered by the lumbar and sacral dermatomes (▶ Fig. 21.1, ▶ Fig. 21.2, ▶ Fig. 21.3, ▶ Fig. 21.4). L1 covers the upper part of the lower extremity, hip girdle, and the skin overlaying the back over the L1 vertebrae. L2 covers the anterior and medial aspect of the thigh. L3 represents the anterolateral part of the thigh, down to the medial part of the knee, and the medial aspect of the posterior part of the lower leg. L4 covers the posterolateral thigh, down to the lateral part of the knee and the anterior aspect of the anterior part of the lower leg. L4 also covers the plantar part of the foot and the 2nd, 3rd, and 4th digits. S1 is distributed over the lateral aspect of the thigh down to the posterior part of the lower leg, heel, and lateral aspect of the foot.

S2 covers the posterior thigh and the medial aspect of the posterior leg. The skin overlying the perineum is covered by S2 to S5. S2 and S3 cover the skin over the penis and the scrotum. S3 covers parts of the penis and scrotum and the perianal region. S4 and S5 cover the perianal region with S5 covering the skin adjacent to the anus.[2]

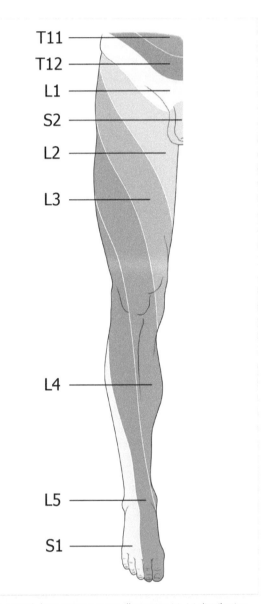

Fig. 21.1 A typical dermatome pattern illustration L1–L4 distribution via branches of the lumbar plexus. (Reproduced with permission from Gilroy AM, MacPherson BR, Ross LM, Schuenke M, Schulte E, Schumacher U. Atlas of Anatomy. 2nd ed. New York, NY: Thieme Medical Publishers; 2012. Illustration by Karl Wesker.)

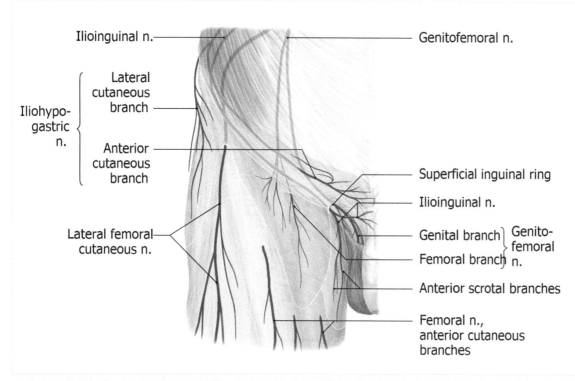

Fig. 21.2 Individual nerve branches of the lumbar plexus and their contributions to regional dermatomes of the upper anterior thigh. (Reproduced with permission from Gilroy AM, MacPherson BR, Ross LM, Schuenke M, Schulte E, Schumacher U. Atlas of Anatomy. 2nd ed. New York, NY: Thieme Medical Publishers; 2012. Illustration by Karl Wesker.)

21.3 The Basis of Various Dermatome Maps

Otfrid Foerster created his dermatome map by isolating single dorsal nerve roots. He accomplished this by surgically sectioning the dorsal nerve roots above and below the ones he wanted to isolate. He was able to individually isolate the nerve roots from L1 to S2. He was only able to map C6 via the isolation method. C3 to C5 and C8 were mapped using a vasodilatory method via electrical stimulation. S3, S4, and S5 were not mapped by data but he mentioned that they covered the perineum, anus, scrotum, and penis.[3] Foerster's map is criticized because it was created on the basis of few subjects, poor documentation, and his failure to document the interval between sectioning the root and testing.[1] Failure to record this time lapse is significant because he did not take into account nerve regeneration and its effect on the extent of sensory loss over that period.[4]

Henry Head created his dermatome map using a study of 450 patients with herpes zoster. He accurately recorded the distribution of the herpetic eruptions, however, tying the eruption to a specific dorsal root proved difficult. His study was limited by the fact that he could only confirm 16 of the 450 cases as involving only a single dorsal root ganglion. Lewis[5] concluded that herpetic eruptions can involve multiple adjacent dorsal root ganglia. The 16 cases that involved a single dorsal root ganglion were used to map C3, C4, T2, T6 to T8, T11, T12, and L1.[5,6]

Keegan and Garrett's map was based on their patients that experienced intervertebral disc prolapse. Disc prolapse leads to spinal root nerve compression and thus decreased tactile sensation. The hypoalgesia that resulted from the disc compression was tested by light pin scratch. Keegan had recognized that the hypoalgesia used to create his map did not completely represent the cutaneous distribution of the spinal nerve in question. Keegan confirmed 707 of 1,264 cases of prolapse between L3–S2 as involving only a single nerve root.[7] The map is criticized for various reasons. There are no data on L1 and L2, yet they are represented on the map. The lack of advanced imaging in diagnosis of cervical root compression also posed a problem.[1] Davis et al conducted a study that contradicted the results of Keegan's map.[8] He reported difficulty in demonstrating a narrow band of hypoalgesia extending from the spine to the distal end of the extremity the way Keegan had.

21.4 The Evidence-Based Dermatome Map

Lee et al conducted a literature review of 14 different dermatomes, and through his analysis he was able to create his own evidence-based dermatome map.[1] These authors transferred

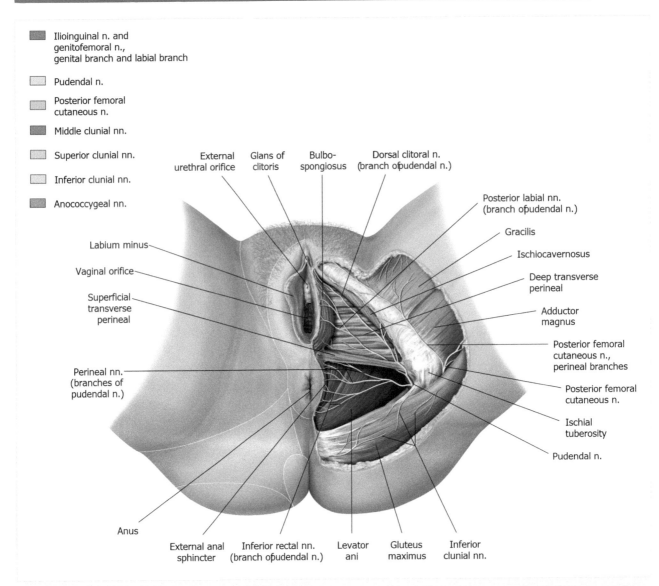

Ilioinguinal n. and genitofemoral n., genital branch and labial branch

Pudendal n.

Posterior femoral cutaneous n.

Middle clunial nn.

Superior clunial nn.

Inferior clunial nn.

Anococcygeal nn.

External urethral orifice

Glans of clitoris

Bulbo-spongiosus

Dorsal clitoral n. (branch of pudendal n.)

Posterior labial nn. (branch of pudendal n.)

Gracilis

Ischiocavernosus

Deep transverse perineal

Adductor magnus

Posterior femoral cutaneous n., perineal branches

Posterior femoral cutaneous n.

Ischial tuberosity

Pudendal n.

Labium minus

Vaginal orifice

Superficial transverse perineal

Perineal nn. (branches of pudendal n.)

Anus

External anal sphincter

Inferior rectal nn. (branch of pudendal n.)

Levator ani

Gluteus maximus

Inferior clunial nn.

Fig. 21.3 Although the perineum is largely supplied by the pubdental nerve in regard to cutaneous innervation, note the significant aspects of it innervated by branches of the lumbar plexus here illustrating the ilioinguinal nerve and genitofemoral branches. (Reproduced with permission from Gilroy AM, MacPherson BR, Ross LM, Schuenke M, Schulte E, Schumacher U. Atlas of Anatomy. 2nd ed. New York, NY: Thieme Medical Publishers; 2012. Illustration by Karl Wesker.)

Foerster's map onto Head's dermatomal map. The areas that were common were kept and the areas that were not were deleted. He used this as the template for his new map. Inouye and Buchthal's research with cervical spinal nerves and Cole et al's study with the lumbosacral dermatomes yielded better evidence for those regions.[9,10] Lee et al used Inouye and Buchthal's data to map C6, C7, and C8 and Cole et al's data for L4, L5, and S1. The map shows large blank areas that signify areas overlap and variability. Lee et al states that this variability could be a result of several factors.[1] Moriishi et al reported that intrathecal intersegmental anastomoses of dorsal spinal rootlets existed in his study of 100 cadavers.[11] This is another reason that could lead to distribution variability. Lee et al concluded that the strength in their systematic review of literature that led to his evidence-based dermatomal map is not only attributed to the areas of the defined dermatomes, but also because of the large blank areas that represent overlap and variability.[1]

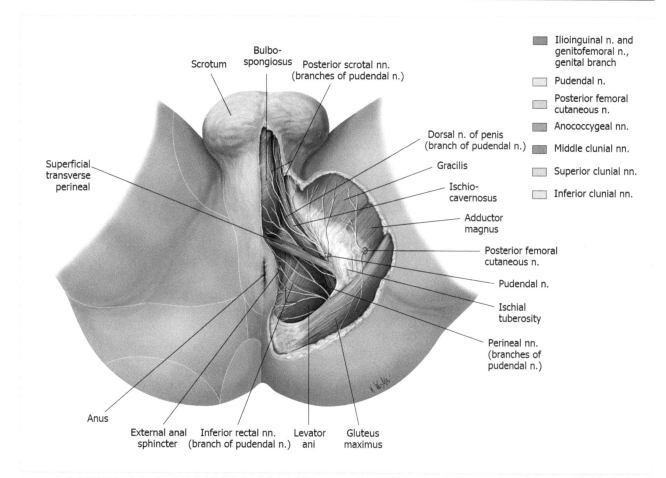

Fig. 21.4 Male perineum noting contributions from the ilioinguinal and genitofemoral nerves. (Reproduced with permission from Gilroy AM, MacPherson BR, Ross LM, Schuenke M, Schulte E, Schumacher U. Atlas of Anatomy. 2nd ed. New York, NY: Thieme Medical Publishers; 2012. Illustration by Karl Wesker.)

References

[1] Lee MW, McPhee RW, Stringer MD. An evidence-based approach to human dermatomes. Clin Anat. 2008; 21(5):363–373

[2] Gray H. Gray's Anatomy. 39th ed. Philadelphia: Elsevier; 2006

[3] Foerster O. The dermatomes in man. Brain. 1933; 56(1):1–39

[4] Apok V, Gurusinghe NT, Mitchell JD, Emsley HC. Dermatomes and dogma. Pract Neurol. 2011; 11(2):100–105

[5] Lewis GW. Zoster sine herpete. BMJ. 1958; 2(5093):418–421

[6] Head H. The pathology of herpes zoster and its bearing on sensory localisation. Brain. 1900; 23(3):353–562

[7] Keegan JJ. Relations of nerve roots to abnormalities of lumbar and cervical portions of the spine. Arch Surg. 1947; 55(3):246–270

[8] Davis L, Martin J, Goldstein SL. Sensory changes with herniated nucleus pulposus. J Neurosurg. 1952; 9(2):133–138

[9] Inouye Y, Buchthal F. Segmental sensory innervation determined by potentials recorded from cervical spinal nerves. Brain. 1977; 100(4):731–748

[10] Cole JP, Lesswing AL, Cole JR. An analysis of the lumbosacral dermatomes in man. Clin Orthop Relat Res. 1968; 61(61):241–247

[11] Moriishi J, Otani K, Tanaka K, Inoue S. The intersegmental anastomoses between spinal nerve roots. Anat Rec. 1989; 224(1):110–116

22 Anesthetic Blockade of the Femoral Nerve

Prasanthi Maddali, Marc D. Moisi, Parthasarathi Chamiraju

Abstract

Anesthetic blockade of the femoral nerve requires a good understanding of its overall anatomy and landmarks. Although ultrasound guidance has made this technique more precise, the variants and detailed morphology in relation to the nerve should be known by the clinician. This chapter discusses both the anatomy of the femoral nerve and techniques for is anesthetic blockade.

Keywords: anesthesia, block, anatomy, thigh, femoral triangle

22.1 Introduction

The femoral nerve is the largest branch of the lumbar plexus. It arises from the dorsal branches of the second to fourth ventral rami (▶ Fig. 22.1), descends on the iliopsoas muscle, and enters the thigh deep to the inguinal ligament at the lateral edge of the femoral sheath, which separates it from the femoral artery.[1] The inguinal ligament is a convergent point of the transversalis fascia (fascial sac lining the deep surface of the anterior abdominal wall) and iliac fascia (fascia covering the posterior abdominal wall). As the femoral nerve passes beneath the inguinal ligament, the nerve is positioned lateral to and slightly deeper than the femoral artery between the psoas and iliacus muscles (▶ Fig. 22.2). At the inguinal crease, it is on the surface of the iliacus muscle and covered by the fascia iliaca or sandwiched between two layers of fascia iliaca.

Conventionally, the femoral nerve passes behind the inguinal ligament and divides into anterior and posterior divisions in the thigh.[2] The femoral nerve block is performed on the main trunk of the femoral nerve just below the inguinal ligament.[3] The higher division of the nerve in the iliac fossa results in incomplete femoral nerve block.

The pectineus nerve is the most medial branch of the femoral nerve in the thigh. A branch to the pectineus muscle is given off as the femoral nerve enters the femoral triangle, beyond the inguinal ligament, innervating the anterior thigh muscles, hip and knee joints, and skin on the anteromedial thigh.[3,4] The origin of this nerve from the femoral nerve in relation to the pectineus is more important morphologically than clinically.

There are instances in which the femoral nerve[5,6,7] is split by an aberrant slip of the iliacus or psoas major muscle. The branches from the anterior divisions are mainly to the sartorius muscle and two cutaneous branches: the medial cutaneous nerve of the thigh and the intermediate cutaneous branch of the thigh. The branches from the posterior division[8] are the saphenous nerve, the nerve to quadriceps femoris, and the branch to the knee joint.

22.2 Variations

The femoral nerve can arise from the ventral rami of T12 to L4 (prefixed) or from L1 to L5 (postfixed). It is rarely found within the iliopsoas muscle or between the femoral vessels.

Aizawa reported that the medial cutaneous nerve branch and the adductor longus branches were the first two branches to leave the femoral nerve in the thigh.[1]

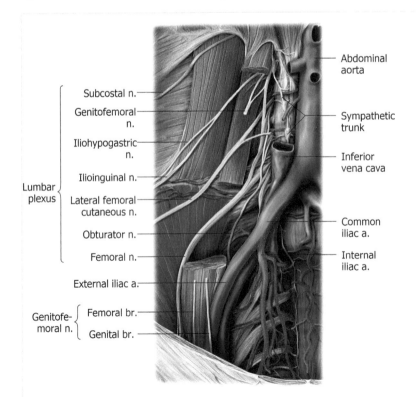

Fig. 22.1 Proximal portion of the right femoral nerve and its relationships. (Reproduced with permission from Gilroy AM, MacPherson BR, Ross LM, Schuenke M, Schulte E, Schumacher U. Atlas of Anatomy. 2nd ed. New York, NY: Thieme Medical Publishers; 2012. Illustration by Karl Wesker.)

Subcostal n.

Genitofemoral n.

Iliohypogastric n.

Ilioinguinal n.

Lumbar plexus

Lateral femoral cutaneous n.

Obturator n.

Femoral n.

External iliac a.

Genitofemoral n. { Femoral br.
                   Genital br.

Abdominal aorta

Sympathetic trunk

Inferior vena cava

Common iliac a.

Internal iliac a.

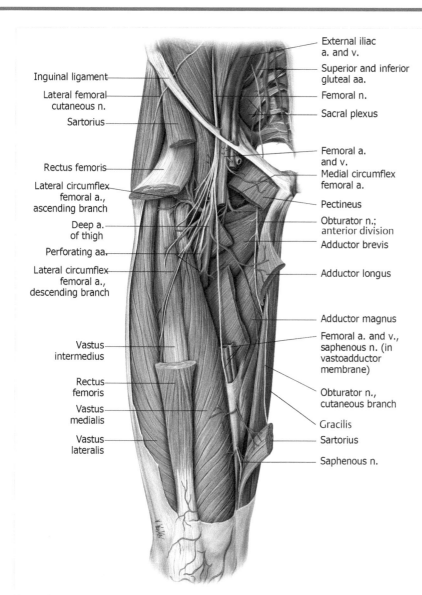

Fig. 22.2 Distal portion of the right femoral nerve and its relationships. (Reproduced with permission from Gilroy AM, MacPherson BR, Ross LM, Schuenke M, Schulte E, Schumacher U. Atlas of Anatomy. 2nd ed. New York, NY: Thieme Medical Publishers; 2012. Illustration by Karl Wesker.)

Labels on figure:
- Inguinal ligament
- Lateral femoral cutaneous n.
- Sartorius
- Rectus femoris
- Lateral circumflex femoral a., ascending branch
- Deep a. of thigh
- Perforating aa.
- Lateral circumflex femoral a., descending branch
- Vastus intermedius
- Rectus femoris
- Vastus medialis
- Vastus lateralis
- External iliac a. and v.
- Superior and inferior gluteal aa.
- Femoral n.
- Sacral plexus
- Femoral a. and v.
- Medial circumflex femoral a.
- Pectineus
- Obturator n.; anterior division
- Adductor brevis
- Adductor longus
- Adductor magnus
- Femoral a. and v., saphenous n. (in vastoadductor membrane)
- Obturator n., cutaneous branch
- Gracilis
- Sartorius
- Saphenous n.

The medial cutaneous nerve branches and vastus medialis, vastus intermedius, vastus lateralis, and rectus femoris branches are arranged medially to laterally, respectively.[1] Gustafson et al[9] reported this pattern except in two specimens where the sartorius branch from the femoral nerve was located between two cutaneous branches.

22.2.1 Applied Anatomy: Dermatomal Innervations

The femoral nerve innervates the skin over the anteromedial aspect of the thigh and knee, and the medial border of the leg and medial malleolus (via the saphenous nerve).

22.2.2 Myotomal Innervations

The femoral nerve innervates the following muscles: sartorius, quadriceps femoris (rectus femoris, vastus lateralis, vastus intermedius, and vastus medialis), iliopsoas, and pectineus.

22.2.3 Articular Innervations

The femoral nerve innervates the anterior wall of the hip joint, the anterior aspect of the femur, and the anteromedial walls of the knee joint.

22.2.4 Femoral Nerve Block

Indications

Indications for a femoral nerve block include operations on the anterior thigh (i.e., lacerations, skin graft, muscle biopsy), pin or plate insertion/removal (femur), and femur fractures.

Analgesia

The block confers anesthesia of the skin on the medial aspect of the leg below the knee joint (saphenous nerve, a superficial terminal extension of the femoral nerve) and can be used to provide surgical anesthesia, usually in combination with a sciatic nerve block. This can be advantageous in situations where it would be preferable to avoid general or neuraxial anesthesia.

22.2.5 3-in-1 Nerve Block

Indications

The 3-in-1 nerve block refers to a block involving the femoral nerve, the lateral cutaneous nerve of the thigh, and the obturator nerve. Indications are the same as those for femoral nerve block, including applicability in operations on the anterior thigh (i.e., lacerations, skin graft, muscle biopsy), pin or plate insertion/removal (femur), and femoral fractures. The 3-in-1 nerve block is also helpful when analgesia and anesthesia are needed for the hip (i.e., dislocations, femoral neck fractures) and when analgesia of the knee is required.

Depending on the surgical procedure, femoral/3-in-1 nerve blocks can cover only part of the knee joint. The knee joint is innervated by the femoral, obturator, and sciatic nerves. Portions of the knee innervated by the sciatic nerve will not be covered. The hip joint is primarily innervated by the femoral, obturator, and lateral femoral cutaneous nerves with a small contribution from the sciatic nerve and nerve to quadratus femoris.

Analgesia

Analgesia can be used, for example, following total knee arthoplasty (with/without sciatic nerve block) or anterior cruciate ligament repair. Please note that in most patients a femoral nerve block alone will not provide adequate analgesia of the knee owing to significant contributions from the sciatic and obturator nerves. When combined with a sciatic or popliteal block, a femoral nerve block can provide analgesia for amputations above and below the knee.

Adjuvant analgesia can also be used after a hip surgery such as total hip replacement. Please note that a femoral nerve block alone will not provide complete analgesia of the hip owing to contributions from the subcostal, iliohypogastric, lateral femoral cutaneous, sciatic, and obturator nerves. Therefore, it is not commonly used in these cases.

22.2.6 Anesthesia

- Femoral nerve block alone.
- Skin graft or muscle biopsy from the anterior aspect of the thigh.
- In combination with sciatic and obturator nerve blocks: knee surgery.
- In combination with a sciatic/popliteal block: any procedure on the lower leg or foot.

22.2.7 Contraindications

- Burn or infection at injection site.
- Inability to coagulate blood (congenital or acquired).
- Vascular graft of the femoral artery.
- Neurological disease (relative contraindication).
- Local anesthetic allergy.
- Inability to guarantee sterile equipment.

22.2.8 Preparation

Prepare the patient. Obtain a medical history, perform a brief physical exam, and review laboratory/other studies or tests. If elective, the patient should have fasted prior to surgery. General anesthesia may be required if the block fails. Carefully explain the procedure, risks, benefits, and most importantly what to expect after surgery (numbness, weakness, and how long it will take until they regain use of the leg). Obtain consent from the patient to perform the procedure.

Monitor the patient continuously with ECG, blood pressure, and pulse oximetry.

Intravenous access must be gained with a running IV.

Emergency medications, airway/intubation equipment, and an oxygen source should be immediately available.

Assemble local anesthetics, sterile equipment, and antiseptic agents. Consider light sedation. Oversedation can result in an uncooperative patient and can mask signs and symptoms of intravenous injection of local anesthetics and/or intraneural injection.

Technique for femoral nerve block/3-in-1 nerve block: The techniques for both blocks are basically the same, with some minor differences. There are several approaches to this block. Two techniques will be described here.

22.2.9 Position Patient Supine: Identify the Landmarks

The femoral nerve is located just below the inguinal ligament. Locate the anterior superior iliac spine and the pubic tubercle. A line between these two structures is where the inguinal ligament is located. Next, locate the pulsation of the femoral artery. The site for needle insertion is approximately 2 cm lateral to the pulsation. From medial to lateral, the structures are the femoral vein, femoral artery, and femoral nerve. Prepare the site with antiseptic. Using sterile technique, use sterile gloves and drape the area with sterile towels.

Use a 21 to 23 gauge needle (should be blunted because a sharp "cutting" needle can transect a nerve).

22.2.10 Paresthesia Technique

A small skin wheal of local anesthetic is placed at the identified injection site. The needle is inserted slowly in a perpendicular direction. The needle should be blunted to decrease the risk of neural trauma. As the needle is advanced, aspirate for blood. Once a paresthesia is noted in the distribution of the femoral nerve, withdraw the needle slightly and inject the local anesthetic. The patient should not feel pain during the injection. If a depth of 4 to 5 cm has been reached with no paresthesia elicited, then withdraw the needle to the level of the skin and change the angle either slightly medially or laterally. Continue to seek a paresthesia. Always aspirate for blood during needle insertion before, during, and after injection to avoid an inadvertent intravascular injection. Paresthesia techniques carry a higher risk of nerve trauma than the two-pop fascia iliaca technique. Therefore, the availability of ultrasound or nerve stimulators should render the paresthesia technique obsolete.

Stimulation

The nerve stimulator is initially set at 1.0 to 1.2 mA. Use a 22-gauge 2-inch insulated needle, directing it cephalad at an approximately 30° to 45° angle. A brisk "patellar snap" with the current at 0.5 mA or less indicates successful localization of the needle near the femoral nerve. The nerve is usually superficial, rarely beyond 3 cm from the skin. After the injection of 1 mL of local anesthetic, the contractions should start to fade. Always aspirate during needle insertion, before injection, during injection, and after injection to ensure that inadvertent intravascular injection has not occurred.

If the aspiration for blood is negative, inject the local anesthetic. If the patient experiences pain or paresthesia with injection, withdraw the needle slightly. Continue with injection as long as there is no pain or paresthesia.

Studies have demonstrated that the anterior branch of the femoral nerve is usually encountered with the first needle pass, which results in stimulation of the sartorius muscle, often seen as contraction of the lower medial thigh. If this occurs, advance the needle tip until either the sartorius twitch is extinguished or a patellar snap is elicited before redirecting the needle. If the sartorius twitch is extinguished without the patellar snap, withdraw the needle toward the skin (without exiting the skin), and redirect it slightly lateral and slightly deeper than the original needle pass.

The posterior branch of the femoral nerve is typically lateral and deep to the anterior branch.

The anesthetist should resist the urge to use the patient's thigh as a hand rest while directing the needle. Stimulation of the femoral nerve can result in brisk vastus muscle twitching that can disrupt needle positioning.

There are two main differences between femoral nerve block and 3-in-1 nerve block:

1. Volume of local anesthetic. For femoral nerve blocks, the volume of local anesthetic is generally 20 mL or less. For 3-in-1 nerve blocks, the volume of local anesthetic is 25 to 30 mL. This allows the local anesthetic to spread further in the tissue plane resulting in blockade of the femoral, lateral femoral cutaneous, and obturator nerves.
2. Slight alteration in technique. Once the needle has been placed in the correct area, pressure should be applied 2 to 4 cm below the injection site. Next, administer the local anesthetic. Applying distal pressure helps spread the local anesthetic to the obturator and lateral femoral cutaneous nerves, in addition to the femoral nerve.

22.3 Ultrasound Technique

The ultrasound-guided technique of femoral nerve blockade differs from nerve stimulator or landmark-based techniques in several important respects. Ultrasound application allows the practitioner to monitor the spread of local anesthetic and needle placement and make appropriate adjustments, should the initial spread be deemed inadequate. Also, because of the proximity of the relatively large femoral artery, ultrasound can reduce the risk of arterial puncture, which often occurs with this block when no ultrasound techniques are used. Palpating the femoral pulse as a landmark for the block is not required with ultrasound guidance, a process that can be challenging in obese patients. Although the ability to visualize the needle and the relevant anatomy with ultrasound guidance renders nerve stimulation optional, the motor response obtained during nerve stimulation often provides contributory information.

References

[1] Aizawa Y. On the organization of the plexus lumbalis. I. On the recognition of the three-layered divisions and the systematic description of the branches of the human femoral nerve. Okajimas Folia Anat Jpn. 1992; 69(1):35–74

[2] Newell RLM. Pelvic girdel, gluteal region & hip joint. In: Satanding S, Ellis H, Healy JC, Johnson D, Williams A, eds. Gray's Anatomy - The Anatomical Basis of Clinical Practice. 39th ed. Philadelphia: Elsevier Churchill Livingstone; 2005:1455

[3] Ellis H, Feldman SA, Harrop Griffith W. Anatomy for Anaesthetists. 8th ed. Massachusetts: Blackwell Publishing; 2004:188–191

[4] Collins VJ. Principles of Anesthesiology. General and Regional Anesthesia. 3rd ed. Pennsylvania: Lea & Febiger; 1993:1395–1397

[5] Spratt JD, Logan BM, Abrahams PH. Variant slips of psoas and iliacus muscles, with splitting of the femoral nerve. Clin Anat. 1996; 9(6):401–404

[6] Vázquez MT, Murillo J, Maranillo E, Parkin IG, Sanudo J. Femoral nerve entrapment: a new insight. Clin Anat. 2007; 20(2):175–179

[7] Anloague PA, Huijbregts P. Anatomical variations of the lumbar plexus: a descriptive anatomy study with proposed clinical implications. J Manual Manip Ther. 2009; 17(4):e107–e114

[8] Sinnatamby CS. Last's Anatomy. Regional and Applied. London: Churchill Livingstone; 2001:115

[9] Gustafson KJ, Pinault GC, Neville JJ, et al. Fascicular anatomy of human femoral nerve: implications for neural prostheses using nerve cuff electrodes. J Rehabil Res Dev. 2009; 46(7):973–984

23 Anesthetic Blockade of the Lateral Femoral Cutaneous Nerve

Prasanthi Maddali, Marc D. Moisi, Parthasarathi Chamiraju

Abstract

Anesthetic blockade of the lateral femoral cutaneous nerve requires a good understanding of its overall anatomy and landmarks. Although ultrasound guidance has made this technique more precise, the variants and detailed morphology in relation to the nerve should be known by the clinician. This chapter discusses both the anatomy of the lateral femoral cutaneous nerve and techniques for its anesthetic blockade.

Keywords: anesthesia, block, anatomy, thigh

23.1 Introduction

The lateral femoral cutaneous nerve (LFCN) of the thigh is normally a derivative of the posterior divisions of the L2 and L3 spinal nerves. The nerve emerges from the lateral border of the psoas major muscle and runs across the iliacus muscle in the pelvis and travels toward the anterior superior iliac spine (ASIS) (▶ Fig. 23.1).

The LFCN typically exits the lesser pelvis under the inguinal ligament (IL), medial to the ASIS, where it bifurcates into anterior and posterior divisions along the length of the thigh. In the thigh, the nerve runs through its individual fascial tunnel: the LFCN canal.[15] It provides sensory innervation to the skin of the anterolateral and lateral aspects of the thigh[1] (▶ Fig. 23.2).

23.2 Variant Anatomy

Variations in the LFCN's anatomy are common; seven different points of exit from the pelvis have been observed.[2] Four of the variations can be classified into four zones relative to the ASIS,

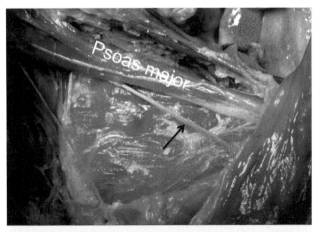

Fig. 23.1 Right posterior abdominal wall illustrating the course of the lateral femoral cutaneous nerve (arrow) exiting lateral to psoas major and traveling toward the anterior superior iliac spine on the iliacus muscle.

through which the LFCN can pass: medial to the ASIS and under the IL, medial to the ASIS and over the IL, directly over the ASIS, and lateral to the ASIS. Three more variations were found in which the nerve passed through another tissue: the ASIS itself, the sartorius muscle, and the IL. Even when the nerve followed the anatomically normal exit pattern—medial to the ASIS under the IL—the distance from the ASIS could vary, creating a zone where the LFCN can be encountered. Furthermore, five branching patterns were observed: the normal single nerve that eventually bifurcates in the area of the thigh, bifurcation within the pelvis, bifurcation near the nerve's exit from the pelvis, trifurcation, and quadrification.[3]

Variations in the anatomy of the LFCN have been known and documented for many years, injury to it having been noted as far back as 1885.[2] Tomaszewski et al assembled all data available on the variations in the anatomy of the LFCN, namely, its points of exit in the pelvis, branching patterns, and distance from other major structures, to provide a better understanding for surgeons operating in its vicinity.[16] Their analysis showed that most nerves follow the pattern of exiting the pelvis medial to the ASIS, under the IL and medial to the sartorius muscle, with an overall prevalence of 86.8%, subgroup analysis showing prevalences above 80% for all groups. When the nerve exited following this pattern, medial to the ASIS and under the IL, it was usually found 1.9 cm medial to the ASIS.

It usually exited as a single nerve, with an overall prevalence of 79.1%. Bifurcation within the pelvis was the second most common pattern with a prevalence of 11.8%. However, it was noted that in studies from South America, there was a much higher prevalence of trifurcation than bifurcation in the pelvis, with prevalences of 24.7 versus 1.2%, respectively.

23.3 Surgery

Several surgeries can cause iatrogenic injury to the LFCN. These include laparoscopic inguinal hernia repair, abdominoplasty, and bone graft harvesting.

Consideration of the variations in the LFCN is especially important in conducting inguinal hernia repairs. Although rare variations of the nerve traveling through the ASIS, the IL, or through the sartorius muscle can actually protect the nerve from injury, the LFCNs of most patients are at a risk of iatrogenic injury. Patients with early bifurcations, including those within the pelvis and in the area of the IL, are at higher risk of iatrogenic injury during surgery as more branches in the area have to be considered than in the normal anatomy. Similarly, trifurcations and quadrifications of the LFCN provide more targets for accidental injury, putting populations from regions of South America, where trifurcations presented with a prevalence of 24.7%, at elevated risk.

Clinical data have shown laparoscopic inguinal hernia repair to be a safer alternative to open repair in terms of incidence of postoperative neuralgias, with a relative risk ratio of 0.66 (95% confidence interval [CI] 0.51–0.87) when compared to open

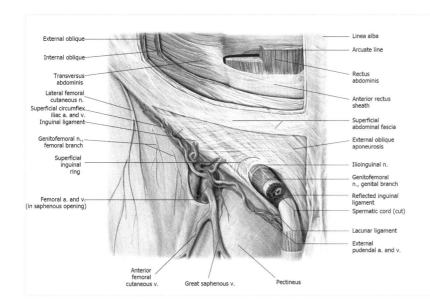

External oblique

Internal oblique

Transversus abdominis

Lateral femoral cutaneous n.

Superficial circumflex iliac a. and v.

Inguinal ligament

Genitofemoral n., femoral branch

Superficial inguinal ring

Femoral a. and v. (in saphenous opening)

Anterior femoral cutaneous v.

Great saphenous v.

Pectineus

Linea alba

Arcuate line

Rectus abdominis

Anterior rectus sheath

Superficial abdominal fascia

External oblique aponeurosis

Ilioinguinal n.

Genitofemoral n., genital branch

Reflected inguinal ligament

Spermatic cord (cut)

Lacunar ligament

External pudendal a. and v.

Fig. 23.2 Schematic drawing of the exit site of the right lateral femoral cutaneous nerve into the skin of the lateral thigh. (Reproduced with permission from Gilroy AM, MacPherson BR, Ross LM, Schuenke M, Schulte E, Schumacher U. Atlas of Anatomy. 2nd ed. New York, NY: Thieme Medical Publishers; 2012. Illustration by Karl Wesker.)

inguinal hernia repair.[4] Regarding a laparoscopic approach, it has been suggested that staples be avoided within 1 cm of the ASIS owing to the proximity of the LFCN.[5] During their subgroup analysis by geographical region, these authors noted very little heterogeneity for the pooled mean distances of the LFCN from the ASIS. Thus, they suspected the cause for heterogeneity in the overall analysis of distance of the LFCN from the ASIS was most likely to be geographical differences. Their analysis revealed that South American populations had LFCNs closest to the ASIS with a mean distance of 0.99 cm (95% CI 0.43–1.55). European and North American populations, in contrast, had LFCNs with mean distances of 2.32 cm (95% CI 1.88–2.81) and 2.31 cm (95% CI 1.54–3.09) from the ASIS, respectively. Asian populations fell between these extremes, with a mean distance of 1.43 cm (95% CI 0.98–1.89). Tomaszewski and Popieluszko suggested that the dangerous zone for staples should be reassessed because their data indicated that the average LFCN passes within 1.9 cm of the ASIS and is highly variable depending on from the patient's geographical location. With other procedures, such as esthetic abdominoplasties, a zone of 4 cm around the ASIS has been demarcated as a potentially dangerous area, requiring careful dissection and preservation to retain proper LFCN structure and function.[6]

Studies have reported that the general rule of thumb used by surgeons is to approximate the LFCN as running two fingerbreadths medial to the ASIS.[7] However, this strategy can grossly miscalculate the location of the nerve depending on the patient and on the surgeon's anatomical knowledge. Ideally, an imaging approach such as ultrasound would help to determine the precise location of the LFCN and confirm the absence of one of the other common variations. However, if a gross estimate must be made, we would suggest 3 cm as a rule of thumb rather than two fingerbreadths, as finger widths can vary. On the basis of our analysis, we ideally suggest a danger zone for all surgical procedures of about 3 cm around the ASIS, which corresponds to the upper limit of the confidence interval of the subgroup with the highest upper limit in the confidence interval (North America), thus minimizing the risk of iatrogenic injury for most populations.

Another procedure where the location of the LFCN is of particular interest is bone graft harvesting. The size of the graft and size of incision can greatly influence the risk of injury. The current suggestions are for grafts to be less than 3 cm in size, and the incisions to be made should be at least 3 cm away from the palpable point of the ASIS.[8] This general guideline could potentially injure patients with an LFCN lateral to the ASIS, which was found in 2.6% of the population studied (95% CI 0.0–6.7). Thus, these studies indicate the value of an imaging study such as ultrasound before graft sampling.

A final consideration of the LFCN is for the anterior approach to hip arthroplasty. In a study in 2010, 81% of patients reported new onset of neurapraxia in the area supplied by the LFCN after a hip resurfacing or total hip arthroplasty performed using the anterior approach.[9] The anterior approach offers many advantages over the posterior approach, which has a higher risk of dislocation, or the lateral approach, which puts the adduction function at risk.[10] Because the anterior approach offers the least damage to a patient's hip function, the loss of sensation provided by the LFCN becomes a larger concern. Current suggestions for minimally invasive anterior approaches involve incisions running parallel to the LFCN.[11] Again, for this approach to be viable and to ensure preservation of the LFCN, the location of the nerve must be strictly determined, not simply estimated, because it is highly variable.

We suggest further analysis of the LFCN and its variations, especially using ultrasound guidance as a quick and effective method, to help surgeons minimize the incidence of meralgia paresthetica due to iatrogenic injury to the LFCN.

23.3.1 Pathology

The most common pathology associated with the LFCN is meralgia paresthetica, a condition entailing pain, a lack of sensation, or dysesthesia of the skin supplied by this nerve.[12] Meralgia paresthetica can have numerous etiologies including pelvic inflammatory disease, pregnancy, various toxicities, tight clothing, and, importantly, iatrogenic injuries from surgical procedures.[3] Detailed knowledge of variations in the pelvic exits and branching patterns of LFCN is crucial for diagnosing meralgia paresthetica and for avoiding injuries during surgical procedures, especially inguinal hernia repair. The incidence of nerve injury in laparoscopic inguinal hernia repair is about 2%.[13] Although this is a relatively small percentage, current studies estimate that close to 20 million hernia repairs are performed annually worldwide.[14]

23.4 Lateral Femoral Cutaneous Nerve Block Anatomical Technique

This block can be performed alone to provide anesthesia of the lateral thigh (e.g., donor area for a skin graft) or to diagnose meralgia paresthetica. It can also be performed along with femoral, obturator, and sciatic blocks to provide anesthesia of the thigh for surgical procedures above the knee and for thigh tourniquet. It is also one of the nerves targeted in a "3-in-1" block, a block of the femoral nerve performed with a higher volume of local anesthetic, with the aim of also blocking the lateral femoral and obturator nerves (not supported by evidence).

23.4.1 Point of Contact with the Nerve

The nerve is approached as it emerges from under the IL, medial, and inferior to the ASIS. The main characteristic of this nerve is a constant relationship to the ASIS, although for several centimeters its trajectory is within the LFCN canal, until it perforates it to become a superficial nerve running on the lateral thigh.[15] It is important to remember this because the fascia lata duplication, forming the anterior and posterior walls of the canal, is thick enough to slow the transfer of local anesthetic to the target nerve.

23.4.2 Patient Position and Landmarks

The patient lies supine. The ASIS is identified by palpation.

23.4.3 Technique

The needle entrance point is identified about 1 cm medial and about 2 cm caudal to the ASIS. The needle is advanced perpendicular to the skin until it enters the LFCN canal where a small volume of local anesthetic is injected. A nerve stimulator with pulse duration of 0.3 to 1 ms (300–1,000 μs) can be used to identify the nerve by eliciting a sensory paresthesia on the lateral thigh.

23.4.4 Local Anesthetic and Volume

A volume of around 5 mL of 1% mepivacaine is frequently used. A long-acting agent such as ropivacaine or bupivacaine can be used if longer anesthesia or analgesia is needed.

23.4.5 Complications

On occasion, some patients complain of dysesthesia on the lateral thigh, which typically resolves within a few days of the procedure without sequelae.

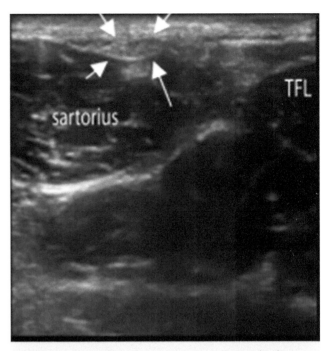

Fig. 23.3 The lateral femoral cutaneous nerve passes under the inguinal ligament medial to the ASIS. In the thigh, the nerve runs through its individual fascial tunnel (the LFCN canal) as shown by the arrows.

23.5 Lateral Femoral Cutaneous Nerve Block

23.5.1 Ultrasound Technique

The use of ultrasound facilitates this block. As previously mentioned, the LFCN passes under the IL medial to the ASIS and in its individual canal as shown in ▶ Fig. 23.3.

A few centimeters distal to the IL, the nerve can still be observed in the LFCN canal and causing a small indentation on the anterolateral surface of the sartorius, as shown by the arrows in ▶ Fig. 23.3.

This nerve is usually superficially located and either an in-plane or an out-of-plane technique can be used, deposing a small volume of local anesthetic around it. In meralgia paresthetica cases, a long-acting corticosteroid can be injected as well, to achieve therapeutic effect.

References

[1] Anloague PA, Huijbregts P. Anatomical variations of the lumbar plexus: a descriptive anatomy study with proposed clinical implications. J Manual Manip Ther. 2009; 17(4):e107–e114

[2] Aszmann OC, Dellon ES, Dellon AL. Anatomical course of the lateral femoral cutaneous nerve and its susceptibility to compression and injury. Plast Reconstr Surg. 1997; 100(3):600–604

[3] Sürücü HS, Tanyeli E, Sargon MF, Karahan ST. An anatomic study of the lateral femoral cutaneous nerve. Surg Radiol Anat. 1997; 19(5):307–310

[4] O'Reilly EA, Burke JP, O'Connell PR. A meta-analysis of surgical morbidity and recurrence after laparoscopic and open repair of primary unilateral inguinal hernia. Ann Surg. 2012; 255(5):846–853

[5] Dibenedetto LM, Lei Q, Gilroy AM, Hermey DC, Marks SC, Jr, Page DW. Variations in the inferior pelvic pathway of the lateral femoral cutaneous nerve: implications for laparoscopic hernia repair. Clin Anat. 1996; 9(4):232–236

[6] Chowdhry S, Davis J, Boyd T, et al. Safe tummy tuck: anatomy and strategy to avoid injury to the lateral femoral cutaneous nerve during abdominoplasty. Eplasty. 2015; 15:e22

[7] Majkrzak A, Johnston J, Kacey D, Zeller J. Variability of the lateral femoral cutaneous nerve: an anatomic basis for planning safe surgical approaches. Clin Anat. 2010; 23(3):304–311

[8] Kosiyatrakul A, Nuansalee N, Luenam S, Koonchornboon T, Prachaporn S. The anatomical variation of the lateral femoral cutaneous nerve in relation to the anterior superior iliac spine and the iliac crest. Musculoskelet Surg. 2010; 94 (1):17–20

[9] Goulding K, Beaulé PE, Kim PR, Fazekas A. Incidence of lateral femoral cutaneous nerve neuropraxia after anterior approach hip arthroplasty. Clin Orthop Relat Res. 2010; 468(9):2397–2404

[10] Bhargava T, Goytia RN, Jones LC, Hungerford MW. Lateral femoral cutaneous nerve impairment after direct anterior approach for total hip arthroplasty. Orthopedics. 2010; 33(7):472

[11] Jameson SS, Howcroft DWJ, McCaskie AW, Gerrand CH. Injury to the lateral femoral cutaneous nerve during minimally invasive hip surgery: a cadaver study. Ann R Coll Surg Engl. 2008; 90(3):216–220

[12] Carai A, Fenu G, Sechi E, Crotti FM, Montella A. Anatomical variability of the lateral femoral cutaneous nerve: findings from a surgical series. Clin Anat. 2009; 22(3):365–370

[13] Rosenberg J, Bisgaard T, Kehlet H, et al. Danish Hernia Database. Danish Hernia Database recommendations for the management of inguinal and femoral hernia in adults. Dan Med Bull. 2011; 58(2):C4243

[14] Bay-Nielsen M, Kehlet H, Strand L, et al. Danish Hernia Database, Collaboration. Quality assessment of 26,304 herniorrhaphies in Denmark: a prospective nationwide study. Lancet. 2001; 358(9288):1124–1128

[15] Hanna A. The lateral femoral cutaneous nerve canal. J Neurosurg. 2017; 126 (3):972–978

[16] Tomaszewski KA, Popieluszko P, Henry BM, et al. The surgical anatomy of the lateral femoral cutaneous nerve in the inguinal region: a meta-analysis. Hernia. 2016; 20(5):649–657

24 Anesthetic Blockade of the Iliohypogastric, Ilioinguinal, and Genitofemoral Nerves

Prasanthi Maddali, Marc D. Moisi, Parthasarathi Chamiraju

Abstract

Anesthetic blockade of the iliohypogastric, ilioinguinal, and genitofemoral nerves require a good understanding of its overall anatomy and landmarks. The variants and detailed morphology in relation to the nerve should be known by the clinician. This chapter discusses both the anatomy of these nerves and techniques for their anesthetic blockade.

Keywords: anesthesia, block, anatomy, thigh, femoral triangle, inguinal, suprapubic

24.1 Anatomical Considerations

The key to understanding nerve blocks of the abdominal wall is knowledge and application of the anatomy. There are three muscle layers within the abdominal wall, each with an associated fascial sheath. From superficial to deep, these are the external oblique, internal oblique, and transversus abdominis. In addition, the paired rectus abdominis muscles form a muscle layer either side of the midline.

The skin and fascia of the anterior abdominal wall overlie the four muscles that help support the abdominal contents and the trunk, the main nerve supply lying in a plane between the internal oblique and transversus abdominis. Between the internal oblique and transversus abdominis muscles lies a plane that corresponds to a similar plane in the intercostal spaces. It contains the anterior rami of the lower six thoracic nerves (T7–T12) and first lumbar nerve (L1), supplying the skin, muscles, and parietal peritoneum.[1] At the costal margins, thoracic nerves T7 to T11 enter this neurovascular plane of the abdominal wall, traveling along it to pierce the posterior wall of the rectus sheath as anterior cutaneous branches supplying the overlying skin. The nerves T7 to T9 emerge to supply the skin superior to the umbilicus. The T10 nerve supplies the umbilicus, whereas T11, the cutaneous branch of the subcostal T12, the iliohypogastric nerve, and the ilioinguinal nerve supply the skin inferior to the umbilicus.

The iliohypogastric nerve originates primarily from the L1 nerve root and supplies the sensory innervations to the skin over the inguinal region (▶ Fig. 24.1). It runs in the plane between the internal oblique and transversus abdominis muscles and later pierces the internal oblique to lie between this muscle and the external oblique before giving off cutaneous branches. The ilioinguinal nerve (▶ Fig. 24.1) also originates from the L1 nerve root and is found inferior to the iliohypogastric nerve, perforating the transversus abdominis muscle at the level of the iliac crest running medially in a deeper plane than the iliohypogastric nerve. The ilioinguinal nerve innervates the inguinal hernia sac and medial aspect of the thigh and anterior scrotum and labia.[2]

24.2 Variations

Al-Dabbagh et al performed a consecutive series of 110 primary hernia patients by mesh repair, and were particular about identifying and following the course of both the ilioinguinal nerve and iliohypogastric nerves and preserving them.[16] In 46 of the 110 patients, the course was consistent with anatomical texts, but in the remaining 64 it was variant. These variations included (1) acute inferolateral angulation of the IIN at its exit behind the superficial inguinal ring (SIR) fibers in 20 cases; (2) similar direction of the IIN but in a plane superficial to the external oblique aponeurosis (EOA) and proximal to the SIR in 18 cases; (3) a single stem for both nerves over the spermatic cord in 24 cases, with variation in the subsequent course; (4) absence of one or both nerves in eight cases; (5) accessory IIN or IHN in three cases; and (6) aberrant origin of the IIN from the genitofemoral nerve (GFN) in two cases. They also observed that none of patients had any sensory disturbances or pain in a dermatomal distribution.

Klaassen et al[2] dissected and analyzed 100 fixed cadavers. All the nerves were documented where they entered the abdominal wall with the point measured in relation to the anterior superior iliac spine (ASIS). The course was followed and the lateral distance from the midline at termination was measured. The ilioinguinal nerve originated from L1 in 130 specimens (65%), from T12 and L1 in 28 (14%), from L1 and L2 in 22 (11%), and from L2 and L3 in 20 (10%). The nerve entered the abdominal wall 2.8 ± 1.1 cm medial and 4 ± 1.2 cm inferior to the ASIS and terminated 3 ± 0.5 cm lateral to midline.

The iliohypogastric nerve originated from T12 on 14 sides (7%), from T12 and L1 in 28 (14%), from L1 in 20%, and from T11 and T12 in 12 (6%). The nerve entered the abdominal wall 2.8 ± 1.3 cm medial and 1.4 ± 1.2 cm inferior to the ASIS, and terminated 4.0 ± 1.3 cm lateral to the midline. For both nerves, the distance between the ASIS and the midline was 12.2 ± 1.1 cm.

The linear course of each nerve was followed, and its lateral distance from the midline at termination was measured.

24.3 Procedure

24.3.1 Ilioinguinal and Iliohypogastric Nerve Blocks

Inguinal herniorrhaphy pain can be significant and difficult to treat without opioid analgesics, but blocking the iliohypogastric and ilioinguinal nerves can provide good analgesia for most operations in the inguinal region. These blocks can be very effective in reducing the need for opioids, and in pediatric patients they have been found as effective as caudal blocks, albeit with a higher failure rate.[2]

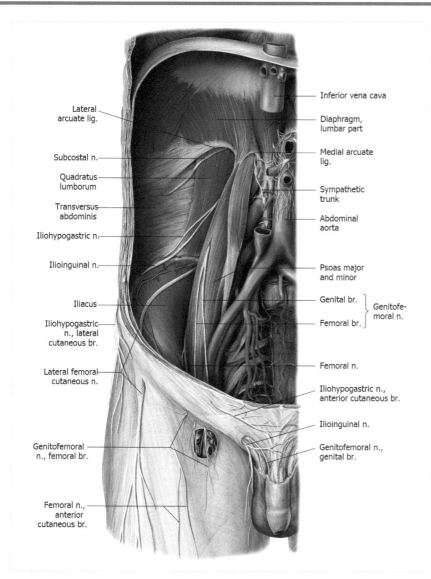

Fig. 24.1 Schematic drawing illustrating the anatomy of the iliohypogastric, ilioinguinal, and genitofemoral nerves. (Reproduced with permission from Gilroy AM, MacPherson BR, Ross LM, Schuenke M, Schulte E, Schumacher U. Atlas of Anatomy. 2nd ed. New York, NY: Thieme Medical Publishers; 2012. Illustration by Karl Wesker.)

The classical approach uses a landmark technique that blocks the nerves once they have separated into the different fascial layers. The injection is made at a point 2 cm medial and 2 cm cephalad to the ASIS using a short-beveled needle advanced perpendicular to the skin. After an initial pop sensation as the needle penetrates the EOA, around 5 mL of local anesthetic is injected to block the ilioinguinal nerve. The needle is then inserted deeper until a second pop is felt penetrating the internal oblique, to lie between it and the transversus abdominis muscle. A further 5 mL of local anesthetic is injected to block the iliohypogastric nerve.[2] A fanwise subcutaneous injection of 3 to 5 mL can be made to block any remaining sensory supply from the intercostals and subcostal nerve. This approach has a success rate of ~70% with failure often due to the local anesthetic being placed more than one anatomical layer away from the nerves.[3]

Ultrasound has been used with increasing success to block the nerves proximal to the ASIS when both nerves can be identified in the fascial layer between the internal oblique and transversus abdominis muscles, before the iliohypogastric nerve has penetrated the internal oblique to lie below the EOA. The ultrasound probe is placed obliquely on a line joining the ASIS and the umbilicus, immediately superior to the ASIS.[4] It is not always possible to identify each nerve exactly on ultrasound; therefore, the most important aspect is to ensure that the needle is in the correct fascial layer. When the correct plane between the internal oblique and transversus abdominis muscles is identified, 10 to 15 mL of long-acting local anesthetic is injected in 5 mL aliquots.

It is worth noting that if used as the sole technique for inguinal herniorrhaphy, the sac containing the peritoneum should be infiltrated with local anesthetic by the surgeon as it is supplied by the abdominal visceral nerves.

Placing the needle and local anesthetic too deep can result in block failure and inadvertent femoral nerve block.[2] Injection into the peritoneal cavity will lead to failure of the block and can risk bowel perforation. Puncture of blood vessels, usually the inferior epigastric vessels, has been described. The use of ultrasound guidance could potentially reduce the incidence of these complications.

24.4 Genitofemoral Nerve

This derives from the ventral rami of spinal nerves L1 to L2 and is formed within the substance of the psoas major muscle (▶ Fig. 24.1). The nerve descends obliquely forward through the muscle to emerge on its abdominal surface opposite the 3rd or 4th lumbar vertebra near the medial border. After that, it descends beneath the peritoneum on the psoas muscle, crosses obliquely behind the ureter, and divides above the inguinal ligament into genital and femoral branches; it often divides close to its origin, in which case its branches emerge separately from the psoas major muscle.

The genital branch of the GFN, also known as the external spermatic nerve in males, is a nerve in the abdomen that arises from the GFN.

The genital branch supplies the cremaster muscle and anterior scrotal skin in males, and the skin of the mons pubis and labia majora in females.

The femoral (crural) branch, also known as the lumboinguinal nerve, descends lateral to the external iliac artery and passes beneath the inguinal ligament entering the femoral sheath anterolateral to the common femoral artery. The nerve pierces the femoral sheath and fascia lata to supply the skin of the groin below the mid-part of the inguinal ligament (the femoral triangle).

24.5 Variant Anatomy

Almost 50% of GFNs examined in cadaveric studies demonstrated anatomical variations[4]:

- Twenty percent bifurcate prematurely at the upper portion (rather than the mid-portion) of the anterior surface of the psoas major muscle.
- Occasionally, the genital and femoral branches do not merge into a common trunk within the substance of the psoas major muscle and remain as distinct nerves as they travel into the pelvis.
- Guérin et al[5,6] dissected cadavers for 60 lumbar plexuses and studied the variations in branches from the lumbar plexus. They divided the intervertebral disc spaces from L1 and L2 to L4 and L5 into four zones. Zone 1, at the level of L2 and L3, contains the sympathetic only. Zone 2 has the GFN. Zone 3 is the safe working zone. All other branches of lumbar plexus lie in Zone 4.
- In a cadaveric study, Gu et al[5,7] determined a safe working zone for performing lateral interbody fusion. This area was located between the anterior border of the lumbar nerve and the posterior border of the sympathetic trunk. The location of the GFN was responsible for a narrowing of the safe zone at the L2 and L3 level.
- McCrory and Bell[5,8] showed that the GFN arises from the rami of the L1 and L2 spinal nerve roots and passes through the psoas major muscle, emerging on its anterior aspect. The nerve divides into the genital and femoral branches. The genital branch enters the inguinal canal and then shares in sensory supply to the scrotal skin or the mons pubis and labium majus. The femoral branch passes under the inguinal ligament to supply a small patch of skin on the anterior thigh.

24.6 Pathology

Injury to the GFN is common when the surgeon uses local infiltration to repair the scrotal skin. Sensory innervation to the scrotum arises from the genital branch of the GFN, traveling with the spermatic cord through the inguinal canal en route to the scrotum. The GFN lies immediately lateral to the spermatic cord as it emerges from the SIR and is involved in the efferent arm of the cremasteric reflex. This causes distortion and apparent shrinkage of the scrotal surface area, and ascent of the ipsilateral testis.

Chronic pain can occur in the inguinal region after repair of an inguinal hernia by the surgeon. This problem was first named by Heise and Starling as "mesh inguinodynia" in 1998.[9] The incidence of chronic pain after inguinal hernial repair has been reported by Poobalan et al[10] to be as high as 54%. Recently, Aroori and Spence[11] suggested that this issue should be included in the informed consent forms for all patients undergoing any type of hernia repair.

The most commonly reported cause of entrapment of the GFN relates to surgical trauma.[12,13] Other rare case reports include wearing tight clothing and direct trauma to the groin resulting in local scarring.[14,15]

Injury to the GFN can affect temperature regulation of the testis.

24.6.1 Technique

The spermatic cord is identified immediately lateral to the pubic tubercle. The area for injection, including the scrotum, is sterilized. The spermatic cord is then stabilized and medialized using the nondominant hand, and 5 mL of 1% lidocaine is injected subdermally immediately lateral to the cord, superficial to the bone.[5] Negative aspiration prior to injection ensures nonpenetrance of the peritoneum or femoral vessels.

24.6.2 Discussion

GFN block provides hemiscrotal anesthesia, allowing manipulation and intervention in an area prone to changes in texture and superficial skin anatomy to be conducted painlessly. This method of regional anesthesia thereby eliminates problems with handling the scrotal skin during anesthetic infiltration, which can occur on stimulation of the cremasteric reflex. This method also minimizes the risk of injury to the male genitalia.

References

[1] McDonnell JG, O'Donnell BD, Farrell T, et al. Transversus abdominis plane block: a cadaveric and radiological evaluation. Reg Anesth Pain Med. 2007; 32(5):399–404

[2] Klaassen Z, Marshall E, Tubbs RS, et al. Anatomy of the ilioinguinal and iliohypogastric nerves with observations of their spinal nerve contributions. Clin Anat. 2011 May; 24(4):454–461

[3] Weintraud M, Marhofer P, Bösenberg A, et al. Ilioinguinal/iliohypogastric blocks in children: where do we administer the local anesthetic without direct visualization? Anesth Analg. 2008; 106(1):89–93

[4] Eichenberger U, Greher M, Kirchmair L, Curatolo M, Moriggl B. Ultrasound-guided blocks of the ilioinguinal and iliohypogastric nerve: accuracy of a selective new technique confirmed by anatomical dissection. Br J Anaesth. 2006; 97(2):238–243

[5] Guérin P, Obeid I, Bourghli A, et al. The lumbosacral plexus: anatomic considerations for minimally invasive retroperitoneal transpsoas approach. Surg Radiol Anat. 2012; 34(2):151–157

[6] Gu Y, Ebraheim NA, Xu R, Rezcallah AT, Yeasting RA. Anatomic considerations of the posterolateral lumbar disk region. Orthopedics. 2001; 24(1):56–58

[7] McCrory P, Bell S. Nerve entrapment syndromes as a cause of pain in the hip, groin and buttock. Sports Med. 1999; 27(4):261–274

[8] Heise CP, Starling JR. Mesh inguinodynia: a new clinical syndrome after inguinal herniorrhaphy? J Am Coll Surg. 1998; 187(5):514–518

[9] Poobalan AS, Bruce J, Smith WC, King PM, Krukowski ZH, Chambers WA. A review of chronic pain after inguinal herniorrhaphy. Clin J Pain. 2003; 19(1):48–54

[10] Aroori S, Spence RA. Chronic pain after hernia surgery–an informed consent issue. Ulster Med J. 2007; 76(3):136–140

[11] Starling JR, Harms BA. Diagnosis and treatment of genitofemoral and ilioinguinal neuralgia. World J Surg. 1989; 13(5):586–591

[12] Laha RK, Rao S, Pidgeon CN, Dujovny M. Genito-femoral neuralgia. Surg Neurol. 1977; 8(4):280–282

[13] Magee RK. Genitofemoral causalgia (a new syndrome). Can Med Assoc J. 1942; 46(4):326–329

[14] O'Brien MD. Genitofemoral neuropathy. BMJ. 1979; 1(6170):1052

[15] Sasaoka N, Kawaguchi M, Yoshitani K, et al. Evaluation of genitofemoral nerve block, in addition to ilioinguinal and iliohypogastric nerve block, during inguinal hernia repair in children. Br J Anaesth. 2005; 94(2):243–246

[16] Al-dabbagh AK. Anatomical variations of the inguinal nerves and risks of injury in 110 hernia repairs. Surg Radiol Anat. 2002 May; 24(2):102–107

25 Microanatomy of the Lumbar Plexus

Miguel Angel Reina, Fabiola Machés, Javier Moratinos-Delgado, Virginia García-García, Manuel Fernández-Domínguez

Abstract

This chapter outlines the microanatomy of the nervous structures that form the lumbar plexus including the nerve roots found at vertebral levels extending from T12 through L1, L2, L3, to L4. A better understanding of the microanatomy of the lumbar plexus can improve patient care and improve surgical outcomes.

Keywords: anatomy, lumbar plexus, morphology, histology

25.1 Introduction

Nerve roots, as well as related motor, sensory, and sympathetic axons, were examined at their origins in the subarachnoid space and along their exits through the intervertebral foramina. Four cross-sectional cuts were obtained at each level. The first consisted of a complete transverse cross-section of the dural sac and its contents, focusing the image exclusively on the anterolateral region of the subarachnoid space called the subarachnoid angle, where nerve root cuffs and their contents can be found. The second cut consisted of a full transverse cross-section of the nerve root cuff at a strategic point between the dural sac and the dorsal root ganglion. The third cut provided a full transverse cross-section of the nerve root cuff at the level of the dorsal root ganglion including the anterior nerve root at that same level. A final fourth cut consisted of a complete transverse cross-section distal to the dorsal root ganglion.

The term "nerve root" can be confusing if used to refer to structures found at different levels as they might not share the same morphology.

Nerve rootlets leave the spinal cord at the ventrolateral and dorsolateral sulci. Anterior rootlets contain predominately efferent fibers from the ventral horn and carry motor signals to voluntary muscles. In the thoracic and upper lumbar regions, they also carry preganglionic sympathetic fibers from the lateral horns. Posterior rootlets are elongations of pseudounipolar nerve cells located in dorsal root ganglions (DRGs).

Different rootlets join together and form the anterior and posterior roots: about 6 to 8 anterior rootlets and 8 to 10 posterior ones. Therefore, the rootlets are formed by successive additions of axonal groups either arriving at or leaving the spinal cord. Cross-sections of nerve roots within the subarachnoid space such as the cauda equina below L2 revealed that each nerve root is formed by multiple units. Each unit appears to be separated from neighboring units by a thin layer of collagen fibers. Similarly, each nerve root of the cauda equina is covered by pia mater. The cerebrospinal fluid is located on the outer aspect of these nerve roots.

Outside the pia mater, the nerve roots are surrounded by arachnoid sleeves. These are formed by arachnoid cells and collagen fibers of the trabeculated arachnoid. At the subarachnoid angle, the arachnoid sleeves delimit and separate the anterior and posterior rootlets, as (▶ Fig. 25.1, ▶ Fig. 25.2, ▶ Fig. 25.3).

Although whether these nerve roots in the cauda equina should be called rootlets or nerve roots can be questioned, the term "subarachnoid nerve root" seems accurate. Subarachnoid nerve roots join together in numbers of 1 to 2 anterior nerve roots and 2 to 5 posterior ones to exit through the anterolateral subarachnoid space toward the nerve root cuffs. Inside the cuffs, these nerves are known as anterior and posterior nerve roots, respectively (▶ Fig. 25.4). In more distal successive cross-sectional cuts of the nerve root cuffs at the level of the DRG, it was observed that the bodies of these ganglia are similar to those of pseudounipolar nerve cells and sensory axons (▶ Fig. 25.5, ▶ Fig. 25.6). At the same cross-sectional level, motor nerves known as anterior nerve roots were present. However, their structural microanatomy does not resemble that of previous and more proximal cross-sectional images. Adjacent to the anterior and posterior nerve roots, structures similar to the pseudo-fascicular type can be found, as the axons contained are not enveloped by epineurium but surrounded by a transitional arachnoid layer with different properties. At the level of the DRG, cross-sectional images demonstrate that the multifascicular appearance of pseudo-fascicles is no longer evident. Whereas axons forming multiple pseudo-fascicles in anterior nerve roots appear in groups of mainly one or two motor units, the axons located in posterior nerve roots are joined either in a single ganglion, one bilobed, or two dorsal nerve ganglia parallel to each other.

In the transverse cross-section obtained beyond and distal to the DRG, fascicles were found. This is the site of origin of fascicles in the peripheral nerve. Successive distal cross-sections at 1 to 2 mm intervals showed different intrafascicular topograms.

Adipose tissue appears sparsely distributed among the dural laminas of the dura mater around the area of nerve root cuffs. The dura mater at this level can be thinner than in the dural sac, although overall the nerve root coverings are thicker.

Details of the microanatomy of the femoral and obturator nerves were included. The microanatomy of the sympathetic chains at the thoracolumbar level was studied, showing the differences between the histology of nerve root and sympathetic ganglia.

25.2 Lumbar Plexus and Associated Structures

The following figures are images of successive cross-sections obtained from same cadaver, where we can see nervous structures of lumbar plexus from subarachnoid space at T12 to L4 level to distal nerves as femoral and obturator nerves, also including sympathetic nervous structures (Fig. 25.1 - Fig. 25.45).

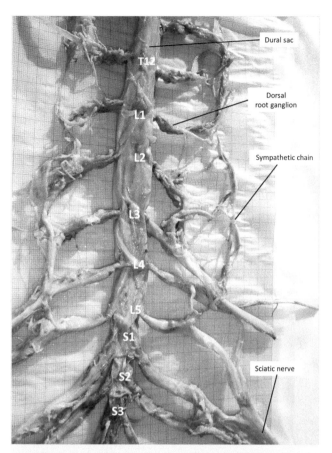

Fig. 25.1 Human dural sac, nerve root cuffs, roots of lumbar plexus, sacral plexus, and sympathetic chain at lumbar level. The dural sac appears flattened owing to loss of cerebrospinal fluid after dissection of the sample.

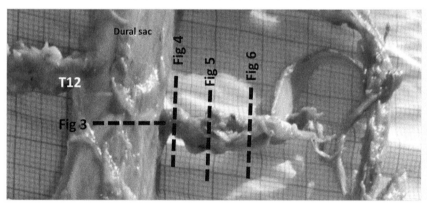

Fig. 25.2 Human dural sac at the 12th thoracic vertebral level. The lines point to the cross-sections and their relationships to the numbers of the succeeding figures.

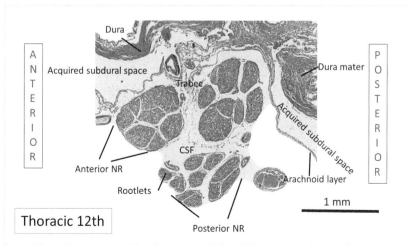

Fig. 25.3 Transverse cross-section of nerve root cuff at 12th thoracic vertebral level. The image shows the 12th thoracic anterior and posterior nerve roots within the subarachnoid space, precisely at the level of the subarachnoid angle. anterior NR, anterior nerve root; CSF, cerebrospinal fluid; posterior NR, posterior nerve root; Trabec, arachnoid trabeculae.

119

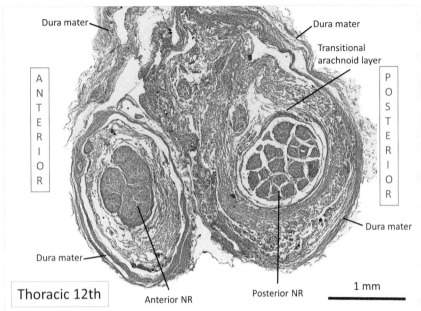

Fig. 25.4 Transverse cross-section of the nerve root cuff between the dural sac and the dorsal root ganglion at the 12th thoracic vertebral level. The image shows the anterior and posterior nerve roots separately enveloped by a transitional arachnoid layer and by dura mater on the outer aspect. In the area of dural cuffs, adipose tissue appears sparsely distributed among the dural laminas that form the dura mater. The dura mater at this level can be thinner than in the dural sac, although the dura covering nerve roots is thicker. Anterior NR, anterior nerve root; Posterior NR, posterior nerve root.

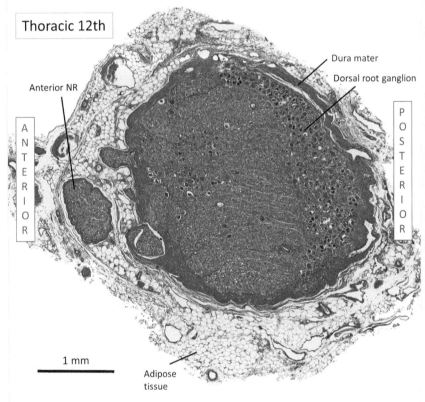

Fig. 25.5 Transverse cross-section of a nerve root cuff at the level of the 12th thoracic dorsal root ganglion. Image includes the anterior nerve root at the same level. Anterior NR, anterior nerve root.

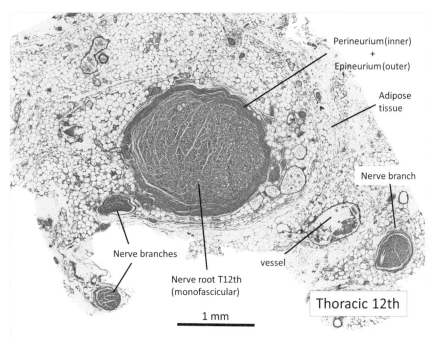

Perineurium(inner)
+
Epineurium(outer)

Adipose tissue

Nerve branch

Nerve branches

Nerve root T12th (monofascicular)

vessel

Thoracic 12th

1 mm

Fig. 25.6 Transverse cross-section of the 12th thoracic nerve root located distal to the dorsal root ganglion, immediately after leaving the spinal cord toward the external orifice of the foramen.

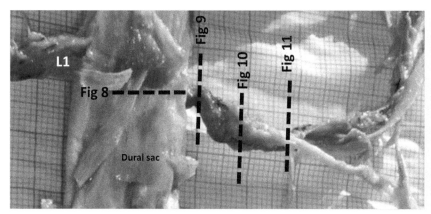

L1

Fig 9

Fig 10

Fig 11

Fig 8

Dural sac

Fig. 25.7 Human dural sac at the first lumbar vertebral level. Lines point toward the cross-sections indicating the relationship to the numbers of the succeeding figures.

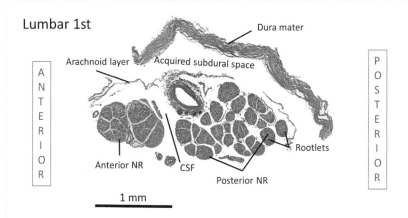

Lumbar 1st

Dura mater

Arachnoid layer   Acquired subdural space

ANTERIOR

POSTERIOR

Anterior NR   CSF

Posterior NR

Rootlets

1 mm

Fig. 25.8 Transverse cross-section of nerve root cuff at first lumbar vertebral level. The anterior and posterior first lumbar nerve roots within the subarachnoid space precisely around the subarachnoid angle. Anterior NR, anterior nerve root; CSF, cerebrospinal fluid; Posterior NR, posterior nerve root.

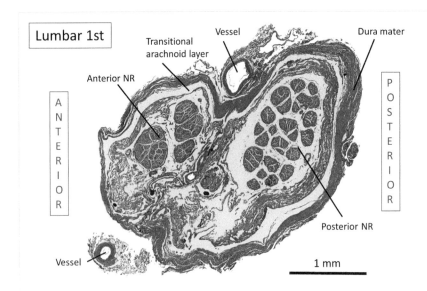

Fig. 25.9 Transverse cross-section of nerve root cuff between the dural sac and dorsal root ganglion at first lumbar vertebral level. The image shows the anterior and posterior nerve roots, each enveloped by a transitional arachnoid layer and outwardly by dura mater. Anterior NR, anterior nerve root; Posterior NR, posterior nerve root.

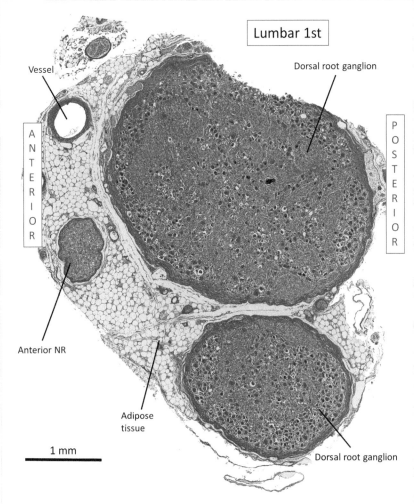

Fig. 25.10 Transverse cross-section of nerve root cuff at the level of the first lumbar dorsal root ganglion, showing the anterior nerve root at the same level. Anterior NR, anterior nerve root. This dorsal root ganglion is bilobed.

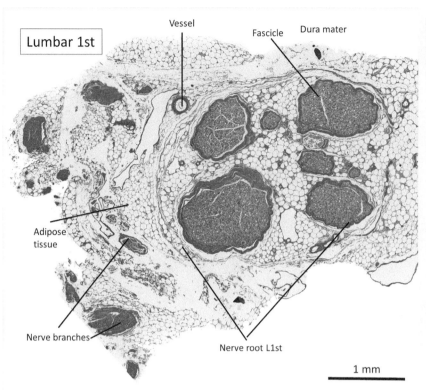

Lumbar 1st

Vessel

Fascicle   Dura mater

Adipose tissue

Nerve branches

Nerve root L1st

1 mm

Fig. 25.11 Transverse cross-section of the first lumbar nerve root beyond and distal to the dorsal root ganglion, immediately after exiting the spinal canal on its way toward the external orifice of the foraminal canal.

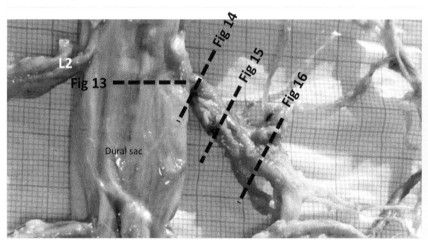

L2

Fig 13

Dural sac

Fig 14

Fig 15

Fig 16

Fig. 25.12 Human dural sac at second lumbar vertebral level. The lines show points of cross-sections and their relationships to the numbers in the succeeding figures.

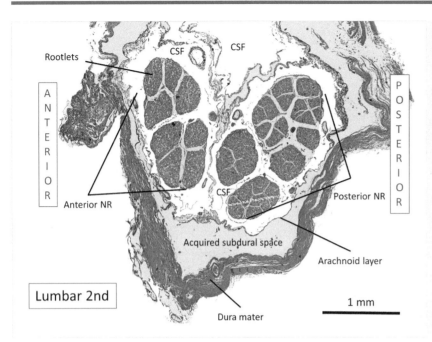

Fig. 25.13 Transverse cross-section of nerve root cuff at second lumbar vertebral level. The anterior and posterior second lumbar nerve roots in the subarachnoid space exactly at the subarachnoid angle. Anterior NR, anterior nerve root; CSF, cerebrospinal fluid; Posterior NR, posterior nerve root.

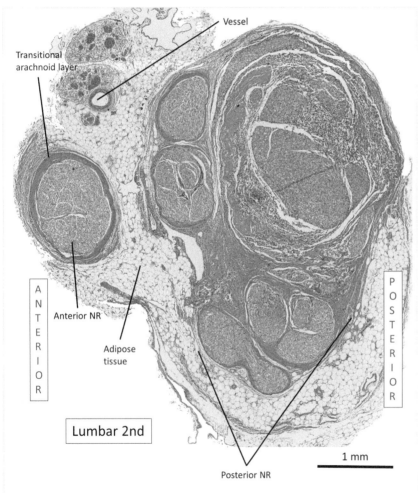

Fig. 25.14 Transverse cross-section of nerve root cuff between the dural sac and dorsal root ganglion at second lumbar vertebral level. The image shows the anterior and posterior nerve roots, each enveloped by a transitional arachnoid layer and outwardly by dura mater. This cross-section was obtained near the dorsal root ganglion. The axons found within pseudo-fascicles of the posterior nerve root are the same as those located within the dorsal root ganglion in ▶ Fig. 25.15. Anterior NR, anterior nerve root; Posterior NR, posterior nerve root.

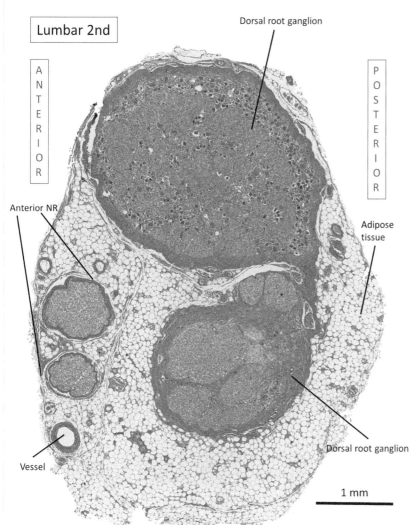

Lumbar 2nd

ANTERIOR

POSTERIOR

Dorsal root ganglion

Anterior NR

Vessel

Adipose tissue

Dorsal root ganglion

1 mm

Fig. 25.15 Transverse cross-section of nerve root cuff at the level of the second lumbar dorsal nerve ganglion including the anterior nerve root at the same level. Anterior NR, anterior nerve root. This dorsal root ganglion is also bilobed.

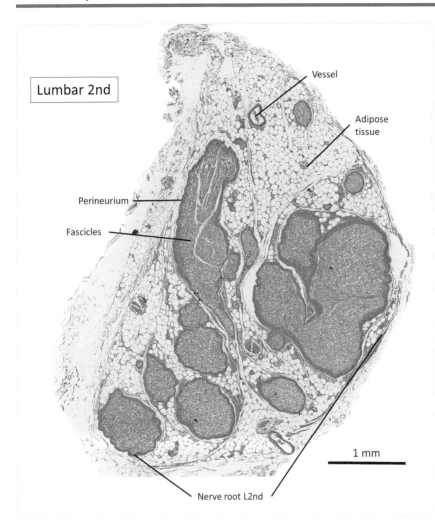

Lumbar 2nd

Vessel

Adipose tissue

Perineurium

Fascicles

1 mm

Nerve root L2nd

Fig. 25.16 Transverse cross-section of second lumbar nerve root beyond and distal to the dorsal ganglion at the exit from the spinal canal, close to the external orifice of the foraminal canal.

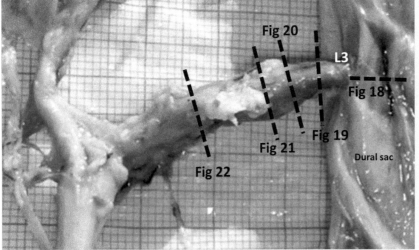

Fig 20

L3

Fig 18

Fig 19

Fig 21

Dural sac

Fig 22

Fig. 25.17 Human dural sac at the third lumbar vertebral level. The lines show the locations of the cross-sections and their relationships to the numbers of the succeeding figures.

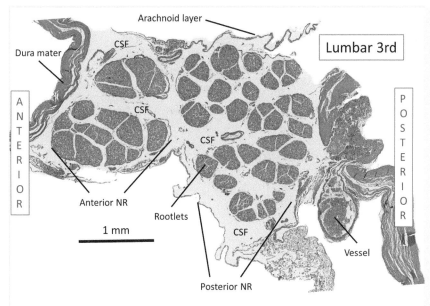

Fig. 25.18 Transverse cross-section of nerve root cuff at third lumbar vertebral level. The anterior and posterior third lumbar nerve roots in the subarachnoid space are exactly at the subarachnoid angle. Anterior NR, anterior nerve root; CSF, cerebrospinal fluid; Posterior NR, posterior nerve root.

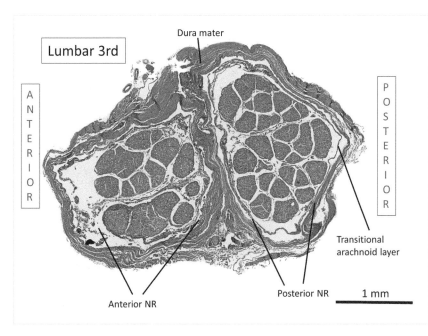

Fig. 25.19 Transverse cross-section of nerve root cuff between the dural sac and the dorsal root ganglion at third lumbar vertebral level. The image shows the anterior and posterior nerve roots each enveloped by a transitional arachnoid layer and outwardly by dura mater. Anterior NR, anterior nerve root; Posterior NR, posterior nerve root.

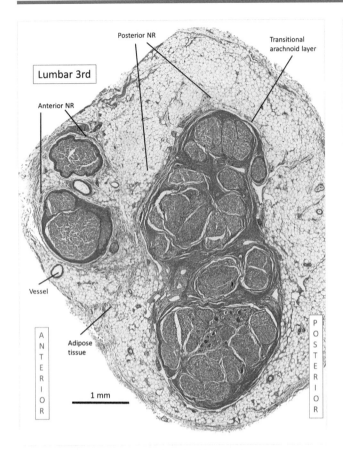

Fig. 25.20 Transverse cross-section of nerve root cuff between the dural sac and the dorsal root ganglion at the third lumbar vertebral level, close to the dorsal root ganglion. This cross-section shows the fusion of some pseudo-fascicles from the dorsal nerve root described in (Fig. 25.19). Anterior NR, anterior nerve root; Posterior NR, posterior nerve root.

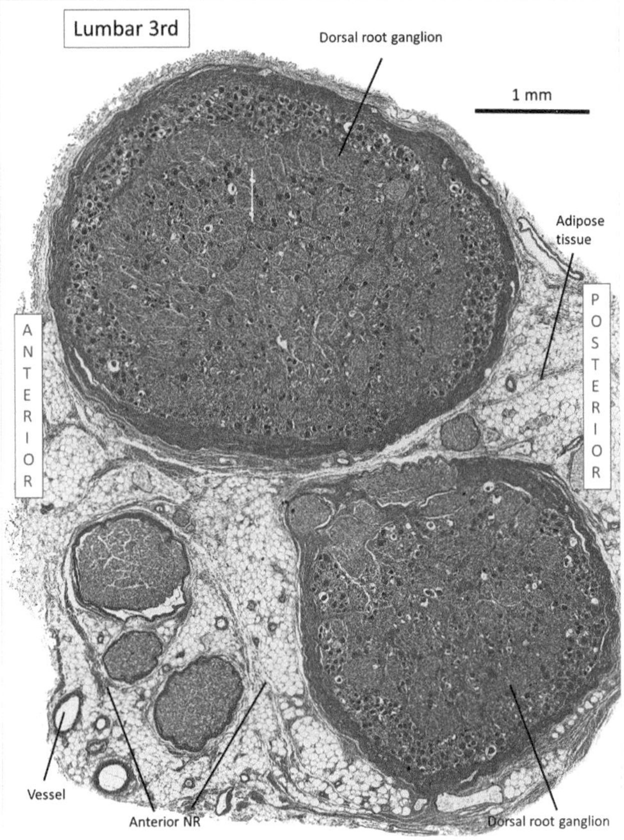

Fig. 25.21 Transverse cross-section of nerve root cuff at the third lumbar dorsal root ganglion including the anterior nerve root at the same level. Anterior NR, anterior nerve root. This dorsal root ganglion is bilobed.

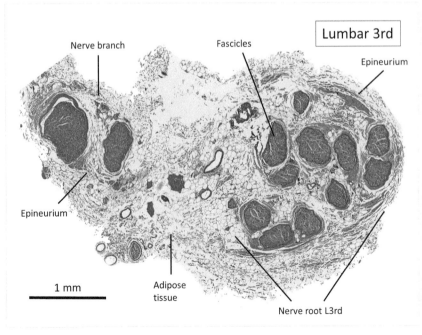

Fig. 25.22 Transverse cross-section of third lumbar nerve beyond and distal to the dorsal root ganglion at the exit from the spinal canal, close to the external orifice of the foraminal canal.

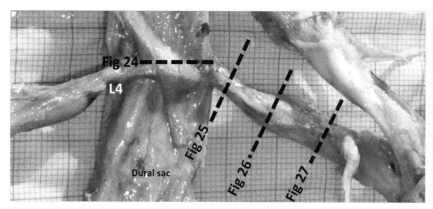

Fig. 25.23 Human dural sac at fourth lumbar vertebral level. The lines mark the cross-sections and their relationships to the numbers of the succeeding figures.

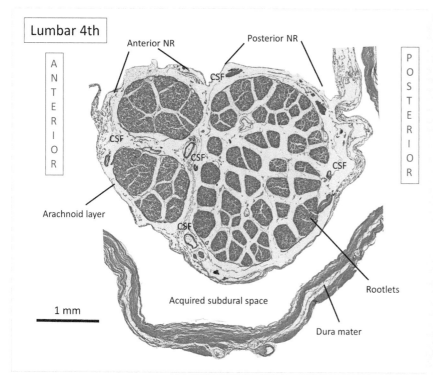

Fig. 25.24 Transverse cross-section of nerve root cuff at fourth lumbar vertebral level. L4 anterior and posterior nerve roots at the subarachnoid space lie exactly at the subarachnoid angle. Anterior NR, anterior nerve root; CSF, cerebrospinal fluid; Posterior NR, posterior nerve root.

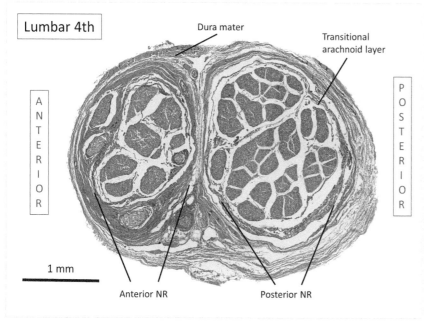

Fig. 25.25 Transverse cross-section of the nerve root cuff between the dural sac and the dorsal root ganglion at fourth lumbar vertebral level. The image shows the anterior and posterior nerve roots each enveloped by a transitional arachnoid layer and outwardly by dura mater. Anterior NR, anterior nerve root; Posterior NR, posterior nerve root.

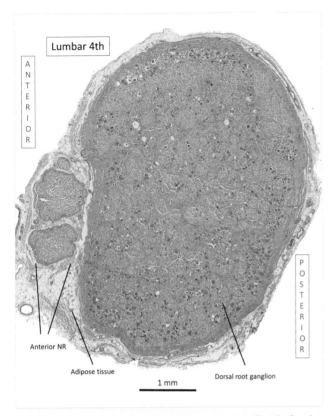

Fig. 25.26 Transverse cross-section of the nerve root cuff at the fourth lumbar dorsal root ganglion level including the anterior nerve root at the same level. Anterior NR, anterior nerve root.

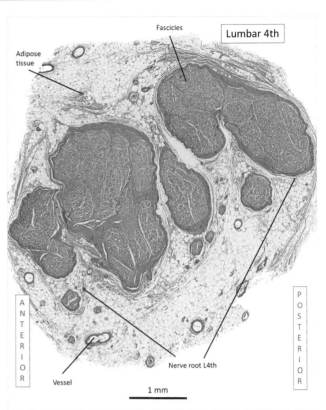

Fig. 25.27 Transverse cross-section of fourth lumbar nerve beyond and distal to the dorsal root ganglion, immediately after leaving the spinal canal on its way toward the external orifice of the foraminal canal.

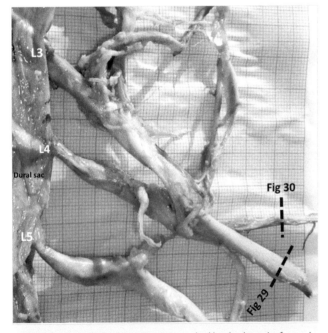

Fig. 25.28 Human dural sac at L3–L4 vertebral level, where the femoral and obturator nerves originate. The lines pinpoint the cross-sections and their relationships to the numbers of the succeeding figures.

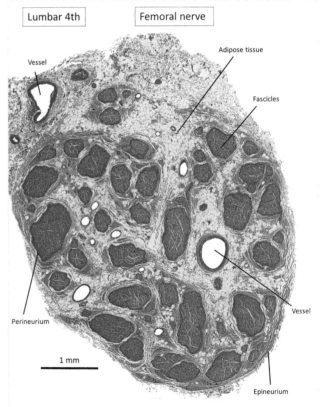

Fig. 25.29 Transverse cross-section of femoral nerve. Details of numbers and sizes of fascicles.

Lumbar 4th   Obturator nerve

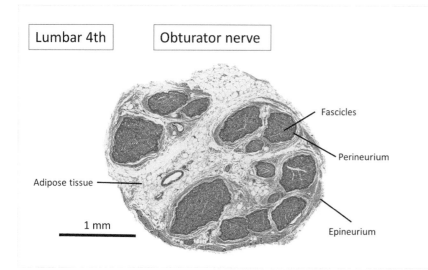

Fascicles

Perineurium

Adipose tissue

Epineurium

1 mm

Fig. 25.30 Transverse cross-section of obturator nerve. Details of numbers and sizes of fascicles.

Lumbar 4th   Anterior nerve root . Detail fig. 25

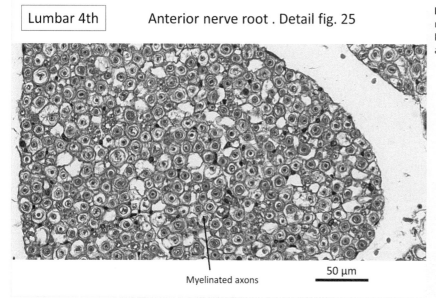

Myelinated axons

50 µm

Fig. 25.31 Transverse cross-section of anterior nerve root at fourth lumbar vertebral level. Details of (Fig. 25.25). Details of myelinated axons.

Lumbar 4th   Posterior nerve root . Detail fig. 25

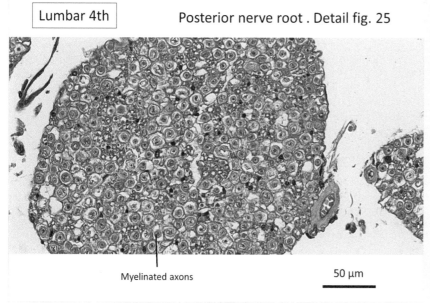

Myelinated axons

50 µm

Fig. 25.32 Transverse cross-section of posterior nerve root at fourth lumbar vertebral level. Details of (Fig. 25.25). Details of large and small myelinated axons.

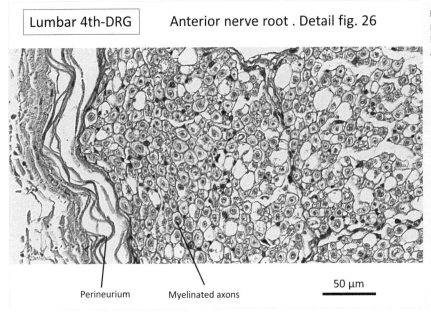

Lumbar 4th-DRG   Anterior nerve root . Detail fig. 26

Perineurium   Myelinated axons

50 μm

Fig. 25.33 Transverse cross-section of anterior nerve root at fourth lumbar vertebral level. Details of (Fig. 25.26). Details of myelinated axons.

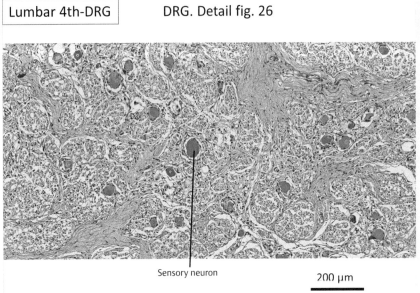

Lumbar 4th-DRG   DRG. Detail fig. 26

Sensory neuron

200 μm

Fig. 25.34 Transverse cross-section of dorsal root ganglion (DRG) at fourth lumbar vertebral level. Details of (Fig. 25.26). Details of axons and bodies of pseudounipolar nerve cells.

Lumbar 4th-DRG   DRG. Detail fig. 26

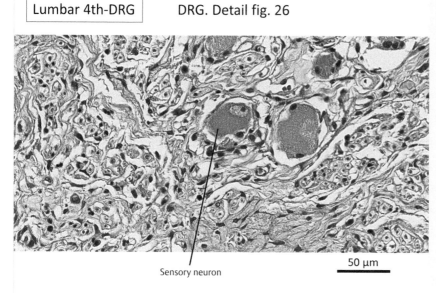

Sensory neuron

50 µm

Fig. 25.35 Transverse cross-section of dorsal root ganglion (DRG) at fourth lumbar vertebral level. Details of (Fig. 25.26) at higher magnification. In this image, the nucleus and nucleolus within the bodies of pseudounipolar nerve cells are visible.

Lumbar 4th-DRG   DRG. Detail fig. 26

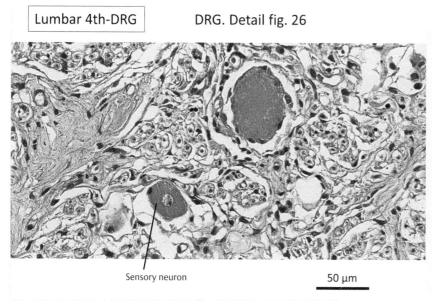

Sensory neuron

50 µm

Fig. 25.36 Transverse cross-section of dorsal root ganglion (DRG) at fourth lumbar vertebral level. Details of (Fig. 25.26) at higher magnifications. In this image, the nucleus and nucleolus of other bodies of pseudounipolar nerve cells are visible.

| Lumbar 4th-outer DRG | Anterior fascicles. Detail fig 27 |

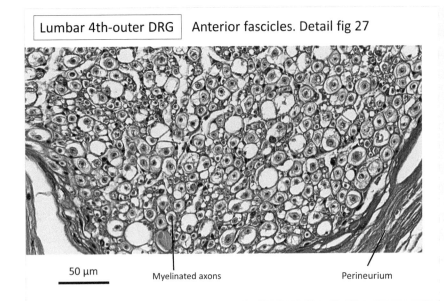

50 µm

Myelinated axons   Perineurium

Fig. 25.37 Transverse cross-section of fourth lumbar nerve beyond and distal to the dorsal root ganglion, immediately after exiting the spinal canal toward the external orifice of the foraminal canal. Details of fascicles located in anterior place of (Fig. 25.27) are shown at higher magnification.

| Lumbar 4th-outer DRG | Posterior fascicles. Detail fig 27 |

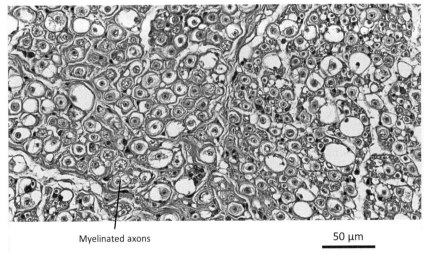

Myelinated axons   50 µm

Fig. 25.38 Transverse cross-section of fourth lumbar nerve beyond and distal to the dorsal root ganglion, immediately after exiting the spinal canal, towards the external orifice of the foraminal canal. Details of fascicles located in posterior place of (Fig. 25.27) are shown at higher magnification.

Lumbar 4th	Femoral nerve. Details of fascicles fig 29

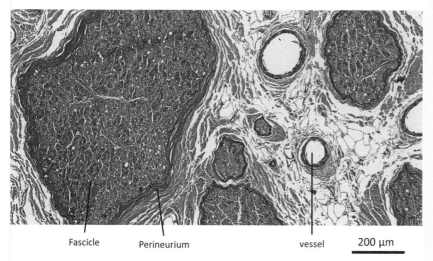

Fascicle   Perineurium   vessel   200 μm

Fig. 25.39 Transverse cross-section of femoral nerve. Details of (Fig. 25.29) are shown at higher magnification.

Lumbar 4th	Femoral nerve. Details of a fascicle fig 39

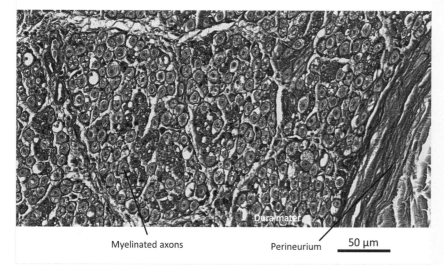

Myelinated axons   Perineurium   50 μm

Dura mater

Fig. 25.40 Transverse cross-section of femoral nerve. Details of (Fig. 25.39) are shown at higher magnification.

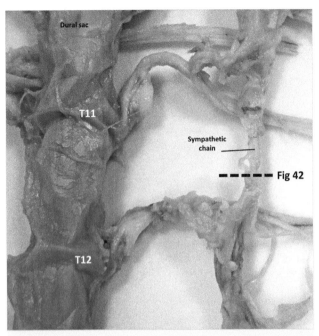

Fig. 25.41 Human dural sac at 11–12th vertebral level. The lines pinpoint the cross-section of a sympathetic chain.

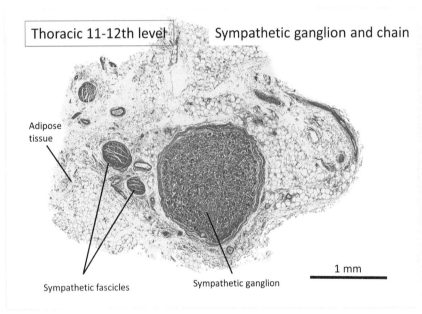

Fig. 25.42 Transverse cross-section of a sympathetic chain. Fascicles of the sympathetic nerve roots and sympathetic ganglion within the thoracic sympathetic chain are visible.

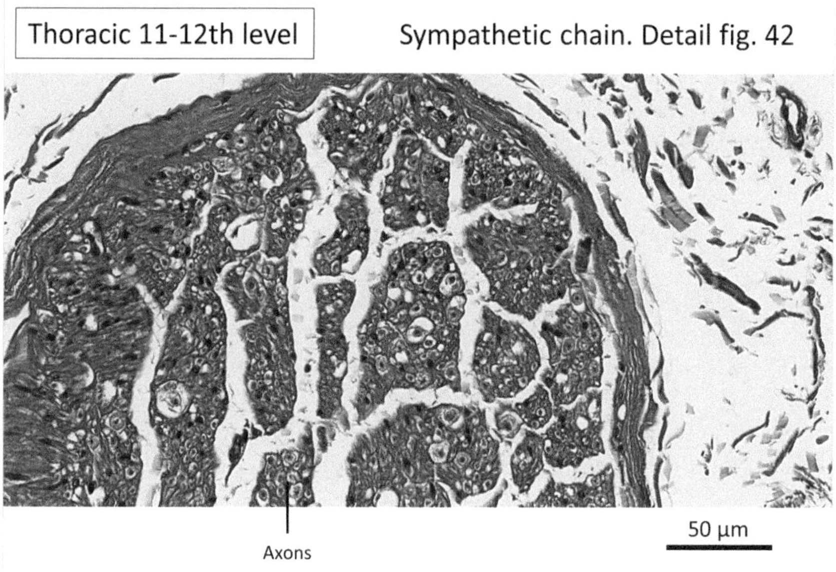

Thoracic 11-12th level	Sympathetic chain. Detail fig. 42

Fig. 25.43 Details of sympathetic axons of the sympathetic nerve roots from (Fig. 25.42) are shown at higher magnification.

Axons

50 µm

Thoracic 11-12th level	Sympathetic ganglion. Detail fig. 42

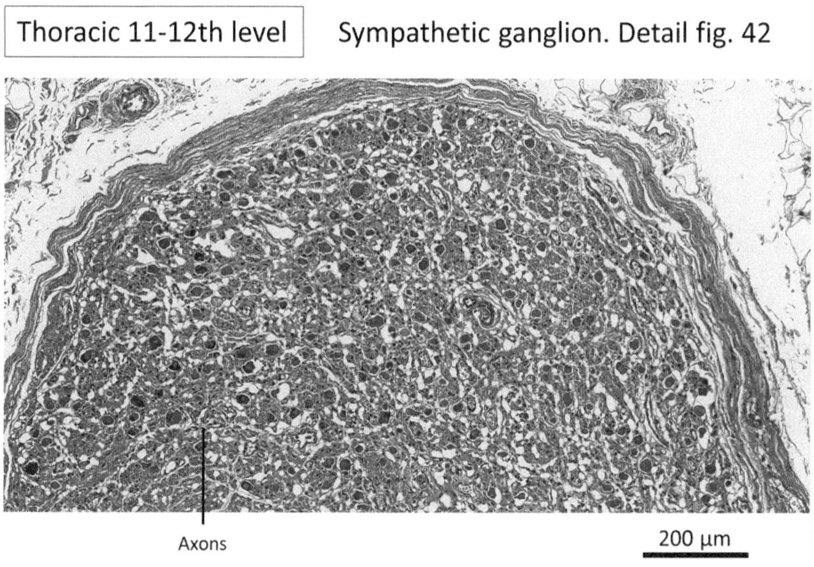

Fig. 25.44 Details of sympathetic axons and bodies of sympathetic neurons within the ganglion of (Fig. 25.42) are shown at higher magnification.

Axons

200 µm

Thoracic 11-12th level	Sympathetic ganglion. Detail fig. 42

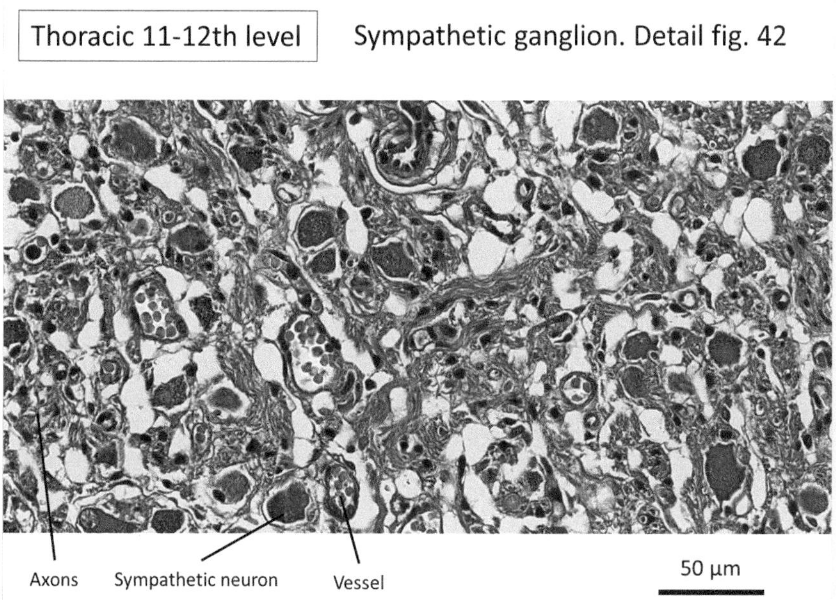

Fig. 25.45 Details of sympathetic axons and bodies of sympathetic neurons of (Fig. 25.42) are shown at higher magnification.

Axons   Sympathetic neuron   Vessel

50 µm

26 Surgical Anatomy of the Lumbar Plexus with Emphasis on Landmarks

Shehzad Khalid, R. Shane Tubbs

Abstract

Surgical landmarks for identifying the branches of the lumbar plexus as found on the posterior abdominal wall are lacking in the English literature. Many surgical complications have involved these nerves, highlighting the significance of the development of a clear topographical map for use in their identification. The surgeon who operates in this region needs a good working knowledge of the nerves of the lumbar plexus on the posterior abdominal wall. Our measurements will hopefully aid the surgeon who wishes to expose or most certainly avoid these nerves, thus lessening patient morbidity.

Keywords: complications, operative, exposure, surgery, nervous, lumbosacral

26.1 Introduction

Although much less common than injuries of the brachial plexus, injuries to the lumbar plexus do occur and the surgeon must be familiar with this region in order to evaluate and potentially treat such problems. Lesions of the lumbar plexus are most commonly iatrogenic but can be due to birth trauma,[9] hematoma, entrapment in fibrous or muscular bands,[13] tumors both intrinsic and extrinsic, or wounds such as incurred by a sharp object or gunshot. Additionally, ablative procedures for pain involving any branch of the lumbar plexus demands a thorough knowledge of this anatomy.[2,4,14,22]

Peripheral nerve surgery is a common neurosurgical procedure. However, the lumbar plexus and its branches are dealt with infrequently. One reason for this is the relative inaccessibility of this region and the infrequency with which the neurosurgeon performs deep dissections within the abdominal and pelvic cavities. Benzel[2] referred to the lumbosacral plexus and lesions of these nerves as a "no-man's-land" and stated that "unfortunately, an inappropriately conservative approach is often undertaken in patients harboring these lesions because of the suspected degree of difficulty of the surgical approach." However, there has been a recent increase in the use of endoscopic approaches to the retroperitoneum for various spinal disorders.[20] Congruently, injury to branches of the lumbar plexus has been estimated at approximately 2% for laparoscopic hernioplasties.[23] Approaches to the lumbosacral plexus in the abdomen and pelvis include a lateral extracavitary approach to the spine,[3] an anterolateral extraperitoneal approach to the spine,[12] a pelvic brim extraperitoneal approach,[12] a Pfannenstiel infraperitoneal approach,[11] and a transperitoneal approach.[1] The anterolateral extraperitoneal approach is essentially the same corridor used by surgeons to access the sympathetic trunk in the lumbosacral region. The lumbar veins and arteries can be obstacles to very medial dissections.[2] The pelvic brim extraperitoneal approach allows the lower branches of the lumbar plexus (e.g., the obturator nerve) to be accessed. The Pfannenstiel infraperitoneal approach also allows for access to lower branches of the lumbar plexus such as the femoral nerve. The transperitoneal approach to the lumbar plexus is perhaps the best method to use when a wide exposure is needed such as for tumors of neural origin.[2]

26.2 General Anatomy

The lumbar plexus is formed in the retroperitoneal abdomen from the ventral rami of spinal nerves T12 to L4 (▶ Fig. 26.1).[30] This pattern can be different if the plexus is pre- or postfixed (i.e., fiber contributions are moved cranially or caudally, respectively).[7,24] Most of these branches traverse the psoas major muscle proximally. They include the subcostal (T12), iliohypogastric (T12–L1), ilioinguinal (L1), lateral femoral cutaneous (L2–L3), genitofemoral (L1–L2), femoral (L2–L4), and obturator (L2–L4) nerves (▶ Fig. 26.1, ▶ Fig. 26.2). The subcostal, iliohypogastric, and ilioinguinal nerves innervate the abdominal wall musculature and aid in supplying the dermatomes of T12 through L1. The iliohypogastric nerve can also innervate the pyramidalis muscle when present. As implied, the lateral femoral cutaneous supplies the skin of the lateral thigh. The genitofemoral nerve innervates a small patch of skin over the proximal anterior thigh, scrotum and labia majora, and also the cremaster muscle. The femoral nerve innervates most of the anterior thigh musculature, much of the skin of the anterior thigh and medial leg, and both the hip and knee joints. The obturator nerve innervates a small patch of skin of the medial thigh, provides most of the motor innervation to the medial thigh muscles, and sends articular branches to the hip and knee joints. An accessory obturator nerve is also encountered in up to 30% of individuals.[29] Each of these branches has both a sensory and motor component with the exception of the lateral femoral cutaneous, which as its name implies, has no somatic motor component.

26.3 Landmarks

In a previous anatomical study, mean distances from the midline at their emergence through or lateral to the psoas major muscle to the subcostal, iliohypogastric, ilioinguinal, lateral femoral cutaneous, genitofemoral, and femoral nerves measured 5.5, 6, 6.5, 6, 4.5, and 4.5 cm, respectively (▶ Table 26.1, ▶ Fig. 26.2).[29] ▶ Fig. 26.2 illustrates these and the following distances. The obturator nerve had a mean distance of 3 cm lateral to the midline. At a vertical line through the anterior superior iliac spine, the subcostal, iliohypogastric, and ilioinguinal nerves were superior to the supracristal plane by mean distances of 8, 4, and 5 cm, respectively. Inferior to the supracristal plane and in a vertical line through a midpoint between the anterior superior iliac spine and midline, the lateral femoral cutaneous and femoral nerves had mean distances of 5 and 5.5 cm, respectively. The lateral femoral cutaneous nerve (LFCN)

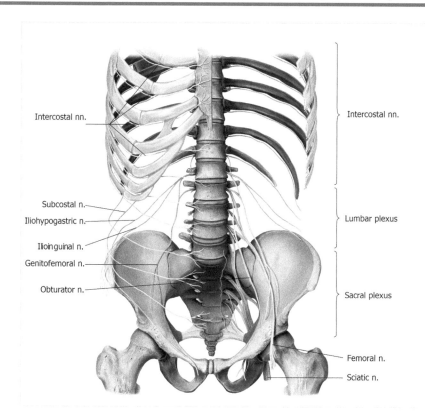

Intercostal nn.

Subcostal n.

Iliohypogastric n.

Ilioinguinal n.

Genitofemoral n.

Obturator n.

Intercostal nn.

Lumbar plexus

Sacral plexus

Femoral n.

Sciatic n.

Fig. 26.1 Schematic view of the branches of the lumbar plexus. (Reproduced with permission from Gilroy AM, MacPherson BR, Ross LM, Schuenke M, Schulte E, Schumacher U. Atlas of Anatomy. 2nd ed. New York, NY: Thieme Medical Publishers; 2005. Illustration by Karl Wesker.) (From THIEME Gilroy Atlas of Anatomy, 2e, © Thieme 2005, Illustration by [Karl Wesker])

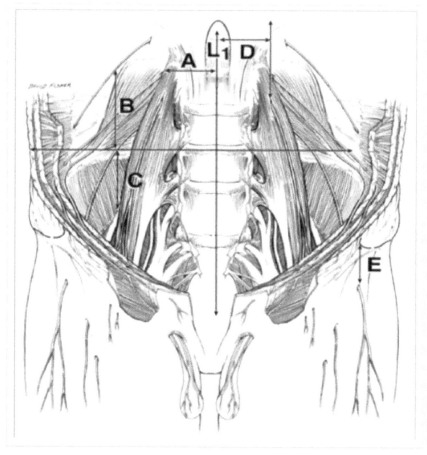

Fig. 26.2 Schematic representation of the posterior abdominal wall with the distances measured in this study. A = distance from midline to branches of the lumbar plexus at their emergence site through the psoas major muscle (the nerve in this example is the lateral femoral cutaneous nerve), B = distance superior to the supracristal plane (the tips of the iliac crests are connected with the horizontal line to create this plane) on a vertical line through a midpoint between the anterior superior iliac spine and midline for nerves of the lumbar plexus (the nerve in this example is the subcostal nerve), C = distance inferior to the supracristal plane on a vertical line through a midpoint between the anterior superior iliac spine and midline for nerves of the lumbar plexus (the nerve in this example is the femoral), D = distance inferior to L1 vertebra that GF emerges through the psoas major muscle, E=distance inferomedial from the anterior superior iliac spine for LFC. L1, first lumbar vertebra.

Table 26.1 Distances from the Nerves of the Lumbar Plexus to Surrounding Bony Landmarks from the Study by Tubbs et al.[29]

Nerve	Distance	Range (cm)	Mean (cm)	SD
Subcostal	A	4.5–7	5.5	1.7
Iliohypogastric	A	5–8	6	1.5
Ilioinguinal	A	5.5–8.5	6.5	1.9
Genitofemoral	A	3.5–6.5	4.5	2.1
Lateral femoral cutaneous	A	5–7.5	6	1.3
Femoral	A	4–5.5	4.5	1.1
Obturator	A	2.5–4	3	0.9
Subcostal	B	5–10	8	2.2
Iliohypogastric	B	3–6	4	1.5
Ilioinguinal	B	4–7	5	1.7
Lateral femoral cutaneous	C	4–7	5	1.2
Femoral	C	4.5–7.5	5.5	0.9
Genitofemoral	D	4–8	6.5	2.3
Lateral femoral cutaneous	E	0.5–3.5	1.5	0.8

Abbreviations: GF, genitofemora; LFC, lateral femoral cutaneous; SD, standard deviation.
Note: See ▶ Fig. 26.2 for a depiction of the following measurements: A = distance from midline to branches of the lumbar plexus at their emergence site through the psoas major muscle, B = distance superior to the supracristal plane on a vertical line through a midpoint between the anterior superior iliac spine and midline for nerves of the lumbar plexus, C = distance inferior to the supracristal plane on a vertical line through a midpoint between the anterior superior iliac spine and midline for nerve of the lumbar plexus, D = distance inferior to L1 vertebra that GF emerges through the psoas major muscle, E = distance inferomedial from the anterior superior iliac spine for LFC.

had a mean distance 1.5 cm inferomedial to the anterior superior iliac spine. The subcostal nerve had a mean distance of 1 cm inferior to the 12th rib. The genitofemoral nerve emerged from the center of the psoas major in all specimens and divided into its genital and femoral components at a mean distance of 6 cm inferior to its exit from the psoas major, which had a mean distance of 6.5 cm inferior to the attachment of the psoas major to the L1 vertebra.

26.4 Iliohypogastric and Ilioinguinal Nerves Surgical Anatomy

The iliohypogastric nerve is a branch of the anterior division of the first lumbar nerve. It can also receive fibers from the 12th thoracic nerve. It passes through the upper portion of the lateral border of the psoas major muscle and crosses the crest of the ileum, where it pierces the transversus abdominis muscle. It then divides into lateral cutaneous and anterior cutaneous branches. The lateral branch supplies the skin of the gluteal region. The anterior branch pierces the internal oblique muscle and exits at the aponeurosis of the external oblique about 2.5 cm above the superficial inguinal ring. Motor branches supply the rectus abdominis and pyramidalis muscles. Sensory cutaneous branches are sent to the suprapubic and hypogastric regions.

Injuries to the nerve are most often associated with surgical procedures including inguinal herniorrhaphy, appendectomy, and pelvic surgery using a low transverse incision. Symptoms of injury are a burning sensation along with pain and numbness in the inguinal and suprapubic regions. The symptoms mostly result from nerve entrapment. Motor loss with nerve injury is minimal since the primary function of the innervated muscles

is to maintain intra-abdominal pressure and to aid the process of forced expiration.

The ilioinguinal nerve is a branch of the first lumbar nerve. In roughly 25% of cases, it originates as a common trunk with the iliohypogastric nerve. It emerges from the lateral border of the psoas major and passes obliquely across the quadratus lumborum. It then perforates the transversus abdominis muscle, becomes closely associated with the iliohypogastric nerve, and pierces the internal oblique muscle. The nerve then accompanies the spermatic cord through the superficial external ring. Some of its fibers are distributed to the skin of the upper, medial thigh. In the male, the nerve terminates as the anterior scrotal nerve, which supplies sensations to the skin over the root of the penis and upper scrotum. In the female, the nerve terminates as the anterior labial nerve, providing sensory input to the skin of the mons pubis and labia majora.

Injury to the nerve is most commonly associated with blunt trauma and damage incurred during inguinal hernia repair. The symptoms of this can be quite significant. Division of the nerve will result in sensory loss to the proximal medial thigh, anterior scrotum, labia majora, and mons pubis. Sensory deficits will diminish over time and are usually minimal after 1 year. A more serious problem arises when nerve entrapment results from hernia repair. This can cause debilitating pain in the proximal medial thigh, groin, labia majora, and scrotum. Motor loss from nerve injury is insignificant.

The iliohypogastric and ilioinguinal nerves, as they cross anterior to the quadratus lumborum muscle and lateral to the psoas major muscle, are situated posterior to the kidneys and posterior to the ascending or descending colon on the right and left sides, respectively. They then travel superior to the iliac crest to run between the internal oblique and transversus abdominis muscles.[15] The iliohypogastric nerve has been cited to emerge approximately 3 cm medial to the anterior superior iliac spine.[19,31] Whiteside et al[31] stated that the second most common neuropathy following gynecological surgery involves the ilioinguinal and iliohypogastric nerves, with a reported incidence of 3.7%. Nephrectomy is also a common cause of injury to these two nerves.[27] We found that the iliohypogastric nerve had a mean distance from the midline of 6 cm in line with the anterior superior iliac spine. Our data showed that the ilioinguinal nerve had a mean distance of 6.5 cm from the midline in line with the anterior superior iliac spine and a mean distance of 1.5 cm inferomedial to the anterior superior iliac spine. Furthermore, we found that at a vertical line through the anterior superior iliac spine the iliohypogastric and ilioinguinal nerves were superior to the supracristal plane by mean distances of 4 and 5 cm, respectively. In one study, 100 adult formalin-fixed cadavers were dissected producing 200 iliohypogastric and ilioinguinal nerve specimens.[32] The linear course of each nerve was followed and its respective lateral distance from the midline at termination was then appropriately measured. It turns out that the ilioinguinal nerve originated from L1 in 130 specimens (65%), from T12 and L1 in 28 (14%), from L1 and L2 in 22 (11%), and from L2 and L3 in 20 (10%). The nerve entered the abdominal wall 2.8 ± 1.1 cm medial and 4 ± 1.2 cm inferior to the anterior superior iliac spine and ended 3 ± 0.5 cm lateral to the midline. The iliohypogastric nerve originated from T12 on 14 specimens (7%), from T12 and L1 in 28 (14%), from L1 in 20 (10%), and from T11 and T12 in 12 (6%). The nerve entered the abdominal wall 2.8 ± 1.3 cm medial and 1.4 ± 1.2 cm inferior to the anterior superior iliac spine and terminated 4 ± 1.3 cm lateral to the midline. For both nerves, the distance between the anterior superior iliac spine and the midline was estimated to be at 12.2 ± 1.1 cm.[32] For sufficient anesthetic for nerve block during surgery and to minimize nerve damage, the exact anatomical location and spinal nerve contributions of the iliohypogastric and ilioinguinal nerves need to be fully considered.[32]

26.5 Genitofemoral Nerve Surgical Anatomy

The genitofemoral nerve usually traverses the substance of the psoas major in a somewhat vertical course. In its course, this nerve crosses posterior to the ureter. The right nerve is posterior to the ileum and the left nerve is posterior to the sigmoid colon. Genitofemoral neuralgia has been treated successfully with ablation techniques and is most common following entrapment at a hernia repair site.[16,22] Laha et al[18] used an extraperitoneal approach for sectioning the genitofemoral nerve for intractable groin pain. Both ilioinguinal and genitofemoral neuralgia must be considered in all cases of intermittent or continuous pain radiating into the genitalia and medial thigh.[22] Moro et al,[20] with respect to retroperitoneal endoscopic surgery, found a relative safety zone for the lumbar plexus excluding the genitofemoral nerve at the L4 to L5 vertebral bodies and above.

The genitofemoral nerve most often arises from the second lumbar nerve; however, in some cases it receives input from the first and third lumbar nerves. It pierces the psoas major muscle and subsequently divides into the genital and femoral branches. The genital branch enters the inguinal canal through the deep ring supplying motor input to the cremasteric muscle.

Sensory input is sent to the scrotum in males and labia majora in females. The nerve also sends fibers to the adjacent proximal medial thigh. The femoral branch enters the femoral sheath lateral to the femoral artery, turns anterior, and supplies the skin overlying the femoral triangle.

Injury to the nerve is most commonly associated with blunt trauma and damage incurred during inguinal herniorrhaphy and pelvic surgery. Injury to the genital branch will result in numbness and burning pain at the bottom of the scrotum in men and the labia majora in women. These symptoms will also be seen in the proximal medial thigh. Pain will increase with extension of the lumbar spine putting traction on the nerve. Motor loss in the cremasteric muscle will be noted. This results in loss of the cremasteric reflex that elevates the testicles. Injury to the femoral branch of the nerve will result in sensory loss and possibly burning pain in the skin overlying the femoral triangle. Although the genitofemoral nerve is mixed, it chiefly functions as an afferent nerve.

This nerve has often been found to emerge near the medial border of the psoas major muscle opposite the L3 to L4 vertebral bodies.[22] We found that it always pierced the psoas major more or less in its midline and divided into its genital and femoral components at a mean distance of 6 cm inferior to its exit from this muscle and a mean distance of 6.5 cm inferior to the attachment of the psoas major to the L1 vertebra.[5]

26.6 Femoral Nerve Surgical Anatomy

The femoral nerve arises principally from the second, third, and fourth lumbar nerve roots. It can occasionally receive a contribution from the fifth lumbar nerve. It is a major nerve that innervates the lower limb and is the largest nerve to exit the lumbar plexus. It descends inferiorly from the lumbar plexus in a groove located between the psoas major muscle and the iliacus before exiting the lateral aspect of the psoas muscle, then sends off its first branch within the abdomen to supply motor input to the iliacus muscle, which functions as a hip flexor. The nerve continues into the pelvis to approximately the mid portion of the inguinal ligament. It then travels under the inguinal ligament through the femoral triangle, lateral to the femoral vessels. This is an important external landmark in which the nerve can be located. The location can be identified by palpating the pulse of the femoral artery and then moving laterally to the adjacent tissue. The nerve then splits into anterior and posterior divisions, which further divide into many branches throughout the thigh.

The anterior division divides into medial and intermediate branches. The medial cutaneous branch delivers sensory input to the skin of the medial thigh through its anterior branch and the medial leg through its posterior branch. The intermediate branch supplies sensory input to the anterior thigh. Muscular branches of the anterior aspect of the femoral nerve supply the pectineus and sartorius muscles, which are responsible for flexion, adduction, and abduction of the thigh.

The posterior division of the femoral nerve forms branches that serve the leg and are vital to the function of knee extension. Its muscular branches innervate the four quadriceps muscles, the rectus femoris, vastus lateralis, vastus medialis, and vastus intermedius. The quadriceps muscles are responsible for extension of the leg at the knee joint, and to a lesser extent flexion of the thigh at the hip. The longest branch of the femoral nerve coming off the posterior division is the saphenous nerve. This is considered to be the terminal branch of the femoral nerve. Distally, it runs parallel to the saphenous vein in the subcutaneous tissue of the medial thigh and continues into the lower leg, giving off sensory cutaneous branches to the anterior and medial surface of the leg. The femoral nerve is a mixed nerve combining afferent and efferent fibers. One of the major outflows of the lumbar plexus, it has an 8- to 10-cm course within the pelvis.[15] Within the pelvis it is found at the lateral border of or under cover of the psoas major muscle and innervates the iliacus muscle. On the right side, it rests posterior to the ileocecal junction, and on the left side, posterior to the sigmoid colon.[27] Injury to it primarily interferes with a normal gait.[15] Interestingly, there are case reports of patients who have had their right femoral nerve inadvertently transected while undergoing appendectomy.[27] We found that the femoral nerve had a mean distance of 5.5 cm inferior to the supracristal plane on a vertical line through the anterior superior iliac spine. It has been found in axial scans of cadavers to lie approximately 9 cm from the skin surface of the back.[8] Neuropathy of the femoral nerve as a result of hemorrhage in hemophiliac patients and patients on anticoagulant therapy has been known for some time.[13,17,25] Spratt et al[26] posited that anomalous slips of the psoas major and iliacus muscles that split the femoral nerve can cause undiagnosed tension in the nerve and result in referred pain to the hip and knee joints and lumbar dermatomes L2 to L4. Kline and Hudson[15] reported patients with injury to this nerve from femoral artery manipulation for angiography, following aortofemoral bypass, and packing of the pelvis for bleeding of pelvic contents associated with surgery. This nerve can also be mistaken for the LFCN and can inadvertently be resected during treatment of meralgia paresthetica, or it can be injured with methyl methacrylate during hip repair or total hip replacement.[15]

26.7 Lateral Femoral Cutaneous Nerve Surgical Anatomy

On emergence from the psoas major muscle, the LFCN extends laterally and crosses the iliacus muscle obliquely. En route to the lateral thigh, it exits the abdomen in or in juxtaposition to the inguinal ligament near the anterior superior iliac spine. While in the iliac fossa, the LFCN is posterior to the cecum on the right side and posterior to the sigmoid colon on the left. It can become entrapped at the inguinal ligament resulting in meralgia paraesthetica.[28] However, it can be injured iatrogenically with autogenous iliac bone grafts.[6,21] Hospodar et al[10] found that it is commonly located 10 to 15 mm medially from the anterior superior iliac spine, although it can emerge lateral to the anterior superior iliac spine.[21] We found that it had a mean distance of 1.5 cm inferomedial to the anterior superior iliac spine.

Lesion of the LFCN represents the chief complication during minimally invasive anterior approach dissection to the hip joint. There was a study done to describe the different presentation features of the LFCN at the thigh and primarily to determine the potential location of damage during minimally invasive anterior approaches for total hip replacement. The LFCN divided proximal to the inguinal ligament in 13 cases and distal to it in 21 cases. In the distal group, the mean distance from the anterior superior iliac spine to the nerve division was 34.5 mm (10–72 mm).[33] The gluteal branch crossed the anterior margin of the tensor fasciae latae 44.5 mm (24–92 mm) distally to the anterior superior iliac spine. In 18 cases, the femoral branch did not cross the tensor fasciae latae and was located in the intramuscular space between tensor fasciae latae and sartorius. In the remaining 16 cases, this branch crossed the anterior margin of the tensor fasciae latae ligament 46 mm (27–92 mm) distally to the anterior superior iliac spine. During minimally invasive anterior approach along the anterior border of the tensor fasciae latae, the LFCN was found to be potentially at risk between 27 and 92 mm below the anterior superior iliac spine. It was therefore suggested to position the skin incision as lateral and distal to the anterior superior iliac spine as possible to avoid this particular danger zone.[33]

The origin of the LFCN is variable. It can arise from the second lumbar nerve root, the third lumbar nerve root, or, less frequently, the second and third lumbar nerve roots. It emerges at the lateral border of the psoas major muscle and passes beneath the iliac fascia and the inguinal ligament lateral to the femoral nerve, and then divides into anterior and posterior branches. The anterior branch supplies sensory input to the skin of the anterior and lateral thigh. The posterior branch supplies the skin of the lateral portion of the thigh from the greater trochanter distally to the mid-thigh.

Injury to the nerve most commonly results from compression as it passes under the inguinal ligament. Meralgia paresthetica is the term used to describe the clinical syndrome of pain, dysesthesia, or both. Dysesthesia is defined as the unpleasant sensation that occurs when touching a body part results in pain, burning, or tingling. The area of skin involved with meralgia paresthetica is located on the anterior and lateral thigh. The most common causes of the syndrome are obesity, diabetes mellitus, tight clothing, pregnancy, and surgical procedures. Most cases respond to weight loss and decreasing pressure on the inguinal ligament. In the most severe cases, the symptoms can be quite debilitating. Surgery is sometimes needed but pain medications and nerve blocks are often considered. The nerve is afferent, so no motor dysfunction results from injury.

26.8 Obturator Nerve Surgical Anatomy

The obturator nerve originates from the third and fourth lumbar nerves. It occasionally receives input from the second lumbar nerve. It descends through the psoas major muscle and emerges at its medial border, running posterior to the common iliac arteries. It continues downward and forward on the lateral wall of the pelvis and enters the thigh through the obturator foramen, then bifurcates into anterior and posterior divisions. The anterior division descends between the adductor longus and brevis muscles, giving off major branches to them and to the gracilis muscle. The posterior division descends through the obturator externus muscle before passing anterior to the adductor magnus muscle and sending branches to supply it.

The obturator nerve innervates the muscles in the medial compartment of the thigh along with a sensory component to the skin of the medial thigh. The adductor longus, adductor brevis, and gracilis adduct the thigh. The adductor magnus consists of an adductor portion and a hamstring portion. The adductor component flexes and adducts the thigh and is supplied by the obturator nerve. The hamstring component is supplied by the tibial nerve and is responsible for thigh extension. The obturator nerve innervates the obturator externus, which laterally rotates the thigh.

Injuries to the obturator nerve are most frequently seen in direct trauma, and to a lesser extent, surgical procedures involving the pelvis. Nerve injury will result in weakness or loss of adduction of the thigh. Weakness in external rotation of the thigh will be seen along with a slight loss of hip flexion. Pain and numbness of the medial thigh will be seen with injuries to the obturator nerve. Injury to the obturator nerve results in a gait that is mildly disturbed because the lower extremity is externally rotated and swings outwardly. This nerve is most frequently injured iatrogenically or following a pelvic fracture.[15] In our earlier anatomical study, we normally found it at a mean distance of 5 cm inferior to the supracristal plane on a vertical line through the anterior superior iliac spine, and it had a mean distance of 3 cm lateral to the midline.[29]

References

[1] Abernathey CD, Onofrio BM, Scheithauer B, Pairolero PC, Shives TC. Surgical management of giant sacral schwannomas. J Neurosurg. 1986; 65(3):286–295

[2] Benzel EC. Surgical exposure of the lumbosacral plexus and proximal sciatic nerve. In: Benzel EC, ed. Practical Approaches to Peripheral Nerve Surgery. 1993. Park Ridge, IL: AANS:153–169

[3] Benzel EC. The lateral extracavitary approach to the spine using the three-quarter prone position. J Neurosurg. 1989; 71(6):837–841

[4] Benzel EC, Barolat-Romana G, Larson SJ. Femoral obturator and sciatic neurectomy with iliacus and psoas muscle section for spasticity following spinal cord injury. Spine. 1988; 13(8):905–908

[5] Ducic I, Dellon AL. Testicular pain after inguinal hernia repair: an approach to resection of the genital branch of genitofemoral nerve. J Am Coll Surg. 2004; 198(2):181–184

[6] Erbil KM, Sargon FM, Sen F, et al. Examination of the variations of lateral femoral cutaneous nerves: report of two cases. Anat Sci Int. 2002; 77(4):247–249

[7] Mine Erbil K, Onderoğlu S, Başar R. Unusual branching in lumbar plexus. Case report. Folia Morphol (Warsz). 1998; 57(4):377–381

[8] Farny J, Drolet P, Girard M. Anatomy of the posterior approach to the lumbar plexus block. Can J Anaesth. 1994; 41(6):480–485

[9] Hope EE, Bodensteiner JB, Thong N. Neonatal lumbar plexus injury. Arch Neurol. 1985; 42(1):94–95

[10] Hospodar PP, Ashman ES, Traub JA. Anatomic study of the lateral femoral cutaneous nerve with respect to the ilioinguinal surgical dissection. J Orthop Trauma. 1999; 13(1):17–19

[11] Ingram AV. Miscellaneous affections of the nervous system. In: Edmonson AS, Crenshaw AH, eds. Campbell's Operative Orthopaedics. 6th ed. St. Louis, MO: Mosby-Yearbook;1980:1567–1641

[12] Johnson RM, Southwick WO. Surgical approaches to the lumbosacral spine. In: Rothman RH, Simeone FA, eds. The Spine. 2nd ed. Philadelphia: WB Saunders Co;1982:171–187

[13] Kashuk K. Proximal peripheral nerve entrapment syndromes in the lower extremity. J Am Podiatry Assoc. 1977; 67(8):529–544

[14] Kempe LG. Surgery of peripheral nerves. In: Kempe LG, ed. Operative Neurosurgery. New York: Springer-Verlag;1970:203–232

[15] Kline DG, Hudson AR. Nerve Injuries: Operative Results for Major Nerve Injuries, Entrapments, and Tumors. Philadelphia: W.B. Saunders;1995:326–339

[16] Krähenbühl L, Striffeler H, Baer HU, Büchler MW. Retroperitoneal endoscopic neurectomy for nerve entrapment after hernia repair. Br J Surg. 1997; 84(2):216–219

[17] Kumar S, Anantham J, Wan Z. Posttraumatic hematoma of iliacus muscle with paralysis of the femoral nerve. J Orthop Trauma. 1992; 6(1):110–112

[18] Laha RK, Rao S, Pidgeon CN, Dujovny M. Genito-femoral neuralgia. Surg Neurol. 1977; 8(4):280–282

[19] Moore DC. Regional Block: A Handbook for Use in the Clinical Practice of Medicine and Surgery. Springfield, IL: Charles C Thomas;1965:206–210

[20] Moro T, Kikuchi S, Konno S, Yaginuma H. An anatomic study of the lumbar plexus with respect to retroperitoneal endoscopic surgery. Spine. 2003; 28(5):423–428, discussion 427–428

[21] Murata Y, Takahashi K, Yamagata M, Shimada Y, Moriya H. The anatomy of the lateral femoral cutaneous nerve, with special reference to the harvesting of iliac bone graft. J Bone Joint Surg Am. 2000; 82(5):746–747

[22] Perry CP. Laparoscopic treatment of genitofemoral neuralgia. J Am Assoc Gynecol Laparosc. 1997; 4(2):231–234

[23] Rosenberger RJ, Loeweneck H, Meyer G. The cutaneous nerves encountered during laparoscopic repair of inguinal hernia: new anatomical findings for the surgeon. Surg Endosc. 2000; 14(8):731–735

[24] Rosse C, Gaddum-Rosse P. Hollinshead's Textbook of Anatomy. 5th ed. Philadelphia: Lippincott-Raven;1997:607

[25] Seijo-Martínez M, Castro del Río M, Fontoira E, Fontoira M. Acute femoral neuropathy secondary to an iliacus muscle hematoma. J Neurol Sci. 2003; 209(1–2):119–122

[26] Spratt JD, Logan BM, Abrahams PH. Variant slips of psoas and iliacus muscles, with splitting of the femoral nerve. Clin Anat. 1996; 9(6):401–404

[27] Sunderland S. Nerves and Nerve Injuries. 2nd ed. Edinburgh: Churchill Livingstone;1978:999–1020

[28] Sürücü HS, Tanyeli E, Sargon MF, Karahan ST. An anatomic study of the lateral femoral cutaneous nerve. Surg Radiol Anat. 1997; 19(5):307–310

[29] Tubbs RS, Salter EG, Wellons JC, III, Blount JP, Oakes WJ. Anatomical landmarks for the lumbar plexus on the posterior abdominal wall. J Neurosurg Spine. 2005; 2(3):335–338

[30] Urbanowicz Z, Zaluska S. Formation of the lumbar plexus in man and macaca. Folia Morphologica. 1969; 28:256–271

[31] Whiteside JL, Barber MD, Walters MD, Falcone T. Anatomy of ilioinguinal and iliohypogastric nerves in relation to trocar placement and low transverse incisions. Am J Obstet Gynecol. 2003; 189(6):1574–1578, discussion 1578

[32] Klaassen Z, Marshall E, Tubbs RS, Louis RG, Jr, Wartmann CT, Loukas M. Anatomy of the ilioinguinal and iliohypogastric nerves with observations of their spinal nerve contributions. Clin Anat. 2011; 24(4):454–461

[33] Ropars M, Morandi X, Huten D, Thomazeau H, Berton E, Darnault P. Anatomical study of the lateral femoral cutaneous nerve with special reference to minimally invasive anterior approach for total hip replacement. Surg Radiol Anat. 2009; 31(3):199–204

27 Comparative Anatomy of the Lumbar Plexus

Malcon Andrei Martinez-Pereira, Denise Maria Zancan

Abstract

In this review, the anatomy of the lumbar plexus is compared between humans and other mammals that are commonly used as experimental models in studies of plexopathies and peripheral nerve injuries. The differences in topography, origin, and distribution of the spinal nerves that constitute the lumbar plexus are discussed. A brief description of the lumbar plexus in lower tetrapods (birds, reptiles, and amphibians) is also included. The descriptions of the lumbar plexus in nonhuman primates are based on three genera of Hominidae, the genus *Hylobates*, and other primate species of experimental interest. The major anatomical differences between humans and the animals more widely used for experimental plexopathies and peripheral nerves injuries (rat, guinea pig, dog, cat, and pig) are examined.

Keywords: lumbar plexus, comparative anatomy, peripheral nervous system, experimental models

27.1 Introduction

Peripheral nerve lesions and plexopathies are common in routine clinical practice and surgery. Injuries to the lumbar spinal cord and *cauda equina* can compromise quality of life and incapacitate the individual. Therefore, knowledge of the origin, route, and destination of the plexus components is needed for intravenous or intramuscular injections and locoregional anesthesia and surgical interventions in order to diminish the risk of iatrogenic injury and to help in the examination and diagnosis of injuries. The mapping provided can correlate each nerve to the target organ, allowing the neurological injury to be identified and treatment and rehabilitation managed.

In this review, the topography, origin, and distribution of the nerves of the lumbar plexus are compared among vertebrates. This comparative approach to the neuroanatomy of the peripheral nervous system helps us to understand the functional aspects of neural structure design. For this reason, the anatomical descriptions in this review include mammals used as experimental models for studies of plexopathies and peripheral nerve injuries, such as the rat (*Rattus norvegicus*), the guinea pig (*Cavia porcellus*), the chinchilla (*Chinchilla lanigera*), the rabbit (*Oryctolagus cuniculus*), dogs, cats, pigs, and nonhuman primates. The comparative perspective on mammalian plexus design includes an analysis of lower tetrapods, although fewer available reports are available on amphibians and reptiles or even birds than on mammals. These descriptive analyses elucidate the remarkable variation of limb anatomy and modes of locomotion among tetrapods.

27.2 Lumbar Spinal Cord and Nerves

The topography of the caudal end of the spinal cord (*intumescentia lumbalis* and *conus medullaris*) varies widely among mammals and other species and is of considerable interest in clinical and surgical medicine. These portions are important in procedures for epidural anesthesia or analgesia,[1,2] collection of cerebrospinal fluid,[3] and injection of radiopaque substances during radiographic procedures.[4] This explains why there are morphological and morphometric descriptions of this structure in many animals. Precise descriptions of the spinal cord end in terms of the characteristics of each species are necessary for refining the aforementioned procedures. However, the topographies of the *intumescentia lumbalis* and *conus medullaris* between the last lumbar vertebra (basis) and the first sacral one (apex) vary with species and age. The topographies of these structures in different species are compared in ▶ Table 27.1.

Owing to the differential growth rates of vertebral column and spinal cord, the more caudal lumbar nerves constitute the *cauda equina*. This consists of nerve roots located inside the spinal canal of the lumbar and sacral spine, together with the medullar cone and terminal filament, the location varying among species. The *cauda equina* is located laterocaudally to the *conus medullaris*. An injury in this region can involve several nerves, since the *cauda equina* contains numerous nerve

Table 27.1 Level of *lumbar intumescentia* and *conus medullaris* in spinal cords of some vertebrates

Species	Lumbar intumescentia	Conus medullaris
Human	T11–L1	L1–L3
Nonhuman primates		
Ateles	L1–L4	L5–S2
Cebus	L1–L4	L5–S3
Chimpanzee	T11–L1	L1–L3
Cynomolgus	L1–L4	L5–S3
Gibbon	L1–L4	L3–S3
Gorilla	T11–L1	L1–L3
Lagothrix	L1–L4	L1–S2
Orangutans	T11–L1	L1–L3
Rhesus macaque	L1–L4	L1–S3
Other mammals		
Cat	L3–L5	L5–S3
Chinchilla	L2–L5	L6–S2
Dog	L4–L6	L3–L7
Guinea pig	T12–L2	L5–S2
Swine	L6–L7	L5–S3
Rabbit	T12–L2	L5–S4
Rat	T11–L1	L1–L3
Other tetrapods		
Birds	Synsacrum	Synsacrum
Iguana	PS25–PS28	PS28–S2
Varanus	PS28–PS30	PS30–S2
Tortoise	T6–S1–S5–C1	No information
Anurans	SN7–SN10	S1–urostyle

roots in the small area between L3 and S3 and includes the main nerves of the lumbar and sacral plexuses.

Unlike the spinal cord in mammals, the spinal cord in birds extends along the length of the vertebral canal including the coccygeal region; it is as long as the whole vertebral column and decreases in diameter caudally.[5,6] Although its segmentation is the same as in mammals, the cervical portion is longer and variable among avian species, while the thoracic portion is very short and the sacral cord is also longer, as in the coccygeal region. There are two intumescences in birds, cervical and lumbar, and only birds display a glycogen body lying in the spinal cord in the area of the lumbosacral sinus.[5,6] Glycogen body cells are of glial origin, possibly from astrocytes, and have undergone extreme differentiation, but neither the origin of these cells nor the function of the glycogen body is wholly clear.

The reptilian spinal cord extends throughout the vertebral canal, filling only 50% of the lumen in alligators and 29 to 34% in several lizard species.[7] Although the reptilian spinal cord has a segmented organization as in other vertebrates, it lacks some of the functional regionalization seen in mammals. It tends to be larger near the brainstem, and the cervical and sacral regions are larger in cross-section, corresponding to the brachial and lumbosacral plexuses, though there is no lumbar region in turtles,[8,9] lizards, or crocodiles.[7,10] The cords in snakes and limbless lizards lack the brachial and sacral intumescences.[7] The spinal cord varies among amphibians, being more differentiated in anurans than in urodeles. Anurans have a relatively short spinal cord with 11 segments and conspicuous *intumescentiae cervicalis* and *lumbalis*.[11] The spinal cord terminates in a relatively long and slender cone, which represents the remnant of the premetamorphosis caudal portion.[11,12] In reptiles, no lateral horn can be distinguished, but the large area of gray matter between the horns is composed of interneurons.[7] In chelonians, the ventral horn is reduced in the midtrunk because there are fewer motor neurons since trunk musculature is lacking.[9]

The number of spinal nerves varies among species according to the number of vertebrae. However, the numbers of segments and nerves in the cervical spinal cord are the same in almost all species. For example, humans have five lumbar segments and nerves[13]; nonhuman primates vary between four and seven[14,15,16]; dogs have seven.[17] From T1, all spinal nerves emerge below their corresponding vertebrae, even those that constitute the *cauda equina*. The numbers of lumbar spinal nerves that correspond to spinal segments for some species are shown in ▶ Table 27.2. Although the neuroanatomy and cytoarchitecture of the mammalian cerebral cortex (pallial domains) differs considerably from that of birds, the peripheral nervous system is very similar in cytoarchitecture features and anatomical arrangement. In birds, the spinal segments and nerves are identified in relation to the cervical, thoracic, lumbar, sacral, and coccygeal regions. However, as stated in the *Nomina Anatomica Avium*,[18,19] the best way to determine the spinal nerves is to count the number of vertebrae, starting at the base of the skull and proceeding caudally. Because the number of vertebral segments varies widely across taxa and distinct regional boundaries are lacking, this same method is used for other tetrapods such as amphibians and reptiles (▶ Table 27.2).

The lumbar nerves comprise five pairs of spinal nerves (the last thoracic and the first four lumbar) emerging between the last thoracic vertebra and, eventually, the first lumbar vertebra,

Table 27.2 Numbers of vertebrae, medullary segments, and lumbar spinal nerve ventral rami in the lumbar region in some vertebrates

Species	Lumbar region		
	Vertebrae	Spine segment	Lumbar nerves
Human	5	5	5
Nonhuman primates			
Ateles	4	4	6
Cebus	5–6	5–6	5
Chimpanzee	4	4	6
Cynomolgus	6–7	6–7	5
Gibbon	5	5	6
Gorilla	4	4	6
Lagothrix	4	4	6
Orangutans	4	4	5
Rhesus	6–7	6–7	6–7
Tarsius	6	6	6
Other mammals			
Cat	6	7	7
Chinchilla	6	6	7
Dog	7	7	7
Guinea pig	6	6	6
Swine	6–7	6	6
Rabbit	7	7	7
Rat	6	6	6
Other tetrapods			
Crocodylia	5 last PSV	5 last PSS	5
Iguana	6 last PSV	6 last PSS	4
Varanus	6–7 last PSV	6 last PSS	5
Anurans	4 PSV	4 PSS	5 PSSN

Abbreviations: PSS, presacral medullary segments; PSSN, presacral spinal nerve; PSV, presacral vertebrae.

but there are species differences. Each lumbar nerve is organized as a typical spinal nerve divided into anterior and posterior primary divisions and a visceral communicating branch to the sympathetic trunk. The primary posterior or dorsal division emits a medial branch to the multifidus muscles and skin, a lateral superior branch to the sacrospinalis muscles and skin of the gluteal region, and a lateral inferior branch to the sacrospinalis muscles. The primary anterior (or ventral) division constitutes the *iliohypogastricus*, *ilioinguinalis*, *genitofemoralis*, *cutaneus femoris lateralis*, *femoralis*, *obturatorius*, and *truncus lumbosacralis* nerves, constituted by the last lumbar and the first two sacral nerves. Small recurrent branches innervate the spinal dura mater.

The lumbar autonomic innervation to the abdominal and pelvic viscera is complex. The sympathetic lumbar nerves (*nervi splanchnici lumbales*) originate from L1–L2 but receive contributions of neurons from the last lumbar ganglia. Because of this, intestinal and renal pain can be a source of lower back pain and, if the intestines or uterus are involved, the pain signal can manifest in the pelvic limb via the *ischiadicus* nerve, although a visceral dysfunction is responsible.[13,20] On the other hand, severe caudal lumbar lesions block the central inhibition of micturition and result in urinary incontinence, since the parasympathetic reflex of bladder emptying usually persists.[13, 20] The sympathetic innervation should survive parasympathetic loss; detrusor sphincter dyssynergy can result in the loss of detrusor muscle activity and abnormally strong contractions of the urethra sphincter muscle.

Because the lumbar plexus formation varies in the location of the *medullary conus* and *cauda equina* (▶ Table 27.1), occasional lesions cranial to L4–L5 can produce signs of lumbosacral disease. For example, a lesion affecting the L4–L6 roots is likely to produce sensory-motor deficit in the extensors and adductors of the thigh (femoral and obturator nerves, respectively) and partially affect the cranial and caudal gluteus nerves. However, authors disagree about the formation and division of the lumbar and lumbosacral nerves, especially in nonhuman animals. Anatomy textbooks mention three possible configurations: (1) a lumbar plexus (*nervi iliohypogastricus, ilioinguinalis, genitofemoralis, cutaneus femoris lateralis, femoralis,* and *obturatorius*); (2) a sacral plexus (*nervi gluteus cranial, gluteus caudal, ischiadicus, pudendus,* and *rectales caudales* or *inferiores*); and (3) the lumbar nerves and the *ischiadicus* constituting the lumbosacral trunk.[17,21,22,23] Another difference is the presence of unisegmentary nerves (*iliohypogastricus* and *ilioinguinalis*: 22) in nonhuman species, while in humans all lumbar nerves comprise two or more spinal segments.[24] However, some axon fibers that innervate the pelvic limb via the lumbar and/or sacral nerves could originate from various cord segments, allowing each segment to participate more in the formation of nerve trunks and terminal nerves. Thus, axonal tracing has frequently been used to determine the exact axons and cell bodies that constitute each nerve.

On the other hand, several studies describe variations in the formation and distribution of the lumbar nerves. Since the terms prefixed (proximal or superior or cranial), ordinary (normal or median-fixed), and postfixed (distal or inferior or caudal) were introduced by Sherrington,[25] the variations in lumbar plexus and nerve origins in humans have been extensively revised. The ordinary form comprises the L1 to L4 nerves. When a communicating branch from T12, also known as the subcostal nerve, joins the first lumbar trunk (L1), it constitutes a prefixed plexus,[26,27,28] while the postfixed includes L5 in the formation of the more lumbar caudal nerves, the *femoralis* and *obturatorius*.[26, 27,28] In animals, the lumbar plexus is highly variable irrespective of species and sex. A prefixed model is described as including the participation of a cranial nerve in this ordinary formation. For example, in dogs, the *genitofemoralis* nerve is prefixed when L3 constitutes a more cranial root in its origin, while it is postfixed when it includes the more caudal nerve, as observed when L5 or L6 gives rise to the femoral nerve.[29]

27.2.1 Lumbar Plexus in Humans and Nonhuman Primates

As mentioned above, human anatomy textbooks describe the caudal medullary innervation as divided into three main trunks: (1) first trunk or lumbar plexus (T12 and L1–L4); (2) second trunk or sacral or lumbosacral plexus (L4–L5 and S1–S3); and (3) third trunk or pudendal plexus (S2–S5 and C1).[13] The first trunk originates from the ventral rami of the L1–L4 nerve roots and projects laterally and caudally from the intervertebral foramina, posterior to the psoas major muscle. A communicating branch

from T12, also known as the subcostal nerve, often joins the first lumbar trunk and constitutes a prefixed plexus.[30] Primary divisions give rise to six peripheral nerves: T12–L1 (*iliohypogastricus* and *ilioinguinalis*), L1–L2 (*genitofemoralis*), and L2–L4 (*cutaneus femoris lateralis, femoralis,* and *obturatorius*).[30]

Despite the functional correspondence between the lumbar innervation in humans and some nonhuman primates, certain differences can be explored in relation to the variable number of thoracic and lumbar vertebrae. The existence of 13 thoracic vertebrae is considered a primitive feature for primates[16,31]; this is based on the number of vertebrae in arboreal shrews, which is considered the common ancestor of all primates. In fact, the number of thoracic vertebrae ranges from 11 to 18 in modern primates. Twelve thoracic vertebrae are described in orangutans, as in humans. Therefore, starting from 13, the number of thoracic vertebrae in modern primates has increased or decreased. Arboreal shrews have five or six lumbar vertebrae. The original number in primates seems to be six, as observed in *Platyrrhines, Alouattinae, Atelinae,* and higher primates, although many new world and old world primates have seven.[31]

The degrees of pre- and postfixation are more variable in nonhuman primates than in humans owing to their numbers of presacral vertebrae and the probable shortening of the thoracic region. The lumbosacral plexus tends to show inferior displacement in all primate genera except the Hominoidea, indicating a postfixed plexus.[16] In fact, orangutans and other primates that show a reduced presacral vertebral column have more prefixation. In this type, the last thoracic or subcostal nerve (T12 or T13) participates in forming the lumbar plexus.[31] As result, the displacements of bones change the number of roots and the nerve topography, giving rise to a relationship among plexus structure, lower limb development, and body posture.

Although the medullary segments show no numerical correspondence between humans and nonhuman primates, the nerves and plexus configuration are very similar in all species. For example, chimpanzees and orangutans have four lumbar nerves, while gorillas and gibbons have five.[14,15] The medullar segment L2 of *Macaca* corresponds to L1 in humans,[32,33] but while the first root can be L1, L2, or L3, as in chimpanzees and gorillas,[14,15,34,35] the first root in humans is T12 or L1. Therefore, it can be assumed that the lumbar plexus in apes is formed by the subcostal nerve (last thoracic or first lumbar nerve) and the L1–L4 nerves, and has more marked progressive traits than in humans. In prosimians and primates, a bifurcated nerve usually connects the lumbar and sacral plexuses. This nerve is described in apes (L5: 14; 36, 37; 53) and *Cebus*[36] but is absent in rhesus macaque,[37] *Cynomolgus,*[33] and *Ateles.*[38,39,40]

The lumbar and sacral plexuses are formed as a single unit from L1–L7–S1–S2 in *Cynomolgus*[33] and the rhesus macaque,[37] and from L3–L5 and S1–S2 in *Ateles,* but in other primates the two are distinct. In general, the lumbar plexus is formed from L2–L3 in chimpanzees,[41] orangutans,[14,15] and gorillas,[42] while in the gibbon, as in humans, it arises from L2–L4[14,15]; in *Cebus,* it arises from L3–L4.[36] Functionally, the lumbar and sacral nerves are classified into flexor (iliohypogastric, ilioinguinal, genitofemoral, anterior branches of the femoral, obturator, flexor branches of the tibial and common fibular, pubioisquiofemoral, and pudendal) and extensor (lateral femoral cutaneous, femoral, piriformis, superior and inferior gluteal, sciatic, and posterior femoral cutaneous) nerve groups.[40] However, there is no distinct division between the flexor and extensor nerves in primates, because nonhuman primates have hindlimbs of both pickup and load-carrying types, while humans have only the load-carrying type.

The iliohypogastric, ilioinguinal, and genitofemoral nerves occur in most prosimians and all primates, and they can originate from the lumbar plexus (primates) or separately (prosimians).[43] However, the ilioinguinal nerve is generally absent in apes, probably because the thoracic region is shortened and there are fewer nerves in the lumbar segment. The organization of the upper lumbar nerves in apes, particularly the gibbon,[14,15] is similar to that in humans. However, L1 and L2 do not form a common trunk for the iliohypogastric nerve in the gibbon, as in humans, whereas T12–L1–L2 in the chimpanzee[41] and orangutan,[14,15] and L1–L3 in the gorilla,[14,15] join together and form the iliohypogastric and genitofemoral nerves; the latter rises from L2 in the gibbon. In addition, in Hominoidea (apes and gibbons), the lateral femoral cutaneous nerve arises from the union of L2 and L3.[14,15] However, in *Cebus*[36] and *Ateles*,[38,39,40] the iliohypogastric, ilioinguinal, and genitofemoral nerves originate from the union of T12 and L1, while the lateral femoral cutaneous nerve arises from L2–L3. These nerves belong to the lumbar plexus in neither species.

In monkeys, the lumbar plexus gives rise to the femoral and obturator nerves and, in some cases, the lateral femoral cutaneous nerve (mentioned earlier). The femoral nerve arises from L2–L3 in the gibbon[14,15] but has a more cranial origin in the chimpanzee and the orangutan, emerging from L1–L3.[14,15,41] It arises from a common trunk with the obturator nerve in the gorilla,[14,15,34,35] rhesus, and *Cynomolgus*,[33,37] *Cebus*,[36] and *Ateles*.[38,39,40] In the rhesus and *Cynomolgus*, an inferior femoral nerve is described as originating from L5–L6. The obturator nerve emerges from L3–L4 in gibbons,[14,15] from L2–L4 in chimpanzees[41] and gorillas,[35,42] and from L1–L2 in orangutans.[14,15] The subcostal nerve can form the obturator nerve in chimpanzees,[12,14,15] while in *Macaca*[32] and in *Pongo pygmeu*[40] it is formed by the more cranial lumbar nerves (L2–L3), and in *Mandrillus* by the more caudal ones (L3–L6).[44]

27.2.2 Other Mammals

Different animals can be used to study injuries to peripheral nerve fibers, simulating the different conditions of injury in humans. Several descriptions indicate species differences in the formation of the lumbar innervation. However, the distance between the nerve and its target organs is shorter in small mammals, which makes it easier to observe the pathophysiology of injury and reduces the neural recovery period. Among the methods widely studied are those that produce mechanical trauma, with special reference to the sciatic nerve.

In rodents, rabbits, and domestic mammals, as in nonhuman primates, it can be inferred that the more cranial lumbar innervation does not arise through the formation of a common trunk as it does in humans.[13] Nevertheless, the lumbar plexus is formed from a junction of the ventral rami of the L3–L5 nerves in dogs.[45] The more cranial lumbar ventral rami (L1–L4) constitute the iliohypogastric (L1), ilioinguinal (L2), lateral femoral cutaneous (L4), and genitofemoral (L3) nerves, the latter relying on a contribution from L4 in some cases.[17,21,22] On the other hand, in the prefixed plexus of rabbits[46,47,48] and rodents,[49,50,51]

the iliohypogastric nerve receives a contribution from T13 and the ilioinguinal nerve arises from L1–L2, except in the guinea pig[52] and chinchilla.[53] In species with seven lumbar segments (carnivores and pigs), there are two iliohypogastric nerves, cranial and caudal.[45,54,55,56,57] The latter arises from the ventral branches of L1–L2, and the ilioinguinal nerve arises from the ventral branch of L3. In the chinchilla, which has six lumbar segments, the L1–L2 spinal nerves give rise to the cranial and caudal iliohypogastric nerves and the ilioinguinal nerve arises from L3,[53] while the iliohypogastric nerves emerge from L4 in the guinea pig.[52] In the guinea pig[52] and rat,[49,51] the genitofemoral and lateral femoral cutaneous nerves arise from L3–L4, while in the rabbit they arise from L4–L5.[46,47,48] In the dog, the lateral femoral cutaneous nerve arises mostly from L4, with occasional contributions from L3 or L5 and the genitofemoral from L3–L4.[17,45] In the cat,[55] the lateral femoral cutaneous nerve arises from L4–L5 and the genitofemoral nerve from L3, as in the chinchilla[53] and pig.[54,57,58] In both these species, the lateral femoral cutaneous nerve emerges from L4.

The iliohypogastric nerve emerges between the psoas major and minor muscles and innervates the abdominal wall, *paralumbal fossa*, and *peritoneum*, while the ilioinguinal and the genitofemoral nerves, after emerging between the lumbar muscles, extend subperitoneally and in a caudoventral direction toward the *annulus inguinalis abdominalis*.[17,22] These nerves innervate the internal abdominal oblique and cremaster muscles, the *testicular fascia*, spermatic funiculus and preputium in males, the *mammae* in females, and the skin of the medial side of the femoral region in both sexes. The lateral cutaneous femoral nerve arises from the plexus, projects toward to the caudal iliac region by crossing the abdominal muscles, and innervates the external abdominal oblique, *iliac* and *tensor fasciae latae* muscles, the skin of the femoral region, and the craniomedial side of the knee joint.[17,22]

In many mammals, in contrast to primates, the caudal lumbar nerves (femoral and obturator) are described as originating from a cranial trunk of the lumbosacral plexus.[17,21,22,23] Thus, to allow these nerves to be compared with those described in humans and nonhuman primates, a description of the cranial trunk of the lumbosacral plexus follows. The constitution of the cranial trunk varies among the species described because more caudal lumbar and/or sacral segments are involved in the formation of the obturator nerve in the guinea pig (L5–L6)[19] and rabbit (L5–S3).[7,11,47] However, the cranial trunk in the rat is formed by L2–L4 or L5, and the femoral nerve originates from L2–L4[8] and the obturator from (L2) L3–L5,[49,51] while in the dog,[17,45] pig,[54,56,57,58,59] and chinchilla,[53] both nerves emerge from a common trunk formed by L3–L6 and L3–L4, respectively. The femoral nerve arises from L4–L5 in the guinea pig,[52] mostly from L6 with contributions from L5 and L7 in rabbits,[46,47,48] and from L5–L6 in the cat; and the obturator nerve emerges from L6–L7 in the cat.[55]

The femoral nerve emerges between the psoas major and minor muscles to innervate them together with the deep lumbar muscles, then reaches the femoral space and emits branches to the femoral quadriceps muscle.[17,22] The saphenous nerve arises more caudally and innervates the *gracilis*, *pectineus*, and *sartorius* muscles, branching to supply the skin and fascia in the medial femoral region. The obturator nerve, after leaving the pelvic cavity through the obturator foramen, supplies the branches of the *adductor*, *pectineus*, *gracilis*, and internal and external obturator muscles.[17,22]

27.2.3 Birds

Before the lumbar innervation in birds can be described, it is important to note that the caudal region of the avian vertebral column is differentiated. It is formed from 14–15 vertebrae that are fused to constitute the *synsacrum*.[19] The connection between the synsacrum and the ilium, which reaches far into the thoracic region, is crucial for the shape of the trunk in birds. The bony connection is accomplished cranially by spines and transverse processes and caudally by the transverse processes of the synsacrum, which are fused into a continuous bony plate that permits the passage of nerves and blood vessels.[19] From cranial to caudal, the vertebrae in the synsacrum are differentiated as follows: synsacrothoracic, synsacrolumbar, primary sacral, and synsacrocaudal. If we consider that the lumbar to coccygeal segments of the spinal cord are located in the canal of the synsacrum, the spinal nerves arising from it can be called synsacral nerves (Sy: 46).

In birds, the lumbar and pelvic regions, hindlimb, and tail are innervated by the mixed nerves that constitute the lumbar, sacral, and pudendal plexuses.[5,6,19] The ischiadicus nerve is more important for diagnosing Marek's disease than the other lumbar and pelvic nerves. This pathology is one of the most widespread avian infections. It causes swelling of peripheral nerves, loss of striated muscle mass, and lethargy.[5] The lumbar plexus is described as being formed by the last two lumbar ventral (L6–L7) and first sacral (S1) strands; the latter, also called the forked nerve (*furcalis*), connects the lumbar plexus to the sacral plexus.[5,6,19] The sacral plexus is formed by the ventral strands of spinal nerves S1–S5[26] and the number of roots constituting it ranges from five to seven. Nevertheless, the furcal and *bigeminus* nerves, which connect the sacral to the pudendal plexus, are not always visible. However, these descriptions refer to domestic birds (chicken, duck, and goose: 50). In the ostrich (*Struthio camelus*), the lumbar plexus is formed by the union of four roots (Sy2–Sy5) and the sacral plexus by seven roots (Sy5–Sy11). Sy5–Sy9 form the cranial trunk of the plexus, whereas Sy10–Sy11 constitute its caudal trunk and Sy5 the forked nerve.[60] However, in the Kyrgyz pheasant (*Phasianus colchicus mongolicus*), the plexus sacralis is formed by the ventral branches of S1–S5 and is located between the lumbar and pudendal plexuses. In this species, the sacral plexus originates three trunks: a cranial trunk formed by the union of S1–S3, a medium trunk formed by S4, and a caudal trunk comprising S5 only. The cranial and medium trunks connect in a single root.[61]

The nerves of the lumbar plexus are the iliohypogastricus and ilioinguinalis (both to the ventral muscles of the trunk), obturator (to the external obturator and adductor muscles), cutaneous femoris (to the sartorius muscle and a cutaneous branch in the lateral surface of the thigh), femoral (the thickest branch of the plexus that innervates the iliac, quadriceps femori or femorotibialis, gracilis, and tensor fasciae latae muscles), cranial gluteus (to the medius and profound gluteus muscles), and saphenous (which innervates the knee joint and the inner surface of the shank).[19] However, the cranial femoris nerve in the ostrich originates from the union of Sy2–Sy3, supplies the iliotibialis cranialis muscle, and divides into the lateral and cranial femoral cutaneous nerves that supply the skin of the lateral and cranial surfaces of the thigh.[60] The obturator nerve is the smallest branch of the lumbar plexus formed by Sy3–Sy5 in the ostrich, while in chickens two lumbar roots form it.[60]

27.2.4 Reptiles and Amphibians

The description of the lumbar plexus in *Reptilia* is based on studies of the iguana (*Iguana iguana*) and varanus (*Varanus dumerilii*). Before the lumbar innervations in reptiles are described, it is important to explain the organization of their vertebral column. In Squamata, the vertebral column is divided into cervical, thoracic, sacral, and coccygeal regions. In general, there are eight cervical vertebrae, the last three being joined by ribs to the sternum; 16–17 thoracic vertebrae, which articulate with ribs; and two or three sacral vertebrae, which are fused. The coccygeal vertebrae showed dimorphism, characterized by a hemal arch.[62,63] In view of the wide variation across taxa in the number of vertebral segments and the lack of distinct regional boundaries, the best method to determine the spinal nerves is to count the number of vertebrae, starting at the base of the skull. Thus, the cervical and thoracic (presacral) vertebrae total 22 or 23.[62,63]

Spinal nerves 23–25 (SN23–SN25) constitute the lumbar plexus and nerves 25–30 form the sacral plexus in the iguana,[64,65] while in the varanus the lumbar and sacral plexuses are formed by spinal nerves 27–28 and 28–31, respectively.[64] Nevertheless, it is important to note that these animals have, respectively, 25 presacral and 2 sacral vertebrae, and 29 presacral and 2 sacral vertebrae. However, both species have a distinctive lumbosacral plexus, as described in other animals,[17,21,22,23] which is constituted by three trunks: a cranial trunk formed by SN23–SN25 in the iguana and SN27–SN28 in the varanus; a medium trunk or sacral plexus (from SN25–SN27 in the iguana and SN28–SN30 in the varanus); and a caudal trunk (from 27–28 in the iguana and SN30–SN31 in the varanus).[64,65]

The cranial trunk of the lumbosacral plexus gives rise to the femoral and obturator nerves and two nerve branches to the abdominal wall through the iliohypogastric nerve. The femoral nerve innervates the craniomedial and lateromedial faces of the thigh, through the *cutaneus femoralis cranialis*, *medialis* and *lateralis* nerves, while the obturator nerve innervates the caudomedial surface of the thigh.[64,65] Four nerves arise from the medial trunk: the dorsal (fibularis or peroneus), ventral (tibial), and ventral-most (pubioischiotibilalis) nerves, and the thin caudoiliofemoralis nerve. The fibularis innervates the calf and foot extensor muscles, whereas the tibial nerve supplies the flexor muscles of the same region. The pubioischiofemoralis nerve can be analogous to the ischiadicus nerve described in other vertebrate species, mainly considering their innervation territories (laterocaudal surface and muscles of the thigh, including the flexor muscles of the tibia and the pelvic muscles, excluding the obturator nerve's territory).[64,65] The caudal trunk of the lumbosacral plexus forms the caudofemoralis, pudendal, and caudoischiadicus nerves and the innervation to the musculature of the caudal body wall. The pudendal nerve has a wide innervation territory including the cranial pudendal (muscles of the tail) and caudal pudendal (muscles of the penis and cloaca) divisions.[64,65]

In amphibians, adaptation to terrestrial life entailed the development of limbs and central nervous system modifications subserving tetrapod locomotion. Nevertheless, some species are limbless (the caecilians of order Gymnophiona) or have rudimentary extremities (e.g., *Amphiuma*, a genus of aquatic salamander). SN7– SN10 join to form the lumbosacral plexus, the main component of which is the ischiadicus nerve that gives rise to the iliohypogastric, femoral or crural, tibial, and coccygeal nerves.[11] However, in the Japanese giant salamander (*Megalobatrachus japonicus*), the lumbosacral plexus comprises SN19–SN22 (SN20 is a bifurcated nerve; 2), as in the iguana and varanus.[64,65] In this species, the nerves are organized into four groups[11]: (1) innervating the caudofemoralis muscle (SN19–SN21, peroneus, or common fibular and tibial nerves); (2) passing between the caudofemoralis and caudoischiadicus muscles (SN20–SN22, pubioischiotibilais, and pudendal nerves); (3) following ventrally to the caudoischiadicus muscle (SN21–SN22 and nerve to the caudoischiadicus muscle); and (4) terminal nerves of the limb (ischiadicus from SN20, femoral from SN19–SN20, and obturator from SN19–SN20).

References

[1] Hall LW, Clarke KW. Veterinary Anaesthesia. 9th ed. London: Bailliere Tindall; 1991:183–187

[2] Jones RS. Epidural analgesia in the dog and cat. Vet J. 2001; 161(2):123–131

[3] Elias A, Brown C. Cerebellomedullary cerebrospinal fluid collection in the dog. Lab Anim (NY). 2008; 37(10):457–458

[4] Paithanpagare YM, Tank PH, Mankad MY, Shirodkar K, Derashri HJ. Myelography in dogs. Vet World. 2001; 1(5):152–154

[5] Baumel JJ. Aves nervous system. In: Getty R, ed. Sisson and Grossman's. The Anatomy of the Domestic Animals. 5th ed. Vol. 2. Philadelphia, PA: W.B. Saunders Company; 1975:2044–2052

[6] Dubbeldam JL. Systema nervosum periphericum. In: Baumel JJ, ed. Handbook of Avian Anatomy: Nomina Anatomica Avium. 2nd ed. Cambridge: Nuttall Ornithological Club; 1993:555–584

[7] Wyneken J. Reptilian neurology: anatomy and function. Vet Clin North Am Exot Anim Pract. 2007; 10(3):837–853, vi

[8] Ashley LM. Laboratory Anatomy of the Turtle. Dubuque, IA: WM C. Brown Company Publishers; 1962

[9] Kadota T, Nakano M, Atobe Y, Goris RC, Funakoshi K. The chelonian spinal nerve ganglia are a conglomerate of the spinal nerve ganglia proper and the sympathetic ganglia. Brain Behav Evol. 2009; 73(3):165–173

[10] Rowe T. Homology and evolution of the deep dorsal thigh musculature in birds and other reptilia. J Morphol. 1986; 189:327–346

[11] Underhill RA. Laboratory Anatomy of the Frog. Dubuque, IA: WM C. Brown Company Publishers; 1969

[12] Akita K. An anatomical investigation of the muscles of the pelvic outlet in Japanese giant salamander (Cryptobranchidae Megalobatrachus japonicus) with special reference to their nerve supply. Ann Anat. 1992; 174(3):235–243

[13] Standring S. Gray's Anatomy: The Anatomical Basis of Clinical Practice, Expert Consult. 40th ed. New York, NY: Elsevier; 2009

[14] Hepburn D. The comparative anatomy of the muscles and nerves of the superior and inferior extremities of the anthropoid apes. Part I. J Anat Physiol. 1892a; 26(Pt 2):149–186

[15] Hepburn D. The comparative anatomy of the muscles and nerves of the superior and inferior extremities of the anthropoid apes Part II. J Anat Physiol. 1892b; 26(Pt 3):324–356

[16] Hill WCO. Primates Comparative Anatomy and Taxonomy. Vol. I. Strepsirhini. Edinburgh: Edinburgh University Press; 1953

[17] Dyce KM, Sack WO, Wensing CJG. Textbook of Veterinary Anatomy. 4th ed. New York, NY: Elsevier; 2009

[18] Baumel JJ, Breazile JE, Evans HE, King AS, Vanden-Berge J. Handbook of Avian Anatomy: Nomina Anatomica Avium. 2nd ed. Cambridge: Nuttal Ornithological Society, 1993; 1993:779

[19] Nickel R, Schummer A, Seiferle E. Peripheral nervous system. In: Nickel R, Schummer A, Seiferle E, eds. Anatomy of the Domestic Birds. Berlin: Parey; 1977:131–139

[20] Di Dio LJA. Tratado de anatomia aplicada. 2nd ed. São Paulo: Póluss Editorial; 2002

[21] Frandson RD. Anatomia e fisiologia dos animais domésticos. 2nd ed. Rio de Janeiro: Guanabara Koogan; 1979:61

[22] Getty R. Sisson and Grossman's: The Anatomy of the Domestic Animals. 5th ed. Philadelphia, PA: WB Saunders Company; 1975

[23] Lacerda PMO, Moura CEB, Miglino MA, Oliveira MF, Albuquerque JFG. Origin of lumbar sacral plexus of rock cavy (Kerodon rupestris). Braz J Vet Res Anim Sci. 2006; 43:620–628

[24] Klaassen Z, Marshall E, Tubbs RS, Louis RG, Jr, Wartmann CT, Loukas M. Anatomy of the ilioinguinal and iliohypogastric nerves with observations of their spinal nerve contributions. Clin Anat. 2011; 24(4):454–461

[25] Sherrington CS. Notes on the arrangement of some motor fibres in the lumbo-sacral plexus. J Physiol. 1892; 13(6):621–772, 17

[26] Bardeen CR, Elting AW. A statistical study of the variations in the formation and position of the lumbo-sacral plexus in man. Anat Anz. 1901; 19:209–239

[27] Severeano G. Du plexus lombaire. Bibliogr Anatomique. 1904; 12:299–313

[28] Webber RH. Some variations in the lumbar plexus of nerves in man. Acta Anat (Basel). 1961; 44:336–345

[29] Fletcher TF. Lumbosacral plexus and pelvic limb myotomes of the dog. Am J Vet Res. 1970; 31(1):35–41

[30] Anloague PA, Huijbregts P. Anatomical variations of the lumbar plexus: a descriptive anatomy study with proposed clinical implications. J Manual Manip Ther. 2009; 17(4):e107–e114

[31] Schultz AH, Straus WL, Jr. The numbers of vertebrae in primates. Proc Am Philos Soc. 1945; 89:601–626

[32] Krechowiecki A, Gościcka D, Samulak S. The lumbosacral plexus and lumbar enlargement in Macaca mulatta [in Polish]. Folia Morphol (Warsz). 1972; 31 (1):11–19

[33] Urbanowicz Z, Zaluska S. Arrangement of lumbar plexus in man and macaca [in Polish]. Folia Morphol (Warsz). 1969; 28(3):285–299

[34] Champneys F. The muscles and nerves of a chimpanzee (Troglodytes Niger) and a cynocephalus anubis. J Anat Physiol. 1871; 6(Pt 1):176–211

[35] Raven HC, Hill JE. Regional anatomy of the gorilla. In: Gregory WK, ed. The Anatomy of the Gorilla. New York, NY: Columbia University Press; 1950

[36] Barros RAC, Prada ILS, Silva Z, Ribeiro AR, Silva DCO. Lumbar plexus formation of the Cebus apella monkey. Braz J Vet Res Anim Sci. 2003; 40:373–381

[37] Hartmann CG, Straus WL Jr. Anatomy of the Rhesus Monkey. New York, NY: Editora; 1932

[38] Chang H-T, Ruch TC. Morphology of the spinal cord, spinal nerves, caudal plexus, tail segmentation, and caudal musculature of the spider monkey. Yale J Biol Med. 1947; 19(3):345–377

[39] Chang H-T, Ruch TC. The projection of the caudal segments of the spinal cord to the lingula in the spider monkey. J Anat. 1949; 83(4):303–307

[40] El Assy YS. Beitrage zur morphologie des periphere nervensystems der primaten. Gegenbaurs Morphol Jahrb. 1966; 27:476–567

[41] Sonntag CF. On the anatomy, physiology, and pathology of the chimpanzee. Proc Zool Soc Lond. 1923; 23:323–429

[42] Eisler P. Das Gefass- und Periphere Nervensystem des Gorilla. Halle: Tausch & Grosse; 1890

[43] Zaluska S, Urbanowicz Z. Origin of the sacral plexus in man and in macacus [in Polish]. Acta Biol Med (Gdansk). 1972; 17(2):93–107

[44] Utzchneider E. 1892. Die Lendennerven der Affen und des Menschen. Miincli. Med. Abhand., S. vii, Heft 1

[45] Miller M, Christensen G, Evans H. Anatomy of the Dog. Philadelphia, PA: W. B. Saunders Company; 1964

[46] Barone R, Pavaux C, Blin PC, Cuq P. Atlas of Rabbit Anatomy. Paris: Masson & Cie; 1973

[47] Bensley BA, Craigie EH. Practical Anatomy of the Rabbit: An Elementary Textbook in Mammalian Anatomy. 6th ed. Toronto: The University of Toronto Press; 1938

[48] Mclaughlin CA, Chiasson RB. Laboratory Anatomy of the Rabbit. Dubuque, IA: W. C. Brown Company; 1987

[49] Chiasson RB. Laboratory Anatomy of the White Rat. Dubuque, IA: Brown Company Publisher; 1980

[50] Cook MJ. The Anatomy of the Laboratory Mouse. London: Academic Press; 1965

[51] Greene EC. Anatomy of the Rat. New York: Hafner Publishing Company; 1968

[52] Cooper G, Schiller AL. Anatomy of the Guinea Pig. Cambridge, MA: Harvard University Press; 1975

[53] Martinez-Pereira MA, Rickes EM. The spinal nerves that constitute the lumbosacral plexus and their distribution in the chinchilla. J S Afr Vet Assoc. 2011; 82(3):150–154

[54] Bosa YM, Getty R. Somatic and autonomic nerves of the lumbar, sacral and coccygeal regions of the domestic pig (Sus scrofa domesticus). Iowa State J Sci. 1969; 44:45–77

[55] Ghoshal NG. The lumbosacral plexus (plexus lumbosacralis) of the cat (Felis domestica). Anat Anz. 1972; 131(3):272–279

[56] Miheliae D, Gjurèeiae-Kantural V, Markovinoviae S, Damjanoviae A, Trboje-viae-Vukièeviae T. Variations of formation of n. femoralis, n. obturatorius and n.ischiadicus in pigs. Veterinarski Arhiv. 2004; 74(4):261–270

[57] Swindle MM, Smith ACT, Hepburn BJS. Swine as models in experimental surgery. J Invest Surg. 1988; 1(1):65–79

[58] Ghoshal NG. Spinal nerves of the swine. In: Getty R, ed. Sisson and Grossman's: The Anatomy of the Domestic Animals. 5th ed. Philadelphia: WB Saunders Company; 1975

[59] Chagas RG, Drummond SS, Silva FOC, Eurides D, Alves ECM, Miranda RL. Origem e distribuição do nervo obturatório em suínos (Sus scrofa domesticus – Linnaeus, 1758) da linhagem AG-1050. Arq Ciên Vet Zool. 2006; 9:15–20

[60] El-Mahdy T, El-Nahla SM, Abbott LC, Hassan SAM. Innervation of the pelvic limb of the adult ostrich (Struthio camelus). Anat Histol Embryol. 2010; 39 (5):411–425

[61] İstanbullugil FR, Karadağ Iİ, Scfergil S, Gezer İnce N, Alpak N. Formation of the plexus sacralis in pheasants (Phasianus colchicus mongolicus) and macro-anatomic investigation of the nerves originating from the plexus sacralis. Turk J Vet Anim Sci. 2013; 37:160–163

[62] Estes R, Queiroz K, Gauthier J. Phylogenetic relationships within Squamata. In: Estes R, Predill G, eds. Phylogenetic Relationships of the Lizard Families. Palo Alto, CA: Stanford University Press; 1988:119–281

[63] Veronese LB, Krause L. Esqueleto pré-sacral e sacral dos lagartos Teiídeos (Squamata, Teiidae). Rev Bras Zoologia. 1997; 14(1):15–34

[64] Akita K. An anatomical investigation of the muscles of the pelvic outlet in iguanas (Iguanidae Iguana iguana) and varanus (Varanidae Varanus (dumerillii)) with special reference to their nerve supply. Ann Anat. 1992b; 174(2): 119–129

[65] Arantes RC. Ossos da coluna vertebral e origens dos plexos braquial e lombossacral da iguana Iguana iguana [tese]. Universidade Federal de Uberlândia, Programa de Pós-Graduação em Ciências Veterinárias; 2016

Index

Note: Page numbers set **bold** or *italic* indicate headings or figures, respectively.